Emesis in Anti-cancer Therapy

Emesis in Anti-cancer Therapy

Mechanisms and treatment

Edited by

P.L.R. Andrews
Reader in Physiology
St George's Hospital Medical School
London
UK

and

G.J. Sanger
Director of Gastrointestinal Research
SmithKline Beecham Pharmaceuticals
Essex
UK

CHAPMAN & HALL MEDICAL
London · Glasgow · New York · Tokyo · Melbourne · Madras

Published by Chapman & Hall, 2–6 Boundary Row, London SE1 8HN

Chapman & Hall, 2–6 Boundary Row, London SE1 8HN, UK

Blackie Academic & Professional, Wester Cleddens Road, Bishopbriggs, Glasgow G64 2NZ, UK

Chapman & Hall, 29 West 35th Street, New York, NY10001, USA

Chapman & Hall Japan, Thomson Publishing Japan, Hirakawacho Nemoto Building, 6F, 1–7–11 Hirakawa-cho, Chiyoda-ku, Tokyo 102, Japan

Chapman & Hall Australia, Thomas Nelson Australia, 102 Dodds Street, South Melbourne, Victoria 3205, Australia

Chapman & Hall India, R. Seshadri, 32 Second Main Road, CIT East, Madras 600 035, India

First edition 1993

Typeset in 10/12pt Palatino by Graphicraft Typesetters Ltd, Hong Kong
Printed in Great Britain by Richard Clay Limited, Bungay, Suffolk.

ISBN 0 412 37250 9

A catalogue record for this book is available from the British Library

Library of Congress Cataloging-in-Publication data available

Contents

Contributors

1
P.L.R. Andrews
Department of Physiology
St George's Hospital Medical School
University of London
Cranmer Terrace, Tooting
London SW17 0RE, UK

G.J. Sanger
Research Division
Medicinal Research Centre
SmithKline Beecham
Coldharbour Road
The Pinnacles
Harlow, Essex CM19 5AD, UK

2
M.T. Seymour
Department of Medical Oncology
St Bartholomew's and The Homerton Hospitals
Homerton Row
London E9 6SR, UK

3
I.R. Judson
The Royal Marsden Hospital
The Institute of Cancer Research
Royal Cancer Hospital
Clifton Avenue, Belmont
Sutton, Surrey SM2 5PX, UK

4
M. Tonato
Medical Oncology Division
Policlinico Hospital and Institute of Internal Medicine University of Perugia
06100 Perugia, Italy

F. Roila
as above

A. Del Favero
Institute of Internal Medicine I
University of Perugia, 06100 Perugia Italy

5
H.I.M. Davidson
Department of Physiology and Pharmacology
University of Strathclyde
204, George Street,
Glasgow
G1 1XW, UK

M.-A. Pilot
Gastro-intestinal Science Research Unit
The London Hospital Medical College
26 Ashfield Street
Whitechapel
London E1 2AJ, UK

6
R.A. Leslie
Oxford University SmithKline Beecham Centre for Applied Neuropsychobiology, MRC Unit and University Department of Clinical Pharmacology

Radcliffe Infirmary
Woodstock Road
Oxford OX2 6HE, UK

D.J.M. Reynolds
MRC Unit and University Department of Clinical Pharmacology
Radcliffe Infirmary, as above

7
P.L.R. Andrews
as above

C.J. Davis O.B.E.
c/o Department of the Medical Director General (Naval)
Ministry of Defence
1st Avenue House
High Holborn
London WC1V 6HE, UK

8
R.K. Harding
Directorate of Research and Development, Human Performance, Department of National Defence, Ottawa and
Departments of Physiology and Medicine
Faculty of Medicine
University of Ottawa
Health Sciences Building
451 Smyth
Ottawa, Ontario
Canada K1H 8M5

R.W. Young
Human Response Program Manager
RARP (Radiation Policy Office)
Headquarters, Defense Nuclear Agency
6801 Telegraph Road
Alexandria VA 22310-3398, USA

G.H. Anno
Senior Staff Scientist
Pacific Sierra Research Corporation
12340 Santa Monica Boulevard
Los Angeles CA 90025, USA

9
G.J. Sanger
as above

10
Ann Cull
ICRF Medical Oncology Unit
Western General Hospital
Edinburgh EH4 2XU, UK

11
A.L. Jones
The Institute of Cancer Research
Department of Oncology
Royal Marsden Hospital
Downs Road
Sutton, Surrey SM2 5PT, UK

D. Cunningham
The Institute of Cancer Research and Honorary Consultant Physician, Royal Marsden Hospital,
as above

Preface

The aim of this book is to provide a synthesis of the current state of knowledge of the mechanisms and treatment of two of the most common and distressing side effects of anti-cancer therapy: nausea and vomiting.

The problems of nausea and vomiting are set in a more general context of anti-cancer therapy by a detailed study of the pharmacokinetics and pharmacodynamics of chemotherapeutic drugs and an examination of their general toxicities. Aspects of anti-cancer therapy that are rarely incorporated into reviews of emetic mechanisms. The mechanisms by which anti-cancer therapies induce emesis are examined in detail from several areas. Radiation-induced emesis is discussed in a separate chapter and draws attention to the special problems associated with this type of therapy. Particular attention is focused on the pharmacology and neurochemistry of the emetic mechanisms and the involvement of 5-hydroxytryptamine$_3$ receptors which have only come to light in recent years, are critically reviewed in detail.

More practical aspects of cancer chemotherapy are examined in chapters discussing the measurement of nausea and vomiting in man, an understanding of which is critical to the design of adequate anti-emetic trials. The broad psychological effects of cancer treatment and the care of the cancer patient are evaluated and the impact of behavioural therapies and novel pharmacological anti-emetic therapies assessed.

In compiling this book it is our intention to provide the first comprehensive and forward-looking collection of information and ideas on the mechanisms and treatment of emesis induced by anti-cancer therapies. In doing this it is our hope that this will stimulate research leading to further significant advances in the treatment of this distressing problem.

PLRA
GJS
1992

1

The problem of emesis in anti-cancer therapy: An introduction

P.L.R. ANDREWS and G.J. SANGER

'I had to beg them to stop giving me chemotherapy. I just couldn't face another course. After the second course, I found that thinking about going there made me vomit – in fact it was almost as bad as when I was actually having treatment. Even now (two years later) I start feeling sick when I pass by the hospital. I went there the other day to see a friend who had a baby, but I couldn't stay – that hospital smell brought it all back. I doubt that I could voluntarily put myself through chemotherapy again, even if I knew my life depended upon it'. (From Fallowfield and Clark, 1991.)

1.1 THE SIZE OF THE PROBLEM

The above description of the experience of chemotherapy by a patient well illustrates the unpleasant nature of the treatment and its long lasting effects and emphasizes the pressing need for therapies to combat such side effects.

Some insight into the magnitude of the problem of emesis in anti-cancer therapy can be gained by briefly reviewing some statistics from the United Kingdom. It is estimated that one person in three will develop cancer and cancer is responsible for 25% of all deaths. The major treatments for cancer are surgery, radiotherapy and chemotherapy either alone or in various combinations; treatment may be classified as palliative (intended to improve quality of life or alleviate symptoms) or curative. It is clear from the above that it is likely that a relatively large number of patients will, at some point in their treatment, receive cytotoxic chemotherapy and this number is estimated to be between 40–50,000 in the UK (Kaye, personal communication). Thus alleviating the unpleasant side effects of this and related anti-cancer therapies represents a major clinical challenge. This book focuses on the mechanisms and treatment of the most commonly reported side effects of anti-cancer therapy – namely nausea and vomiting.

1.2 AN INTRODUCTION TO MECHANISMS AND THERAPY

Nausea and vomiting are encountered in a wide variety of clinical contexts; these can be divided into three main categories: (1) induced by natural stimuli, (2) disease induced and (3) treatment induced (Table 1.1).

Typical natural stimuli that can induce emesis are early pregnancy, motion and

Emesis in Anti-cancer Therapy
Mechanisms and treatment
Published in 1993 by Chapman & Hall, London
ISBN 0 412 37250 9

Table 1.1 Examples of stimuli which evoke the vomiting reflex

	Clinical	
Natural	Disease	Therapeutic
Food poisoning	Intestinal obstruction	Cytotoxic chemotherapy drugs
Motion	Diabetic gastroparesis	Radiotherapy
Pregnancy	Labyrinthitis	Oral levodopa
Animal toxins, e.g. snake bite	Vestibular neuronitis	Surgery and anaesthesia
	Raised intra-cranial pressure	
	Pancreatitis	
	Medullary lesions, e.g. Wallenberg syndrome	
	Psychiatric disorders	
	Uraemia	
	Addison's disease	
	Hypercalcaemia	
	Diabetic ketoacidosis	
	Circulatory syncope	
	Mesenteric ischaemia	
	Hypertrophic pyloric stenosis	
	Reye's syndrome	
	Hepatitis	

contaminated food. Included in the disease category are the nausea and vomiting associated with labyrinthine disease, raised intra-cranial pressure and gastro-intestinal tract stasis or obstruction. The treatment-induced category includes post-anaesthetic and some types of post-operative (e.g. dumping syndrome) emesis and of course that induced by a wide variety of therapeutic drugs including those used in the treatment of cancer.

The feature that these disparate groups of stimuli have in common is that they are all able to activate the emetic reflex, one of the body's mechanisms which protect against accidental ingestion of toxins in food in rather the same way that the cough reflex protects the airways (Davis, Harding, Leslie and Andrews, 1986). In view of the diverse nature of the stimuli, the similarity of the symtoms evoked is remarkable.

Understanding the mechanisms by which cytotoxic drugs and radiation activate the emetic reflex is important for several reasons:

1.2.1 IDENTIFYING EMETIC PATHWAYS

Unless the emetic pathways which can be activated by the these stimuli are identified and their neurochemistry characterized, the development of new anti-emetic therapies will rely more on serendipity than targeted drug discovery. Consequently the many new drugs available will represent only small improvements over existing therapies. This has been particularly true in the past for dopamine D_2 receptor antagonists and will no doubt become the case for the new 5HT-3 receptor antagonists. However, with a greater understanding of the emetic pathways more radical improvements in therapy may become possible.

In the absence of a better understanding of the mechanisms by which anti-cancer therapies evoke emesis, inappropriate drug screens will be used. Although these will be predictive of anti-emetic activity against one form of emesis, they may not necessarily predict activity against anti-cancer treatments. For example, even with a single chemotherapeutic agent, a number of emetic mechanisms may operate at different times and this is probably the case with the anticipatory, acute, and delayed phases of cisplatin-induced emesis. Thus it may not be possible to extrapolate mechanisms from one phase to another and hence different anti-emetic regimes may be required.

1.2.2 IDENTIFYING CAUSATIVE FACTORS

Pre-clinical research in emesis has tended to focus on the pathways which may be activated by the various cytotoxic agents and radiotherapy regimes. While this has given important insights, attention must now focus on exactly which aspect of the stimulus causes the primary activation of the pathway and presumably contributes to the well-known differing emetic potential of the various agents used. If this was known it might be possible to 'design out', this feature from the cytotoxic agent. With the demonstration of the involvement of 5-hydroxytryptamine in cytotoxic drug and radiation-induced emesis, for example, attention has focused on the gastro-intestinal enterochromaffin cell as the primary site of action of these stimuli. If this is the case, and it is far from proven, then we could ask ourselves what feature of the enterochromaffin cell makes it so sensitive to these cytotoxic stimuli and are there any parallels with tumour cells?

A greater understanding of the effect of cytotoxic drugs at the tissue level in particular may facilitate better scheduling of current drug administration to minimize the emetic and other side effects and optimize the anti-tumour action. Some empirical evidence for the validity of such an approach has come from studies examining the relationship between the pharmacokinetics and pharmacodynamics of chemotherapeutic agents and their anti-tumour effects (Chapter 2). In addition, studies in mice have demonstrated circadian influences on the toxicity and tissue uptake of cisplatin and carboplatin (Boughattas, Levi, *et al.*, 1990), a feature also seen in cancer patients (Hrushesky and von Roemeling, 1986). In view of this it would be of interest to know whether the magnitude of the emetic response is influenced by the time of therapy. This may become an important issue in the design of clinical trials investigating the impact of $5HT_3$ receptor antagonists on the 'acute' and 'delayed' phases of emesis, particularly with regard to national differences in clinical practice.

1.3 ACTIVATION OF THE EMETIC REFLEX BY ANTI-CANCER THERAPY: THE IMPACT ON THE PATIENT

In a biological as opposed to a clinical context the function of the emetic reflex is to provide a mechanism for the removal from the body of contaminated food. The associated phenomenon of nausea gives an early indication of the presence of a toxin and together with vomiting provides a conditioning stimulus for the development of an aversion to future exposure to the same stimulus. In essence, the reason that cytotoxic drugs and vomiting induce the emetic reflex is because they are able to activate the same systems that have evolved to respond to poisonous contaminants in food. When the pathways are triggered by contaminated food the responses induced may be viewed as 'appropriate', limiting further consumption and leading to the ejection of the food already ingested. In addition, a learned aversion to that food will develop. These responses all have a clear survival value but when this mechanism is activated by a therapeutic agent the response is clearly 'inappropriate' and a number of problems arise.

The significance for the patient of activation of the emetic mechanisms can be appreciated by a brief consideration of the consequences of nausea and vomiting summarized in Figure 1.1. These serve to further highlight the need for an improved understanding of the

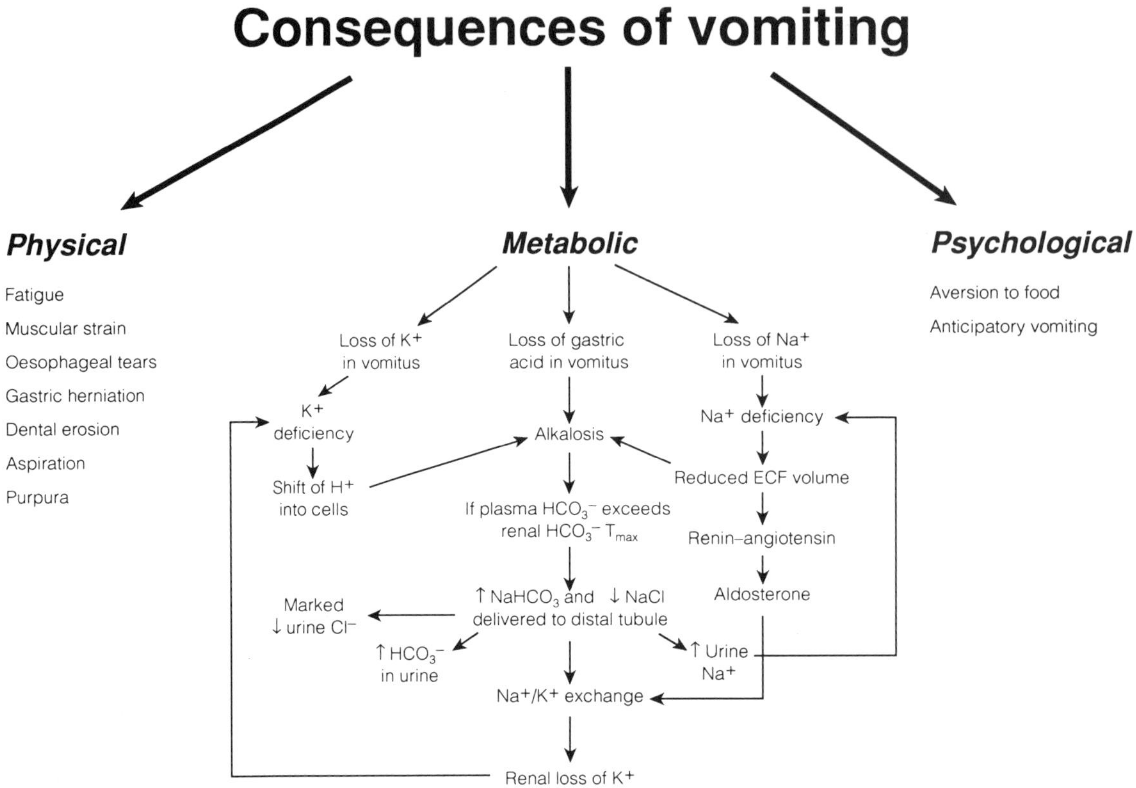

Figure 1.1 A summary of the consequences of nausea and vomiting (adapted from Feldman, 1989). NB: T_{max} = tubular maximum reabsorptive capacity; ECF = extracellular fluid.

causes of this distressing and common side effect of anti-cancer therapy.

1.3.1 RETCHING AND VOMITING

Both of these involve intense activation of the somatic muscles of the diaphragm, chest wall (intercostals) and abdomen which may lead to muscle strain and fatigue. The significance of retching should not be underestimated as the patient may have a number of retches prior to a vomit. In animal studies up to 20 retches have been recorded prior to a vomit although the average number was about six (Chapter 7). If the retching and vomiting are particularly prolonged or intense a number of other physical effects may be induced such as purpura, burst occular vessels, oesophageal tears (Mallory–Weiss syndrome), gastric herniation (Boerhave syndrome) and even fracture of the ribs. The psychological effects of vomiting should also be considered as many people regard it as degrading, particularly in front of others, including medical staff. In addition, the sight of one patient vomiting or the smell of vomitus may trigger a similar response in a susceptible person.

1.3.2 NAUSEA

It is probably true to say that many more patients experience nausea than frank vomiting and yet far less is known of the detailed mechanism involved here. A recent survey of doctors' and patients' perspectives of cytotoxic chemotherapy revealed that nausea was viewed by both groups as more of a problem than vomiting (Cooper and Georgiou, 1992). Although retching and vomiting may continue for several days the episodes are discrete, often with long intervals between episodes. In contrast, the sensation of nausea may be present continually, exerting a greater impact on the patient's quality of life.

The nausea and vomiting induced by therapy will also contribute to the cachexia which may already be present as a result of the cancer. The reduction in food intake may also contribute to the lethargy, fatigue and weakness associated with both radio- and chemotherapy although it is likely that other mechanisms such as cytokines are involved (Kent, Bluthe, *et al.*, 1992).

1.3.3 AVERSION

The development of an aversion to a toxic food makes teleological sense when considered in the context of an animal in the wild. However in a clinical therapeutic context the development of aversion is undesirable. Two types of aversion are particularly associated with anti-cancer therapy. Firstly, the direct association between the nausea and vomiting and the therapy will lead to some form of aversion to future therapy; this is especially a problem in the context of cancer chemotherapy where multiple treatment cycles are required. It is of particular interest that some experimental studies argue that in man nausea is a more potent aversive stimulus than pain (Pelchat and Rozen, 1982). The aversion developed during the first or early courses of therapy may manifest itself as an unwillingness to complete the full number of cycles of therapy although the patient may 'rationalize' their situation and overcome this natural aversion. Secondly and potentially seriously, is the anticipatory syndrome in which the patient experiences nausea and vomiting when they think about the therapy or, more commonly, when they are in the hospital environment and exposed to sights, sounds and smells associated with the therapy. The mechanisms of anticipatory nausea and vomiting are particularly poorly understood and complicated because not all patients develop it and there are no clear predictive factors which provide an insight into the mechanism.

Patients may also develop an aversion to food that is consumed in close association with the therapy (Bernstein, 1978). This is analogous to the conditioned taste aversion that can be readily induced in animals by exposing the animal to a nauseogenic or emetic stimulus shortly after exposure to a particular food. When the animal is exposed to that food in the future it will be rejected after a brief tasting because of the learned association between the food and previous illness (Garcia, Laister, *et al.*, 1985).

1.4 DISCUSSION

From the above brief outline of some of the adverse effects of anti-cancer therapy it is apparent that the identification of rational therapeutic approaches to combat these problems represents a major challenge to both clinicians and basic scientists. Clearly, the discovery that antagonists of the 5-hydroxytryptamine-3 (5-HT_3) subtype of receptor provide substantial protection against the emesis induced by cytotoxic drugs and radiotherapy, has been a major impetus to research into basic emetic mechanisms as an analysis of publications in the field over the past 15 years reveals – (Fig. 1.2). However, further therapeutic advances can only be made by continued research on two fronts in particular: firstly studies of the mechanisms of emesis in appropriate animal models (where limitations are clearly recognized), and secondly by carefully quantified clinical trials so that the information gathered can be used to gain an insight into mechanisms. It is worth

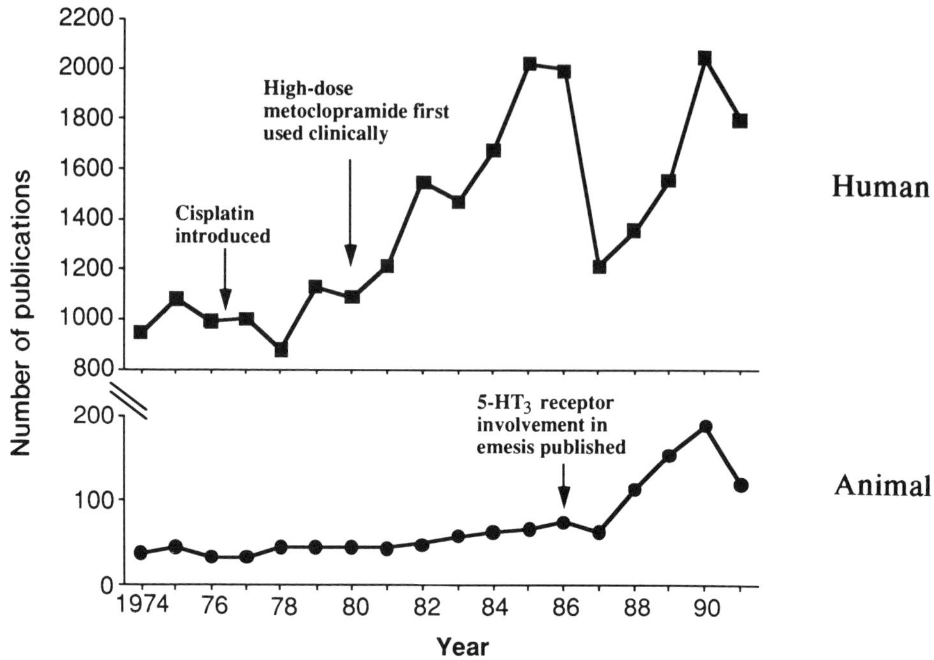

Figure 1.2 Analysis of publications citing research into emesis (vomiting and nausea). (Data from Excerpta Medica).

recalling that the identification of the anti-emetic effects of the 5-HT_3 receptor antagonists was in part due to attempts to explain the pharmacological basis of the effects of 'high dose' metoclopramide which had evolved into clinical use from an empirical base.

An attempt is made in the chapters that follow to provide an insight into how some of these adverse effects may be prevented by adopting a multi-disciplinary approach. The emphasis within chapters is to critically review the various components of the multifaceted problem of emesis induced by anti-cancer therapy.

REFERENCES

Bernstein, I.L. (1978) Learned taste aversions in children receiving chemotherapy. *Science*, **200**, 1302–3.

Boughattas, N.A., Levi, F., Fornier, C. *et al.* (1990) Stable circadian toxicity of two platinum analogs (cisplatin and carboplatin) despite repeated dosages in mice. *J. Pharm. Exp. Ther.*, **255**, 672–9.

Cooper, S. and Georgiou, V. (1992) The impact of cytotoxic chemotherapy-perspectives from patients, specialists and nurses. *Eur. J. Cancer*. 28A, 536–38.

Davis, C.J., Harding, R.K., Leslie, R.A. and Andrews, P.L.R. (1986) The organisation of vomiting as a protective reflex, in *Nausea and Vomiting: Mechanisms and Treatment*. (eds C.J. Davis, G.V. Lake-Bakaar and D.G. Grahame-Smith), pp. 65–75. Springer Verlag, Berlin.

Fallowfield, L.J. and Clark, A. (1991) *Breast Cancer. The experience of illness series*. Series editors: R. Fitzpatrick and S. Newman, Routledge, London.

Feldman, M. (1989) Vomiting, in *Gastrointestinal Disease* (eds M.H. Sleisenger and J.S. Fordtran), pp. 222–38. W.B. Saunders and Co., Philadelphia.

Garcia, J. Laister, P.S., Bermudez-Rattoni, F. and Deems, D.A. (1985). A general theory of aversion learning. *Ann. N.Y. Acad. Sci.*, **443**, 8–21.

Hrshesky, W.J.M. and von Roemeling, R. (1986) Chemotherapy-induced vomiting: circadian drug timing as a source of predictable within-patient variability. *Cancer Treat. Rep.*, **70**, 1347–48.

Kent, S., Bluthe, R.M., Kelly, K.W. and Dantzer, R. (1992) Sickness behaviour as a new target for drug development. *Trends in Pharm. Sci.*, **13**, 24–28.

Pelchat, M.L. and Rozen, P. (1982) The special role of nausea in the acquisition of food dislike in humans. *Appetite*, **3**, 341–51.

2

The pharmacokinetics and pharmacodynamics of chemotherapeutic agents

M.T. SEYMOUR

2.1 INTRODUCTION

There can be little surprise if, when a potentially lethal chemical is introduced into the body, mechanisms are invoked to void the upper gastro-intestinal (GI) tract. This reflex has obvious survival advantage and developed early in our evolutionary history (Borison, 1981): even fish can vomit! Subsequent chapters will deal in detail with the anatomy and physiology of the vomiting reflex; in this chapter an attempt is made to examine how, after administration, a chemotherapeutic agent is distributed around the body, bringing it into contact with the various receptors implicated in acute chemotherapy-induced reflex vomiting. We will see whether knowledge of a drug's movements and elimination (known as its **pharmacokinetics**) helps in predicting the temporal pattern and extent of its effects and side-effects (its **pharmacodynamics**) and whether this knowledge might improve our planning of treatment schedules and anti-emetic prophylaxis.

The sites of the chemosensitive receptors which make up the afferent arms of the vomiting reflex, and their mechanisms, are described in detail in Chapter 7. They are mainly found in the chemoreceptor trigger zone (CTZ) of the hindbrain, in the cerebral hemispheres, and in the gut. To relate a drug's pharmacokinetics with the vomiting it provokes, especially the timing and duration of vomiting, requires thought as to whether the changing concentrations of drug or metabolite at these receptor sites can be inferred from a series of measurements in the accessible body fluids, usually blood and urine. Pharmacokinetic studies allow us to predict the behaviour of the drug in those accessible fluids and may allow us to infer approximately its behaviour in inaccessible 'compartments' such as intracellular water or fat. However, drug behaviour within the central nervous system may be difficult or impossible to infer: the blood–brain barrier (BBB) restricts transit of large or polar molecules into the central nervous system, although its integrity is reduced in the vicinity of the CTZ (Borison, 1986). For data on the behaviour of drugs in the central nervous system and other special sites, one must usually rely on animal studies, or the limited data

Emesis in Anti-cancer Therapy
Mechanisms and treatment
Published in 1993 by Chapman & Hall, London
ISBN 0 412 37250 9

from those occasions when there is access to CSF, bile, serous effusions, tumour tissue or other materials in patients receiving chemotherapy.

If the concentration of drug at the chemoreceptor is one step removed from the measurable plasma concentration, there is another variable which will confound still further our efforts to relate drug pharmacokinetics with vomiting: the delay between receptor stimulation and effect. Even when a drug is rapidly distributed throughout the body, vomiting rarely occurs 'on the end of the needle', but is usually delayed by a period, described as the latency, which may be as long as 12 hours. Several theories have been proposed to explain this phenomenon. One suggestion is that vomiting is triggered not by the cytotoxic drug itself but by the products of cell damage, although this does not fit the observed time patterns nor the wide variation in emetogenic potential between drugs of equal cytotoxicity. Harris (1986) proposed that some cytotoxic drugs may inhibit the synthesis of an enzyme responsible for neurotransmitter degradation, allowing accumulation of the neurotransmitter and leading, after a delay, to triggering of the vomiting reflex. This theory is discussed in detail in Chapters 6 and 7.

2.2 PHARMACOKINETICS

The essence of pharmacokinetics is to measure what happens to a drug when it is administered and to use that information to make predictions: what will happen when the same drug is given a second time; at a different dose; in repeated doses; to different individuals? What is happening to the drug in tissues other than the one we have measurements for? Pharmacokinetic studies therefore examine the changes of drug and metabolite concentration in the different body fluids and tissues in the dynamic system of absorption, distribution, binding, storage, metabolism and excretion, attempting to fit these observations into mathematical equations (i.e. models with predictive power). A summary of pharmacokinetic terms used is given in Table 2.1. (p. 16).

The pharmacokinetics of a drug will be influenced by basic chemical properties such as its molecular weight, solubility in water or lipid and tendency to form ions, all of which affect its passive movement across biological boundaries. More specific biological properties include its affinity for naturally-occurring binding sites on biological molecules, its affinity for transport systems including renal tubular transport and its susceptibility to metabolism by host enzyme systems.

Host factors may vary widely. Obese patients, for example, have an added reservoir for accumulation of lipophilic drugs. Conversely, cancer-related weight loss will deplete the fat compartment. Age may influence the absorption, metabolism and clearance of drugs. Hepatic microsomal enzyme activity is relatively high in children, but also in adults who drink alcohol regularly. Circadian variations in the effect and toxicity of certain drugs (e.g. 5-fluorouracil; cisplatin; adriamycin) are well established and may in part be accounted for by circadian changes in their pharmacokinetics (Fig. 2.1 and section 2.10.3 below).

Absorption from the GI tract may vary widely between patients and from dose to dose in the same patient (Harvey, 1985). Gut disease or previous bowel surgery may disturb enterohepatic cycling. Many cancer patients have impaired hepatic or renal function with alteration in the metabolism and clearance of drugs. Ascites, pleural effusions, oedema and other abnormal collections of fluid may present additional compartments for drug distribution. Tumour involvement of the brain or meninges may disrupt the blood–brain barrier.

2.2.1 PHARMACOKINETIC MODELS

Pharmacokinetic models are mathematical tools for helping to fit observed data, such as drug plasma levels, into predictive equations.

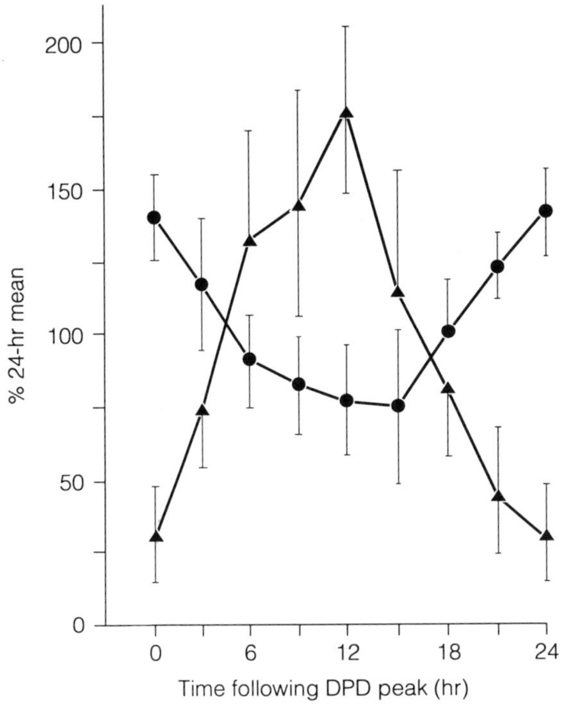

Figure 2.1 Circadian pharmacokinetics, 5-flurouracil (5-FU) is cleared by catabolism, mainly in the liver. The rate depends on an enzyme, dihydropyrimidine dehydrogenase (DPD), which is also present in white blood cells. The diagram shows the results of simultaneous measurement of plasma 5-FU concentration (▲) and white blood cell DPD activity (●) in seven patients receiving the drug by constant-rate continuous infusion. The circadian variation in catabolic enzyme activity is mirrored by circadian variation in drug concentration. (Reproduced from Harris, Song *et al.*, 1990.)

In traditional pharmacokinetic modelling the body is considered as a number of **compartments**, each being an entity of stable volume within which the drug is freely distributed. Drug is introduced into one compartment, after which it will become redistributed amongst the others: movement from one compartment to another depends on the properties of the boundary between them and the concentration on either side of it. If the drug is metabolized, this will occur at a rate defined by enzyme kinetics and dependent on the concentrations of substrate and product, and the metabolite will itself be redistributed among the various compartments. Excretion of the drug or metabolite may occur from one or more compartment; again the rate will depend on its concentration and the properties of the excretion system.

This approach is illustrated by the examples in Figures 2.2–2.3. The blood and those places in rapid equilibrium with it (perhaps the extracellular fluid of various tissues) form the **central compartment** of our model, and from here the drug is cleared, for example, by renal excretion or hepatic metabolism. But the drug might also pass, more slowly, into other places (e.g. the intracellular water). The passage of drug in and out of this second or **peripheral compartment** will affect the pattern of its disappearance measured in the blood: at first the blood level falls quickly as the drug is redistributed, but later drug can leach back into the circulation to replenish what is being cleared (Fig. 2.3). Each of these processes: absorption, distribution, clearance, can be de-fined mathematically, usually (but not always) by simple exponential terms, and each of the compartments has a volume that can be deter-mined. Once we have calculated these para-meters from our observations, we have a model with predictive power.

The model may be as simple or complex as is needed to explain the observed behaviour of the drug. Examples of one- and two-compartment models are given in Figure 2.2 and 2.3. It is important to remember that these compartments do not necessarily correspond with the physical compartments of the body; rather they are mathematical tools, extrapolated from limited observation of just one or two body fluids, usually blood and urine. Indeed, the simplest pharmacokinetic model regards the whole body as a single compartment (Fig. 2.2). Similarly, the rate constants which define the properties of boundaries are derived, not real. Measurement

Figure 2 *A one-compartment model*

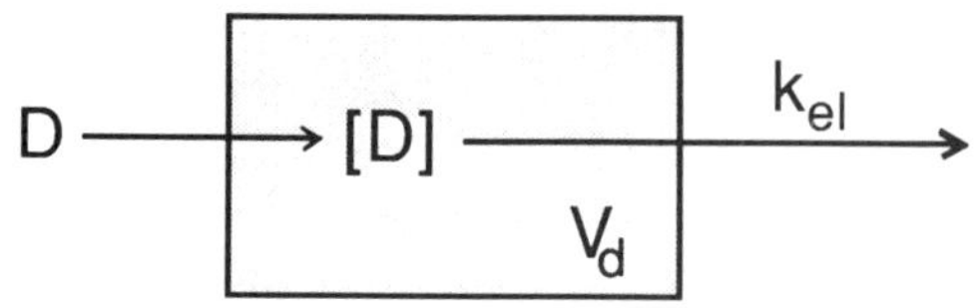

Figure 2.2a Drug (D) is administered and immediately distributed within volume V_d. It is excreted with rate constant k_{el}, and at any time the rate of excretion of drug is directly proportional to its plasma concentration. Therefore, if we know the concentration at time zero, a single exponential equation will tell us the concentration [D] remaining at time *t*:

$$[D]^t = [D]^0 . e^{-k_{el}.t}$$

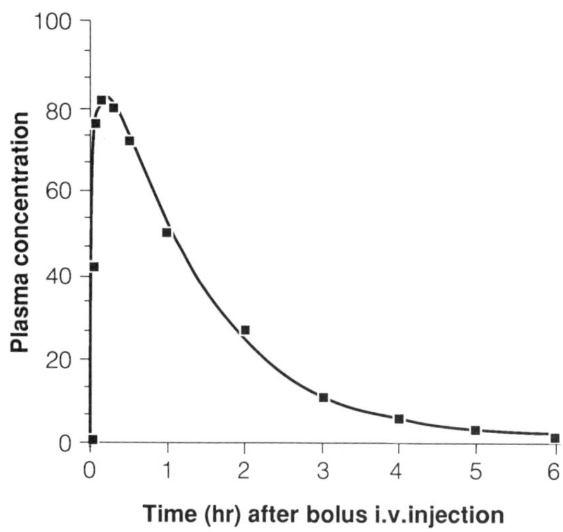

Figure 2.2b Experimental data for a drug following one-compartment pharmacokinetics (see Fig. 2.2a). Even after rapid intravenous bolus administration it will take at least a few minutes for the drug to be distributed around the body. However, after this the drug shows a single exponential fall in plasma concentration.

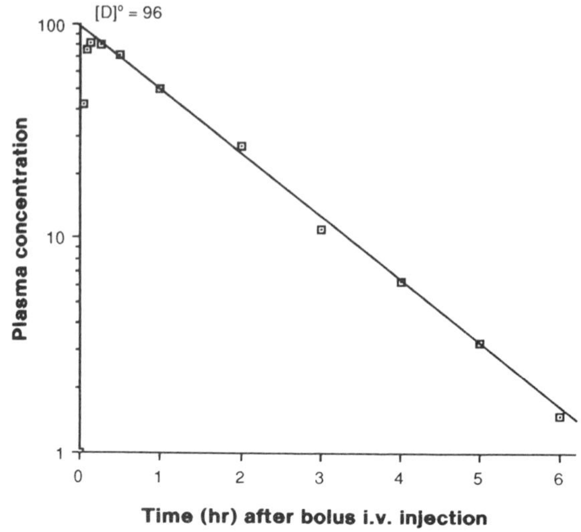

Figure 2.2c The same data given in Figure 2.2b below, plotted on a semi-logarithmic graph. The straight line has a slope of $-k_{el}/e$. The time taken for the concentration to fall by half (i.e. from 50 to 25; from 10 to 5) is constant:

$$\text{half-life}\left(t_{\frac{1}{2}}\right) = \frac{0.693}{k_{el}}$$

By extrapolating the line back to time = 0 we can find out what would have been the plasma concentration had the drug been fully distributed before any elimination had taken place $[D]^0$, and if we know the dose administered, we can now calculate the volume of distribution, V_d:

$$V_d = \frac{\text{dose}}{[D]^0}$$

Figure 3 *A two-compartment model*

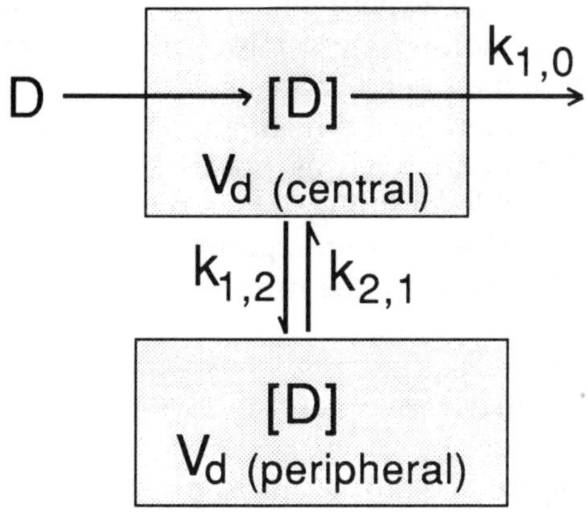

Figure 2.3a Drug (D) is distributed between a 'central' and a 'peripheral' compartment. In this case, drug elimination is renal and occurs only from the central compartment. Rate constants ($k_{1,2}$ and $k_{2,1}$) describe the movement of drug between the two compartments.

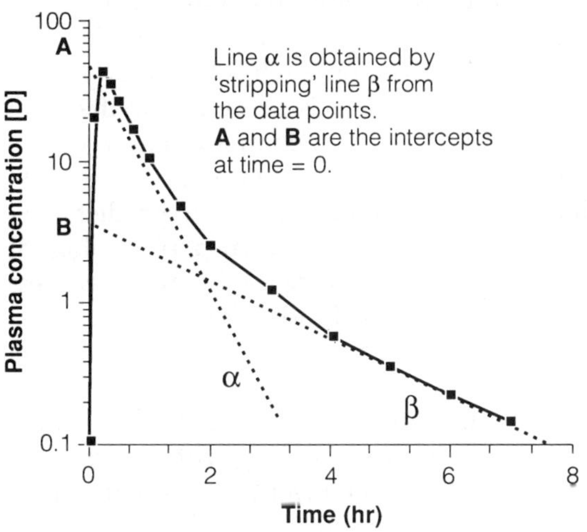

Figure 2.3b Experimental data for a drug fitting the model in Figure 2.4 above have been plotted on a semi-logarithmic graph. The last four points lie on a straight line (β), the terminal or elimination phase, from which are obtained the elimination rate constant and half-life. This line is then extrapolated back, and its values 'stripped' from the earlier points. This leaves another straight line (α) giving a rate constant and half-life for the distribution phase. This process is normally carried out with the aid of a computer.

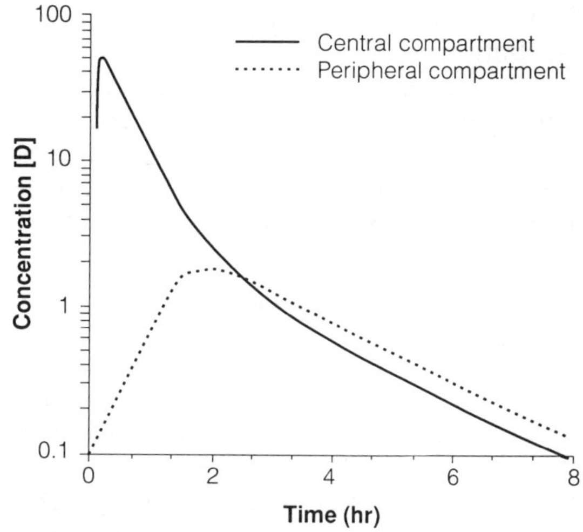

Figure 2.3c Computer-simulated time course of drug concentration in the central and peripheral compartments for the shown data in 2.3b. Since the peripheral compartment is inferred, not real, simulations like this cannot tell us the actual drug concentrations in peripheral tissues. However, they may give an idea of the timing of peak levels in tissues other than blood, as:

$$t_{MAX\ (peripheral)} = \ln\left(\frac{\alpha/\beta}{\alpha - \beta}\right)$$

of plasma levels may allow us to infer the distribution of drug into a composite peripheral compartment of a certain apparent volume, but if we want to know about the drug profile in a real compartment, such as CSF, fat or tumour, we will need to obtain samples from that compartment for analysis.

2.2.2 CHOOSING THE MODEL

It can be seen from Figures 2.2c and 2.3b that when the plasma drug levels after a bolus dose are plotted against time on a semi-logarithmic graph, the one-compartment model gives us a single straight line (Fig. 2.2c), while the two-compartment model results in two lines (Fig. 2.3b), the 'distribution' and 'elimination' phases. A straight line may be drawn through the elimination phase; if this is extra-polated back to time zero and the values obtained are 'stripped' from the curve, we are left with another, steeper straight line representing the rate of distribution from central to peripheral compartments. Indeed, as further compartments are added to the model, so further phases are added to the decay slope. This provides a way of deciding, from experimental data in patients, how many compartments are needed in the pharmacokinetic model.

Thus, using blood sampling alone, it may be possible to infer that the drug is being redistributed into one or more further compartments. It will also be possible to calculate their apparent volume, to derive the concentration/time profile within each of these compartments and to calculate the timing in each of the maximum drug concentration peaks, bearing in mind the constraints mentioned above: namely, that these compartments are derived, not real (Fig. 2.3c).

The appropriate model to choose is the one with the least number of compartments required to give a good fit with the data available and only rarely does the precision of experimental data justify a classical model of more than two compartments. In practice the fitting of experimental data, which was formerly done using semi-logarithmic graph paper and a ruler, is now usually undertaken by computer. Programs of various degrees of sophistication, such as NONLIN and PKMODEL are available for fitting data to compartmental models. Most will fit experimental data to a model defined by the user, and the more sophisticated packages such as ADAPT II allow the model parameters, once established, to be updated continually as further data are accumulated.

Despite the apparent sophistication of computerized pharmacokinetic modelling of this sort, one must remember that the computer's function is to handle the cumbersome exponential equations and regressions that derive from what is conceptually a rather simple mathematical tool. Appropriate use of a computer, then, still demands that the user first defines and understands his model.

An alternative approach is to use **physiological modelling**. This is a response to the main problem of traditional compartmental modelling: that the compartments are not physically defined and so cannot be used to predict drug profiles at target tissues. In a physiological model compartments are used to represent real organs, tissues and fluids. Transport between the compartments is expressed as a function of their known blood flow and a series of distribution ratios that reflect the tissue: plasma partition of the drug within each compartment. The model can be modified to take account of protein binding and known metabolic pathways and non-linear kinetics can be used when information is available. Physiological models are, of course, complicated but they do go some way towards predicting drug concentrations in physical body compartments (Chen, 1979). An example of a physiological model for cisplatin, constructed from detailed measurements in dogs, is shown (Fig. 2.4).

Operational models amalgamate whatever is known of a drug's concentrations in serum,

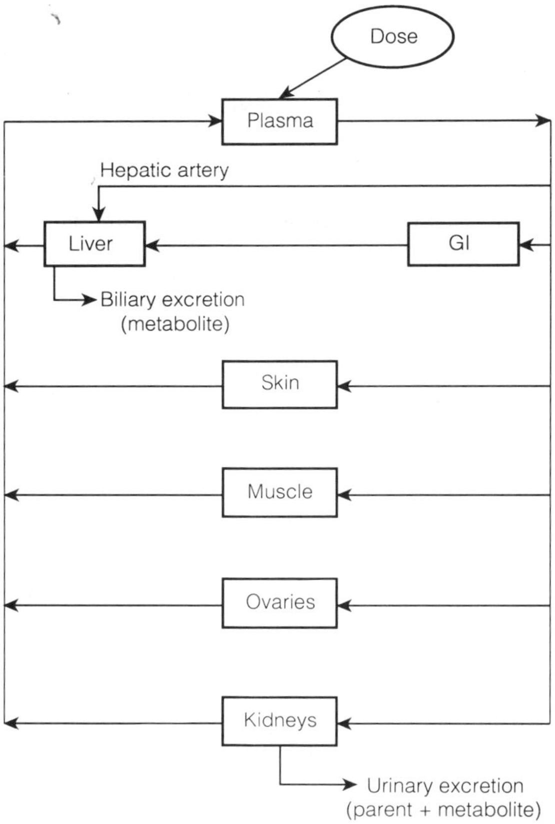

Figure 2.4 A physiological pharmacokinetic model. This model was constructed for cisplatin in beagle dogs. Each box corresponds to a true physiological compartment of known volume, blood flow and platinum distribution coefficient. (From LeRoy *et al.*, 1979.)

body fluids and tissues, metabolic pathways, renal handling, and so on, with the traditional compartmental approach. Where possible, compartments are physical, but extra mathematical compartments are added to fit the experimental data.

2.2.3 USING PHARMACOKINETICS

In the field of drug development, it is essential to establish the pharmacokinetic properties of a new agent. What are the pharmacokinetics in healthy adults; in children; in the elderly? What is the intra- and inter-patient variability? What is the bioavailability when the drug is given by different routes? What are the routes of clearance for the drug and its metabolites and what is the effect of renal or hepatic impairment? These questions should be answered by a combination of studies in animals and humans. Indeed, the comparison of pharmacokinetic parameters in animals and humans may provide an accurate way of extrapolating expected toxicity when deciding on the dose to be used for phase-I clinical trials (Voisin, 1991).

If a drug's toxicity profile is mild, inter-patient variability small and the therapeutic index wide; the above information will be sufficient. However, chemotherapeutic agents have, as a group, the lowest therapeutic indices found in medicine: whereas most drugs are given with the intention of producing their benefits without serious side-effects, the cytotoxic agents are used routinely at doses which are expected to produce dangerous and distressing toxicity. This makes accurate knowledge of their pharmacokinetics of paramount importance, and makes us consider the use of pharmacokinetic data to tailor treatment to individual patients.

Individualized drug dosing of this sort takes two forms, depending on the need for routine drug level measurement. In the first, a pharmacokinetic model is constructed from studies in a sample of patients. The model might include data about patients' size, sex, age and organ function (e.g. measured glomerular filtration rate; serum liver enzymes). This model is then used to predict the pharmacokinetics of the drug in a test population, in whom the dose is calculated to achieve a target drug exposure. Once the model has been tested, it is then used to calculate the dose for all future patients, for whom drug level monitoring is not required. An excellent example of this approach is described in the section on carboplatin (section 2.7).

Table 2.1 Some pharmacokinetic terms

[ ]	Concentration. E.g. $[D]^t$ = the concentration of drug D at time t.
C_{MAX}	Maximum concentration achieved after administration of the drug.
T_{MAX}	Time after administration at which C_{MAX} occurs.
V_d	Volume of distribution. The apparent volume in which the drug is dissolved, expressed as volume per unit body weight or surface area.
k	Rate constant. Used to describe the rate of exponential processes, e.g. k_{el}, elimination rate constant; k_{abs} = absorption rate constant.
$\alpha, \beta, \gamma, \ldots$	(also designated $\lambda_1, \lambda_2, \ldots \lambda_z$). Rate constants for the successive phases of fall in plasma level seen in compartmental models.
$t_{\frac{1}{2}}\alpha$, $t_{\frac{1}{2}}\beta, \ldots$	Half-lives derived from α, β, etc.
$k_{1/2}$, etc	Rate constants for movement between compartments in a model.
C1	Clearance. The rate of drug disappearance expressed as a volume of plasma emptied of drug each minute.
AUC	'Area under the curve'. The area under the plasma concentration versus time curve. A measure of the total amount of exposure to the drug.

However, if bioavailability is unpredictable, if the volume of distribution correlates poorly with the patient's size, or if the clearance correlates poorly with measured organ function, the only way of individualizing drug dosage may be to monitor serum drug levels. This is becoming increasingly widely used thanks to high performance liquid chromatography (HPLC), which provides a relatively simple way of measuring serum levels of a wide variety of drugs and their metabolites. Once again, a pharmacokinetic model must be constructed by studying a test population, but here the time points are determined at which serum drug measurement will provide most information about a patient's pharmacokinetic parameters: a 'limited sampling strategy'. Dosing for individual patients is calculated by feeding their limited sampling information into the model, and calculating the dose required to achieve the target serum concentration or concentration/time product.

This approach may be used after a single test dose, using the information for subsequent dosing of that patient (see melphalan, section 2.5.2, and methotrexate, 2.10.4). Alternatively, further samples may be taken after each dose, and used to continually update the model, a process of feedback control termed 'Bayesian' adaptation.

A good example of adaptive control with feedback is provided by suramin, an anti-helminthic drug which also has activity against prostatic cancer. Suramin has a narrow therapeutic index, with serious neurological toxicity occurring at serum levels only 50% higher than those required for a therapeutic effect. There is also much inter-patient variability in its pharmacokinetics. Jodrell *et al.* (1991), using ADAPT II computerized pharmacokinetic modelling, were able to maintain patients within a narrow target plasma concentration, with consequently reduced toxicity. A major drawback of this approach is the need for rapid HPLC analysis of repeated samples from each patient.

2.2.4 REPORTING PHARMACOKINETIC DATA

When pharmacokinetic data are reported, it is usual to state the model which has been used, the volume of the central compartment (**volume of distribution, V_d**) and of other compartments, and the rate constants for the various phases of the plasma concentration/

time curve, representing one or more distribution rate constants and an elimination constant. These constants are usually expressed in terms of a half-life ($T_{\frac{1}{2}}$ = 0.693/rate constant), which is more easily understood, and are designated α, β, etc. Hence, for a two-compartment model, $t_{\frac{1}{2}}\alpha$ is the **distribution half-life** and $t_{\frac{1}{2}}\beta$ the **elimination** or **terminal half-life**. The rate and route of drug elimination is often expressed in terms of **plasma clearance**. This term expresses the amount of drug disappearing from the body, by whatever route, in terms of the volume of plasma which contains that amount. If, for example, at a time when the plasma concentration is 1 μg/ml, the drug is being eliminated at a rate of 200 μg/min., the total plasma clearance is 200 ml/min. The **renal clearance** is calculated by measuing the rate of appearance of the drug in the urine and comparing this with the plasma concentration at that time. If, in the same example, urine is being produced at the rate of 1 ml/min., and contains 120 μg/ml of the drug, the renal clearance is 120 ml/min., leaving 80 ml/min. for **non-renal clearance** (i.e. by hepatic or other routes).

2.2.5 NON-LINEAR KINETICS

Many biological processes follow **linear** or **first-order** kinetics: the speed of a process (movement across a boundary; metabolism; elimination) is linearly proportional to the concentration of drug, at least over a broad range. Linear functions are expressed by exponential equations and obey the principle of constant half-life ($t_{\frac{1}{2}}$): the time taken for half of the drug to undergo the process is the same, regardless of the starting concentration.

While this may hold true for passive processes, it often does not when active mechanisms are involved, such as renal tubular secretion, active transport and enzymatic metabolism. These processes may be saturable: that is, with increasing drug concentrations, the process becomes gradually saturated. Eventually a point is reached where the enzyme or transport system is operating 'flat out'. This form of kinetics is expressed by the Michaelis Menten equation:

$$\frac{-d\,[D]}{dt} = V_{max} \cdot \frac{[D]}{K_M + [D]}$$

where [D] is the drug concentration, V_{max} is the theoretical maximum rate of the process and K_M (the Michaelis constant) is the drug concentration required to achieve a rate of half the V_{max}. It can be seen from this that when [D] is much less than K_M, the equation reduces to first-order, whilst if [D] far exceeds K_M, the rate becomes constant and independent of [D]: 'zero-order' kinetics. 'Half-life' is no longer a useful term here as the time taken to clear half the drug will increase with increasing dose. Similarly, 'plasma clearance' is no longer a valid measure if the rate of drug elimination is not proportional to its concentration.

Non-linear pharmacokinetics are observed with many anti-neoplastic agents, including ifosfamide, methotrexate, doxorubicin, cisplatin and 5-fluorouracil. In practical terms if, at higher concentrations, the effective half-life of the drug is prolonged, this will mean that the total exposure to the drug increases disproportionately to an increase in dose. The details of this effect will be discussed in the sections on the individual drugs below.

2.2.6 PROTEIN BINDING

Most drugs bind to some extent to plasma proteins, especially albumin, and to tissue proteins. In particular, drugs which are weak acids bind to the basic amino acids arginine, histidine and lysine. This binding is non-specific, competitive and reversible: protein-bound drug may thus buffer the concentration of free drug available for pharmacological interactions. The ratio of bound: unbound drug is often approximately constant over the therapeutic range and between patients, but at high dose protein binding may be saturated giving a disproportionately high free drug concentration. For example, methotrexate at low dose is over 90% protein-bound, but above 5×10^{-5} mol/l the propotion of free drug increases rapidly (Steele, 1981). Not only does this lead to non-linear pharmacokinetics, but similar total plasma methotrexate concentrations may represent different free drug levels in patients with different plasma albumin concentrations. Combinations of protein-bound drugs may lead to competition for binding sites, with similar effects.

2.2.7 BIOAVAILABILITY

When a drug is given by intravenous injection, it is usually safe to assume that 100% of the dose administered is 'available', provided that it has not formed a precipitate or become adsorbed onto the plastic of the syringe. When other routes are used, the drug must be absorbed from the administration site into the circulation: this will take time, and a proportion may not be absorbed at all. The kinetics of this process may be included in a pharmacokinetic model by regarding the administration site (e.g. gastro-intestinal tract) as a separate compartment from which the drug reaches the central compartment with an absorption rate constant.

Bioavailability represents the proportion of the drug absorbed into the circulation after administration by a particular route. The majority of chemotherapeutic drugs are given intravenously so bioavailability is not an issue, but for those given orally or by other routes it is an important factor. For drugs obeying linear kinetics for elimination, the oral bioavailability may be calculated by comparing the total area under the plasma concentration/time curve ('AUC' from time zero to infinity) following intravenous and oral administration of the same dose.

2.2.8 DRUG DOSE DENOMINATORS

Dosage of cytotoxic drugs is most commonly based on body surface area. Because this changes as the square of linear dimensions, while weight changes with the cube of such dimensions, body surface area varies less among individuals than does weight. Surface area correlates well with cardiac output and hepatic and renal blood flow. Its application avoids the relative overdosing of obese patients whose body water (for drug distribution) and hepatic or renal function (for drug elimination) may be low in comparison to their weight. The relationship also holds good between species and the maximum tolerated doses of several cytotoxic drugs, expressed as mg/m^2 surface area, are approximately the same for mouse, rat, dog, monkey and man (Freireich, 1966).

2.3 PHARMACODYNAMICS

If the result of administering a drug is a clinical effect, **pharmacodynamics** is the science of relating the amount of that effect, both useful and toxic, to the drug concentration/time course producing it. Thus pharmacodynamics is the end result of pharmacokinetics (Fig. 2.5).

The crux of pharmacodynamics is whether some aspect of the drug concentration/time course bears more heavily on the therapeutic effect while another relates more to toxicity. For example, if a toxic effect (such as myelotoxicity or vomiting) correlates closely with the peak drug concentration (C_{MAX}) while the therapeutic effect correlates better with the total amount of drug 'seen' by the tumour (the total area under the concentration/time curve; AUC), a divided-dose or slow infusion regimen may be better than single bolus therapy.

The measurable parameters which commonly correlate with a clinical effect are:

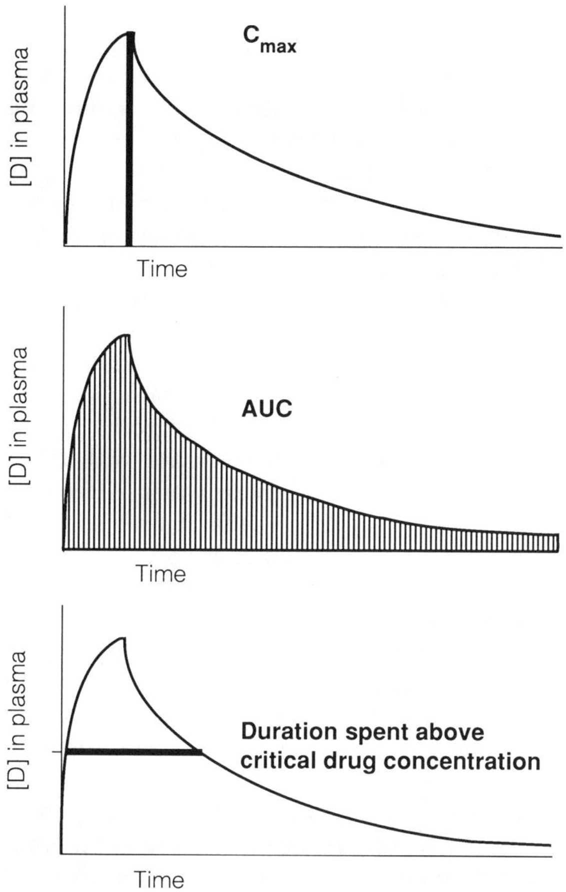

Figure 2.5 The relationship between pharmacodynamics and pharmacokinetics: some of the aspects of the drug concentration/time course which commonly correlate with its effect.

- C_{MAX}
- AUC
- duration of exposure (above a critical concentration)

In addition, if a drug follows first-order kinetics with regard to its absorption, protein binding, distribution, metabolism and elimination, the AUC over a treatment period will be proportional to the total amount of drug given and independent of the dose schedule. This makes valid a fourth and very easily measured parameter, **dose intensity**. Dose intensity is the amount of drug given during the whole treatment course divided by the total length of the course, usually expressed as $mg/m^2/week$.

One might expect that drugs which exert their cytotoxic effect only at a specific phase of the cell cycle, such as antimetabolites (e.g. methotrexate, cytosine arabinoside) or microtubule toxins (e.g. vinca alkaloids), are likely to require prolonged or repeated exposure for maximum clinical effects, while those, such as alkylating agents, which damage DNA at any phase, are more likely to depend on the AUC or dose intensity, independent of schedule.

Etoposide is a phase-specific drug: its activity depends on an interaction with a nuclear enzyme, topoisomerase-II, that is only present during certain phases of the cell cycle. One randomized study in patients with extensive small-cell lung cancer compared etoposide at 500 mg/m^2 as a 24-hour intravenous infusion with the same dose split into five two-hour infusions on consecutive days. Both regimens were repeated three-weekly. Etoposide obeys linear kinetics, and the pharmacokinetic parameters ($t_{\frac{1}{2}}\beta$; clearance (Cl); V_d) were the same for the two groups, but the tumour response rate was 10% for the single-day and 89% for the 5-day treatment, with no difference in haematological or other toxicity. Although the AUC, C_{MAX} and dose-intensity were the same for the two arms, the time spent with more than 1 μg/ml plasma etoposide was twice as long in the 5-day arm, suggesting that prolonged or repeated tumour exposure at this relatively low level was the important determinant of response (Slevin, 1989). Protracted oral administration of etoposide has subsequently been reported to give responses in patients with SCLC (Clark, 1990) and with germ cell tumours which had previously progressed during combination chemotherapy including high-dose intravenous etoposide (Einhorn, 1990; Miller, 1990).

The toxicity and efficacy of the pyrimidine antimetabolite, 5-fluorouracil (5-FU), is schedule-dependent. Widely different patterns of anti-tumour activity and toxicity are found when bolus intravenous injection is compared with protracted infusion (section 2.10.3, below). In this case, it appears that the bone marrow is most sensitive to the C_{MAX} while tumour cells respond more to the duration of exposure or AUC. However, great care is needed when comparing different schedules of this drug since, unlike etoposide, 5-FU's pharmacokinetics are non-linear (section 2.2.5, above). This results in a widely different AUC when the same amount of drug is given by bolus dose or by continuous infusion.

2.4 ANTI-CANCER CYTOTOXIC CHEMOTHERAPY

Anti-cancer cytotoxic drugs constitute a broad collection of cellular poisons that aim to damage cancer cells in preference to the normal body tissues. Like anti-microbial antibiotics, they have to do this by exploiting some difference between the target cell and the host. But while there are fundamental qualitative differences between bacteria and human cells, making possible drugs with high specificity and a wide therapeutic margin, cancer cells by contrast present more subtle targets. Their differences from normal tissue are by and large quantitative: they may undergo mitosis more frequently than usual; they may be poorly responsive to a variety of controlling signals and so fail to differentiate or to die at the appropriate time; they may be relatively incompetent in generating certain chemicals, or in repairing damage to their DNA.

The majority of anti-cancer drugs target the first of these differences, mitosis. However, since many host tissues, notably the bone marrow progenitors and the mucosal epithelia, undergo frequent mitosis as part of their normal function, these tissues are frequently affected by anti-cancer drugs. Clearly, impaired mechanisms for repair and biosynthesis in cancer cells compared with these normal fast-dividing tissues is an important area to exploit, and most anti-cancer drugs are given in cyclical schedules with the aim of allowing a minimum period for recovery of normal tissues between doses.

In the sections that follow, descriptions are given of the commonly used classes of chemotherapeutic drugs, together with a few examples of each. The groupings are based on their proposed sites of action. First are described those drugs which react chemically with nucleic acids, the alkylating agents and platinum compounds. Next, a group of natural compounds which associate with DNA and affect it in a variety of ways. After this, a group of compounds that target some of the proteins and enzymes involved in DNA maintenance and the mechanics of mitosis. Finally, a group of chemicals which inhibit the production of the nucleotide building blocks of nucleic acids, or which imitate them. In many cases, the exact mechanism of action is unknown; in some, several may operate together.

Whatever the particular class of drug, most cytotoxic drugs are capable of inducing vomiting if given in sufficient dose. In practice the drugs for which emesis is a problem, i.e. those for which routine anti-emetic prophylaxis regularly fails, are relatively few in number. Borison and McCarthy (1983) proposed a classification based on the proportion of patients vomiting during the first 24 hours after administration when the drug is given as a single agent without anti-emetic prophylaxis. Inevitably, such a classification is largely conjectural since accurate data on vomiting are frequently omitted from phase-I and II trial reports, many drugs are used only in combination, and anti-emetic prophylaxis is routine. A recent report attempted to update this classification (Lindley, 1989). Table 2.2 lists the commoner cytotoxic agents using this system and while there is room for discussion, it gives at least some idea of the 'league table' of emetogenicity.

Table 2.2 Proportion of patients vomiting during first 24 hours after administration

>90%	60–90%	30–60%	10–30%	<10%
cisplatin (hd)	cisplatin (md)	cyclophosphamide (md)	araC (ld)	melphalan (ld)
DTIC(hd)	carboplatin	doxorubicin (md)	5FU (md)	cyclophosphamide (ld)
cyclophosphamide (hd)	melphalan (hd)	5FU (hd)	methotrexate (hd)	etoposide (ld)
araC (hd)	DTIC (md/ld)	azacytidine	bleomycin	vincristine
BCNU (hd)	araC (md)	etoposide		
CCNU (hd)	BCNU (md/ld)	vinblastine		
streptozotocin	CCNU (md/ld)	methotrexate (md)		
mustine	doxorubicin (hd)	procarbazine		
	methotrexate (hd)	mitomycin C		
	actinomycin D			

Note: Emetic potential of chemotherapeutic agents given alone without anti-emetic prophylaxis.
hd = high-dose; md = medium-dose; ld = low-dose; not stated = standard dose. Abbreviations as in the text. (Adapted from: Lindley, Bernard and Fields, 1989.)

Data on the latency of vomiting are scant for many drugs (Borison 1983), but are important as they have implications for the planning of anti-emetic therapy. It is inappropriate, for example, to give an intravenous bolus of a short-acting anti-emetic such as metoclopramide along with cyclophosphamide, which has an emetic latency of 6–12 hours (see section 2.5.3). In the following sections, data on latency have been included where available.

2.5 ALKYLATING AGENTS

The alkylating agents are a large and diverse group of drugs with the ability to interact with DNA. Most form positively charged alkyl ions in aqueous solution and are able to bond covalently to electron-rich sites such as the N^7 position of guanine bases in DNA. Their different spectra of activity and toxicity depend on their need for host metabolism, their pharmacokinetic properties and the rate of formation, chemcial affinity, and valency of the active ions. Nausea and vomiting are almost universal side-effects of the group, though their severity and time course depend on the route of administration and pharmacokinetics.

2.5.1 MUSTINE

Mustine (a.k.a. mechlorethamine hydrochloride; 'nitrogen mustard') was one of a group of nitrogen mustard compounds first used in patients with lymphomas following the observation of lymphoid aplasia in victims of sulphur mustard gas during World War I. It has now largely been superseded by more stable and less toxic compounds, but is still used in the second-line treatment of Hodgkin's disease as part of the MOPP regimen. Despite its long history, little is known of its pharmacokinetics in humans due to the difficulty of measuring a compound of such reactivity.

The half-life of mustine in plasma *in vitro* is only nine minutes. It breaks down spontaneously in aqueous solution, forming the ethylene ammonium ion, which may react in turn with a nucleophilic group or be inactivated by further reaction with water (hydrolysis). In leukaemia patients, 90–95% of the radioactivity of [^{14}C]-nitrogen mustard had been removed from the blood three minutes after an i.v. injection (Nadkarni, 1956). Data are not available for CSF levels or metabolite pharmacokinetics.

Mustine is a potent and immediate emetic: vomiting may start 'on the end of the needle', though more usually at around ½–2 hrs, and tends to be short-lived. However, vomiting is sometimes delayed for up to three hours and may continue for as long as 24 hours.

Table 2.3 Melphalan

Mode of action:	bivalent alkylation of DNA, etc.
Administration:	low-dose oral; high-dose i.v.
Distribution:	total body water. V_d 0.6 l/kg.
CSF:	CSF levels ≤ 10% plasma, peaking at 30–60 mins.
Pharmacokinetics:	$t_{\frac{1}{2}}\alpha$: 10 mins. $t_{\frac{1}{2}}\beta$: 40–80 mins.
Clearance:	renal clearance low but toxicity increased in renal impairment.
Vomiting:	oral therapy: mild/nausea. high-dose i.v.: moderately severe. latency: 1–3 hours.

2.5.2 MELPHALAN

Melphalan (a.k.a. phenylalanine mustard: L-PAM) is the L-phenylalanine derivative of nitrogen mustard, one of many tested in the search for alkylating agents more stable than the parent compound (Table 2.3). The oral preparation has been used for many years in the treatment of multiple myeloma, ovarian cancer, breast cancer and *polycythaemia rubra vera*. Oral absorption is rapid (C_{MAX} 1–1.2 hr post-dose), but the bioavailability is highly variable and tends to decrease with successive doses (Ehrsson, 1989). Vomiting is rarely a problem at the doses used (usually 10–20 mg/day for 4–7 day courses) but chronic nausea and anorexia may occur.

More recently, melphalan has been used as single high-dose intravenous therapy supported by autologous bone-marrow transplantation. At these doses (up to 220 mg/m^2) emesis is significant, usually occurring with a latency of 2–6 hours.

Like nitrogen mustard, melphalan decays spontaneously in aqueous solution to release the alkylating ion; this may alkylate either water (hydrolysis) or other nucleophiles. However, this process is relatively slow: the half-life of melphalan in plasma *in vitro* is around 2 hours. The AUC of the parent drug is lower in pyrexial patients, possibly because of faster conversion to alkylating ions at higher temperatures (Ehrsson, 1990).

Pharmacokinetics after an i.v. bolus conform to a two-compartment model with $t_{\frac{1}{2}}\alpha$ and $t_{\frac{1}{2}}\beta$ of around 10 and 45 minutes respectively (Gouyette, 1986), though with considerable variability. Indeed, in one study of nine patients, total melphalan clearance ranged from 66–272 ml/min/m^2, renal clearance from 4–188 ml/min/m^2, $t_{\frac{1}{2}}\beta$ from 39–84 min and the fraction of the dose excreted unchanged in the urine from 2½%–93% (Reece, 1988). The clearance of melphalan is delayed in renal dysfunction (Zucchetti, 1988) and a 50% dose reduction has been advocated following the observation of severe myelotoxicity in patients with renal impairment (Cornwell, 1982; Peters, 1989). A method has been proposed for measuring pharmacokinetic parameters in individual patients after a test dose, then calculating the dose required to produce the desired therapeutic AUC (Tranchand, 1989).

CSF levels are about 10% of the plasma levels, reaching their peak 30–60 minutes post-dose (Lazarus, 1983).

2.5.3 CYCLOPHOSPHAMIDE AND IFOSFAMIDE

Cyclophosphamide (Table 2.4) and ifosfamide (Table 2.5) are inactive pro-drugs requiring metabolic conversion to alkylating compounds by mixed function oxidases in hepatic microsomes. Both drugs have wide application in haematological and solid malignancies and low dose cyclophosphamide is used in autoimmune disease as an immunosuppressant. Both are well-absorbed from the GI tract in low doses, but higher doses are given intravenously by bolus injection or short infusion.

Hepatic microsomal oxidation of cyclophosphamide yields 4-hydroxycyclophosphamide

Table 2.4 Cyclophosphamide

Action:	alkylation of DNA
Metabolism:	hepatic microsomal oxidation to 4-HCy then degradation to active species
Administration:	oral or i.v., wide dose range
Distribution:	in total body water
CSF:	active metabolites reach 13–17% of plasma levels in monkeys
Kinetics:	drug $t_{\frac{1}{2}}\alpha$ < 20 min. $t_{\frac{1}{2}}\beta$ $8\frac{1}{2}$ hr active metabolites: C_{MAX} at 0.5–5 hr
Clearance:	renal: 10 ml/min; (only 14% of dose) hepatic: oxidation reactions spontaneous: hydrolysis reactions
Vomiting:	severe with high dose therapy latency: 6–12 hr duration: 6–24 hr

Table 2.5 Ifosfamide

Action: Metabolism: Administration: Distribution: CSF:	similar to cyclophosphamide
Kinetics:	drug: $t_{\frac{1}{2}}\alpha$ < 20 min; $t_{\frac{1}{2}}\beta$ 7–15 hr non-linear kinetics at high doses active metabolites C_{MAX} at 1–3 hr
Clearance:	renal: 20 ml/min. 50% dose lost unchanged in urine hepatic: oxidation + chloroacetylation
Vomiting:	severe with high-dose i.v. therapy latency less than cyclophosphamide toxicity worse in renal impairment

(4-HCy) which has little alkylating activity but acts as a circulating transport compound and spontaneously tautomerizes to aldophosphamide, which generates phosphoramide mustard, the most important alkylator. Both 4-HCy and aldophosphamide are vulnerable to hepatic oxidation, yielding mainly inactive products. So the generation of alkylating activity depends on the balance between the generation and destruction of 4-HCy in the liver, the transport of 4-HCy to the target tissues, and the renal excretion of both parent drug and metabolites.

Ifosfamide undergoes corresponding reactions, but the rate of generation of 4-HIf is slower, especially at higher doses, and an alternative inactivation pathway, dechloroethylation, becomes significant. This yields chloroacetaldehyde, which has been implicated in the neurotoxicity associated with high-dose ifosfamide (Goren, 1986).

Pharmacokinetic studies on the parent drugs show wide variability. Cyclophosphamide levels decline bi-exponentially with $t_{\frac{1}{2}}\alpha$ < 20 mins and $t_{\frac{1}{2}}\beta$ in the range 2–21 hrs (mean 8.5). Renal clearance is only 10.7 ml/min and only 14% of the dose is excreted unchanged in the urine, the rest undergoing metabolic transformation (Cohen, 1971; Egorin, 1989). Ifosfamide is metabolized less quickly at high doses: $t_{\frac{1}{2}}\beta$ at 1.6–2.4 g/m^2 was 6.9 hr, rising to 15.2 hr for doses above 3.8 g/m^2 (Allen, 1975), suggesting that hepatic microsomal metabolism is saturated and Michaelis Menten kinetics apply (see Section 2.2.5 above). Renal elimination of ifos-famide is more important, both because of slower metabolism and higher renal clearance (around 20 ml/min), so that at high doses up to 50% is recovered unchanged in the urine (Nelson, 1976).

V_d for both drugs is around 0.69 l/kg, consistent with distribution in total body water. Penetration of active metabolites into CSF has been studied in rhesus monkeys. After 1 g/m^2 i.v. bolus, the peak CSF concentrations were 13–17% of those found in plasma (Arndt, 1988).

Increased hepatic microsomal activity leads to more rapid metabolism of cyclophosphamide. This has been demonstrated following phenobarbitone and in children, whose microsomal activity is constitutionally higher (Sladek, 1980). Indeed, cyclophosphamide appears to induce its own metabolism: the mean half-life of parent drug fell from 6.3 to 3.7 hours in patients receiving 6–12 months' daily cyclophosphamide therapy (d'Incalci, 1979). Conversely, when pharmacokinetics were studied in seven patients with severe hepatic failure, the mean $t_{\frac{1}{2}}\beta$ of parent drug

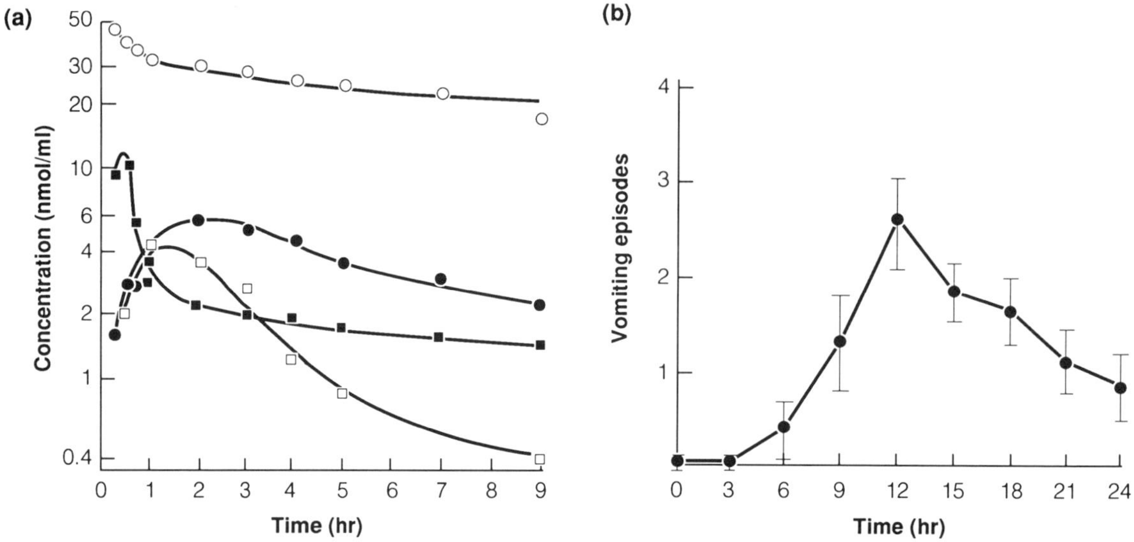

Figure 2.6a Plasma concentrations of cyclophosphamide (O), phosphoramide mustard (■), nor-nitrogen mustard (❑) and overall alkylating activity (●) [nitrobenzyl pyridine assay] in a patient following an intravenous bolus of cyclophosphamide. (From Juma *et al.*, 1980).

Figure 2.6b Mean number of vomits per 3-hr period in patients following high-dose cyclophosphamide. (From Fetting *et al.*, 1982.)

Note: the above two graphs have different time scales.

was 12.5 hr compared with 7.6 hr in controls (Juma, 1984).

Other studies have followed the active metabolites of these drugs. Juma *et al.* (1980) found peak levels of phosphoramide mustard and overall alkylating activity at 30 mins and 2 hrs respectively after an intravenous bolus of cyclophosphamide (Fig. 2.6a). Connors *et al.* (1974) measured plasma alkylating activity after cyclophosphamide and ifosfamide, finding peak levels at 1–5 hr and 1–3 hr respectively.

Both cyclophosphamide and ifosfamide are markedly emetogenic at the higher doses employed clinically. Fetting *et al.* (1982) (Fig. 2.6b) reported nausea and vomiting starting 6–12 hours after high-dose cyclophosphamide with maximum symptoms at 12 hours. Ifosfamide-induced vomiting may persist for several days. While it is tempting to infer that the latency of vomiting for these drugs is due to the need for metabolism to active species, it is also clear that this does not fully explain the length of the delay. There are no published studies which compare the toxicity profile with the pharmacokinetics in individual patients.

2.5.4 NITROSOUREAS

These compounds form two separate reactive moieties in aqueous solution: the chloroethyl carbonium ion (an alkylator) and an isocyanate, which carbamoylates protein. Their clinical usefulness comes partly from their physico-chemical properties: most are highly lipid soluble, allowing penetration of the blood–brain barrier (BBB) and other biological boundaries. Nitrosoureas are used against tumours of the brain and gastro-intestinal tract and in high-dose ablative regimens for lymphomas. Accumulative myelotoxicity is the chief limiting toxicity and has been suggested to be related to drug sequestration in bone marrow fat. The class includes several highly

Table 2.6 BCNU (carmustine)

Action:	alkylation + carbamoylation
Administration:	intravenous
Distribution:	water + fat. V_d = 3 l/kg
CSF/brain:	rapid and full penetration
Kinetics:	$t_{\frac{1}{2}}\alpha$ 5 min; $t_{\frac{1}{2}}\beta/\gamma$ approx. 1–5 hr
Clearance:	spontaneous decomposition + hepatic metabolism; minor renal contribution
Vomiting:	severe latency 2–4 hr; duration 4–24 hr

emetogenic drugs, notably BCNU, CCNU, MeCCNU and streptozotocin.

BCNU (*bis*chloroethylnitrosourea; a.k.a. carmustine) (Table 2.6) decomposes rapidly in serum *in vitro* ($t_{\frac{1}{2}}$ 16 min at 37°C) (El-Yazigi, 1988) and the isocyanate moiety reacts covalently with albumin. Pharmacokinetic studies in humans fit a two- or three-compartment model with $t_{\frac{1}{2}}\alpha$ of approximately 5 min, $t_{\frac{1}{2}}\beta$-γ of 1–4.6 hr and apparent volume of distribution of the tissue compartment around 3 l/kg bodyweight (reviewed in Ames, 1983). The fact that its $t_{\frac{1}{2}}\beta$ *in vivo* far exceeds the half-life in plasma *in vitro* reflects its increased stability in the peripheral compartment, from which it slowly leaches back into the circulation. The serum half-life lengthens with hypertriglyceridaemia, but correlation between body fat and pharmacokinetics was unsuccessful. A recent study of eight patients undergoing high-dose therapy at 200–800 mg/m^2 with autologous bone marrow transplantation gave a mean $t_{\frac{1}{2}}\beta$ of 52 min, ranging from 14 min–10.7 hrs (Mbidde, 1988). The wide variability presents considerable problems in this setting.

BCNU penetrates the BBB well (Meulemans, 1989). While direct data are not available, it would appear likely that BCNU persists at low levels in the brain and other lipid-rich tissues for many hours. Vomiting after BCNU usually starts at 2–4 hr and persists for 4–24 hr. No data are available correlating the severity and duration of vomiting with plasma or CSF levels, nor with body fat content.

CCNU (cyclohexylchloroethylnitrosourea; a.k.a. lomustine) is well absorbed orally. The parent compound is not detected in plasma, but radioactive drug can be traced, with peak plasma radioactivity at 1–4 hr post-dose and elimination half-lives of 27–72 hr for different labelling sites (Sponzo, 1973), though this may represent protein-conjugated or hydrolysed drug rather than an active compound. Distribution to the CSF is rapid (Sponzo, 1973) and when an oral dose of chloroethyl–^{14}C)-CCNU was given at various times prior to brain tumour surgery, tumour tissue radioactivity exceeded plasma by 2–5 hr post-dose. Vomiting commonly occurs between 2 and 12 hours after an oral dose.

Streptozotocin is used against neuroendocrine tumours of the pancreas. It is unusual in having little myelotoxicity but specific toxicity against pancreatic β cells and is used against neuroendocrine islet cell tumours. Its plasma pharmacokinetics fit a two-compartment model with distribution and elimination half-lives of 5 min and 35 min respectively, but when radiolabelled drug is followed in the plasma, a prolonged terminal $t_{\frac{1}{2}}$ of >40 hours is found, presumably representing plasma protein-bound isocyanate (Adolphe, 1975). Streptozotocin is a notoriously potent emetic with latency of 1–4 hours and often causes vomiting for more than 24 hours after administration (Borison, 1983).

2.6 NON-CLASSICAL ALKYLATORS

These are a diverse group of compounds bearing an N-methyl group which may bind covalently to biological macromolecules after metabolic activation. The group includes procarbazine and dacarbazine, both used in curative regimens for lymphomas, and hexamethylmelamine, used particularly against ovarian carcinoma. The precise mechanism of anti-tumour activity of these agents remains

Table 2.7 Procarbazine

Action:	probably alkylation of DNA
Metabolism:	several routes; first-pass hepatic microsomal metabolism to azo-s
Administration:	oral. (severe toxicity when i.v.)
Distribution:	rapid absorption and distribution
CSF:	full, rapid equilibration
Kinetics:	various metabolites have C_{MAX} from 20–200 min, post-dose
Clearance:	renal clearance of metabolites (70% in the first 24 hours)
Vomiting:	moderate initially, becoming less severe with repeated dosing

in doubt. Each may generate alkylating radicals, but there is generally no cross-resistance between their anti-tumour activity and that of the classical alkylating agents.

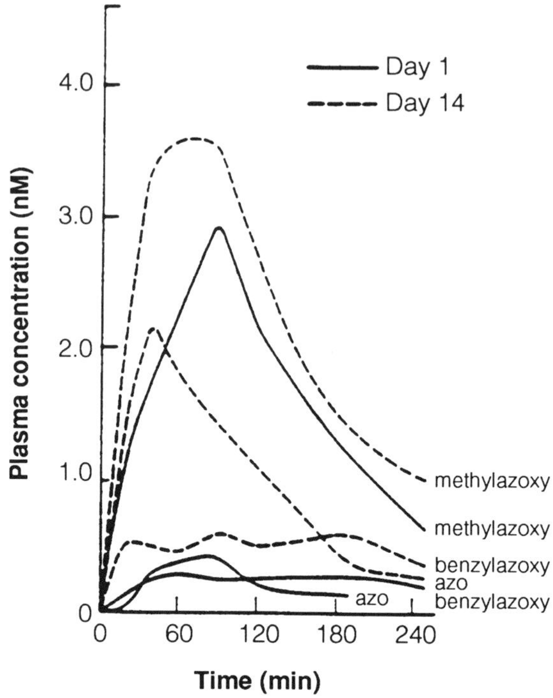

Figure 2.7 Procarbazine induces its own hepatic metabolism. Plasma concentrations of azo-methylazoxy- and benylazoxy-procarbazine in a patient after the administration of 250 mg orally on the first and last days of a 2-week course. (Reproduced from Shiba and Weinkam, 1982.)

2.6.1 PROCARBAZINE

Procarbazine (Table 2.7) was developed as a monoamine oxidase inhibitor antidepressant but was found to have anti-tumour activity during preclinical testing. It is now used as part of MOPP and similar regimens for lymphomas. Serum $t_{\frac{1}{2}}$ after i.v. bolus injection in humans is approximately seven minutes. Given orally, it is rapidly and completely absorbed and probably undergoes 'first pass' hepatic metabolism in a series of cytochrome P-450-mediated oxidation reactions. The active metabolites methylazoxy- and benzylazoxy-procarbazine reach peak plasma levels 40–200 minutes after oral administration (Shiba, 1982) and radiolabelled drug appears in many tissues at 30–60 minutes (Schwartz, 1967). Equilibration with CSF is also rapid (Oliverio, 1964). As with other microsomally metabolized drugs, marked differences in drug handling are noted with repeated dosing. After 21 days of oral treatment the metabolites appeared more quickly and at higher concentration than on day one (Shiba, 1982) (Fig. 2.7). This may be important for the clinical effect: when mice were pretreated with phenytoin or phenobarbitone then implanted with tumours, their subsequent survival on procarbazine treatment was prolonged (Shiba, 1983).

Procarbazine, although used orally, not infrequently induces moderately severe nausea and vomiting over the first week of treatment. However this side-effect subsides as daily treatment continues. It is interesting that high-dose i.v. bolus or five-day i.v. infusion of procarbazine produced neither myelotoxicity nor anti-tumour responses although the patients experienced severe nausea, vomiting and neurotoxicity (Chabner, 1973; Casimir, 1983). These observations suggest that either the

Table 2.8 DTIC (dacarbazine)

Action:	probably mainly alkylation
Metabolism:	hepatic microsomal, generating AIC and methyl cations
Administration:	i.v. infusion, protecting from light
Distribution:	body water. V_d >0.6 l/kg
CSF:	poor. plasma: CSF ratio >7:1
Binding:	20% protein-bound in plasma
Kinetics:	DTIC: $t\frac{1}{2}\alpha$ 3 min; $t\frac{1}{2}\beta$ 41 min
	AIC: C_{MAX} 15 min; $t\frac{1}{2}\beta$ 40–116 min
Clearance:	renal tubular secretion. 50% dose recovered unchanged in urine
Vomiting:	severe
	latency 1–6 hr; duration 6–24 hr

parent drug or an non-hepatic metabolite is responsible for the nausea, vomiting and neurotoxicity and that efficient first-pass hepatic metabolism can prevent its appearance. The likely mechanism for the neurotoxicity is central monoamine oxidase inhibition and pyridoxal phosphate depletion by the parent drug.

A simple practical solution to the problem of procarbazine-induced vomiting is to escalate the dose in a step-wise fashion over the first week of treatment to allow time for hepatic microsomal induction.

2.6.2 DACARBAZINE

5-(3,3-dimethyl-l-triazeno) imidazolely-4-carbox-amide (DTIC; dacarbazine) (Table 2.8) was synthesised in the late 1960s as a purine antimetabolite but appears to function mainly as an alkylating agent. It may have additional biological properties and can cause flu-like symptoms similar to interferon side-effects. It is most frequently used in the treatment of disseminated malignant melanoma, giving responses in about 20% of patients (Luce, 1970) and as part of the ABVD combination for Hodgkin's disease. Its alkylating activity is dependent on metabolism by hepatic microsomal enzymes, yielding an unstable compound which subsequently decomposes spontaneously to release a methyl cation, CH_3^{1+}.

Plasma pharmacokinetics of DTIC after i.v. administration fit a two-compartment model with rapid distribution ($t_{\frac{1}{2}}\alpha$ 3 min) and slower elimination ($t_{\frac{1}{2}}\beta$ 40–75 min) (Skibba, 1969; Breithaupt, 1982). The chief hepatic metabolite 5-aminoimidazole-4-carboxamide (AIC) appears immediately, reaches C_{MAX} at 15 min then declines monoexponentially with $t_{\frac{1}{2}}$ 43–116 min. Of the dose given, 46–52% appears unchanged in the urine and renal clearance exceeds GFR, suggesting active tubular excre tion (Breithaupt, 1982). In the two-compartment model, the volume of distribution in the peripheral compartment is greater than total body water, suggesting accumulation in some tissues. However, the CSF: plasma ratio in dogs did not exceed 1:7 (Loo, 1968) and patients with disseminated melanoma have been observed to have progression of brain meta-stases whilst responding to DTIC elsewhere, suggesting poor CSF penetration in humans as well (Luce, 1970).

DTIC is powerfully emetogenic: vomiting usually starts 0.5–3 hr after administration and lasts up to 12 hours (Cowan, 1971; Luce, 1970). The drug is extremely light-sensitive, decomposing to 4-diazoimidazole-5-carboxamide if exposed to light before administration, and both systemic toxicity and local phlebitis are reported to be reduced in patients treated in subdued light (Koriech, 1981).

As with procarbazine, a notable feature of DTIC-induced vomiting is tolerance: it becomes less severe with successive doses during a five-day course. It has been suggested that, as with procarbazine, this phenomenon is due to induced changes in hepatic microsomal metabolism. However, studies comparing pharmacokinetics on the first and last day of treatment fail to show any consistent pattern in disposition of the parent drug (Skibba, 1969; Breithaupt, 1982). Step-wise escalation of the dose has been advocated as a means of

Table 2.9 Hexamethylmelamine (HMM)

Action:	unknown. ?alkylation, ?antimetabolic
Metabolism:	hepatic hydroxylation and repeated demethylation
Administration:	oral, in prolonged courses
Distribution:	V_d >1 l/kg for metabolites
CSF:	parent drug <10%, but metabolites cross BBB easily, may accumulate
Binding:	95% protein-bound in plasma
Kinetics:	parent drug $t\frac{1}{2}\beta$ 4–10 hr. metabolites variable, prolonged in hepatic failure
Clearance:	metabolites appear in urine
Vomiting:	a problem with cumulative dosing

Table 2.10 Cisplatin

Action:	bivalent bonding with DNA bases
Administration:	i.v. infusion in saline; may be given i.p., ± i.v. thiosulphate
Distribution:	body water; concentrated in kidneys
CSF:	CSF levels <4% plasma
Binding:	mainly irreversible; approx. 60% at 1 hr, 90% at 2 hr
Kinetics:	filterable Pt: $t\frac{1}{2}\alpha$ 30 min; $t\frac{1}{2}\beta$? total Pt: $t\frac{1}{2}\alpha$ 15–20 min; $t\frac{1}{2}\beta$ 50–120 min; $t\frac{1}{2}\gamma$ >24 hr
Clearance:	free drug by glomerular filtration + tubular secretion; protein-bound drug by very slow biliary, renal + non-specific
Vomiting:	severe; worse if given quickly or in morning; latency 1–6 hr; duration 12–24 hr plus delayed (2–5 days)

avoiding nausea and vomiting during a five-day course of treatment.

2.6.3 HEXAMETHYLMELAMINE

Hexamethylmelamine (HMM) (Table 2.9) has some activity against ovarian carcinomas and a number of other solid tumours, although its true value as an anti-cancer remains in doubt (Foster, 1986). Its mode of action is unclear: hepatic oxidation yields a series of demethylated and hydroxylated compounds with N-methyl groups, yet neither parent drug nor metabolites show convincing evidence of alkylating activity (Worzalla, 1973). Hydroxymethyl-pentamethylmelamine, the first metabolite, does however inhibit DNA and RNA synthesis through an unknown mechanism (Rutty, 1979).

HMM is given orally, but peak plasma levels achieved vary enormously, either because of variable absorption or variable first-pass metabolism. $T_{\frac{1}{2}}\beta$ of the parent drug is 4–10 hr (d'Incalci, 1978). The parent drug is largely protein-bound and is not found in the urine, but the metabolites are slowly cleared renally. When methylmelamine metabolites were studied after i.v. pentamethylmelamine injection, marked accumulation occurred in a patient with hepatic dysfunction (Benvenuto, 1981).

CSF penetration of parent drug is poor, but the demethylated metabolites cross the blood – brain barrier readily and may accumulate. This fact is presumably responsible for the high incidence of nausea, vomiting and neurotoxicity with HMM therapy, worsening with cumulative dosing (Wharton, 1979). As expected, these problems are worse in patients with impaired hepatic function.

2.7 PLATINUM COMPOUNDS

The platinum compound *cis*-dichlorodiammine-Pt(II) (cisplatin) (Table 2.10) was identified as an anti-tumour agent by Rosenberg (1969) after his observation of disturbed growth of bacteria grown in an electric current using platinum electrodes. Now, along with its newer analogue carboplatin, it forms the backbone of curative chemotherapy for germ cell tumours, is the most effective single agent for ovarian cancer, and gives high response rates in bladder cancer, head and neck cancer and small cell lung cancer. It is also the most potently emetogenic drug in common use.

Platinum's anti-tumour activity relates to its

high atomic number, with a large total number of electrons. This makes the orbitals of the outer electrons tend to polarize, resulting in bonding of a covalent and stereospecific nature; indeed, covalent bonding with nitrogen is effectively irreversible under physiological conditions. In extracellular fluids with their chloride concentration around 100 mM, cisplatin remains in the un-reactive *cis*-dichloroform but on passive diffusion into cells, with a low chloride concentration, the molecule slowly dissociates (initial reaction $t_{\frac{1}{2}}$ 2.5 hours at 37°C) to form unstable charged complexes with water molecules (Rosenberg, 1985). It can then form two covalent bonds with nucleophilic groups and, like the bivalent alkylating agents, this enables it to cross-link DNA bases, particularly guanosine, and to form links between DNA and protein. There is some doubt as to which of the various types of possible linkage are responsible for platinum's cytotoxicity, but cross-strand DNA links are probably the most important (Fichtinger-Schepman, 1987). Cisplatin has also been shown to stimulate monocyte cytotoxicity and increase the ratio of T-cytotoxic (CD8) to T-helper (CD8) lymphocytes (Kleinerman, 1980; Onsrud, 1986).

Distribution studies in animals and man show that the highest concentration of platinum is found in the kidneys, with some concentration of drug also in liver, gonads, spleen and adrenals (Litterst, 1976). Little is found in brain tissue and CSF levels measured in rhesus monkeys did not exceed 4% of the plasma level at any point after an i.v. injection of cisplatin (Gormley, 1981).

Renal handling of cisplatin and carboplatin are quite different. Free cisplatin is filtered at the glomerulus but is also actively excreted by renal tubules, so that the renal clearance exceeds the GFR (Reece, 1985). However, since a high proportion of the drug becomes irreversibly bound to tissues and plasma proteins, only 30% of the dose of cisplatin is excreted in the urine in the first 24 hours (Patton, 1983; Thatcher, 1982). Renal tubular damage occurs frequently and its incidence is lessened by maintaining a high urine flow with forced diuresis. Carboplatin, on the other hand is less avidly protein-bound (24% at 4 hr) and is cleared by glomerular filtration without renal tubular secretion. In consequence, 65% of an administered dose is excreted in the urine in the first 24 hr (Harland, 1984).

Table 2.11 Carboplatin

Action:	bivalent bonding to DNA bases
Administration:	i.v. infusion in 5% dextrose; may also be given i.p.
Distribution:	total body water
CSF:	poor penetration
Binding:	less than cisplatin: 25% at 4 hr; 87% at 24 hr
Kinetics:	free drug: $t\frac{1}{2}\alpha$ 90 min; $t\frac{1}{2}\beta$ 6 hr total Pt: $t\frac{1}{2}\alpha$ 100 min; $t\frac{1}{2}\beta$ 6–24 hr
Clearance:	glomerular filtration of free drug
Vomiting:	moderate–severe; less than cisplatin

After cisplatin administration, the pharmacokinetics of serum total platinum are reported as showing one or two early exponential phases followed by a prolonged late elimination phase: $t_{\frac{1}{2}}\alpha$ 15–20 min; $t_{\frac{1}{2}}\beta$ 50–120 min; $t_{\frac{1}{2}}\gamma$ > 24 hours (Patton, 1983; Thatcher, 1982). Broadly, the first two phases represent distribution to the tissues and renal excretion of free cisplatin and its free hydrolysis products while the final phase represents the slow elimination irreversibly bound drug. When ultrafilterable (i.e. non-protein-bound) platinum was measured, the pharmacokinetics were monoexponential with $t_{\frac{1}{2}}$ around 30 minutes [Patton 1983; Corden 1985], although one report using a sensitive HPLC assay detected a second phase [Reece 1985].

Carboplatin's pharmacokinetics conform more closely to a two-compartment model (Table 2.11). For ultrafilterable platinum, mean $t_{\frac{1}{2}}\alpha$ was 87 min; $t_{\frac{1}{2}}\beta$ 354 min and renal clearance 69 ml/min, correlating closely with measures of glomerular filtration rate (GFR) (Harland, 1984). Calvert *et al.* (1989) measured GFR and carboplatin pharmacokinetics in a test population, and found that they were able to develop a model to predict the AUC following a carboplatin dose using only the measured GFR. This model has been tested and refined, and proves accurate over a wide range (target AUC 4–28 min.mg/ml; GFR = 33–135 ml/min):

$$\text{Dose (mg)} = \text{Target AUC (min. mg/ml)} \times (\text{GFR [ml/min]} + 25)$$

Thus dosing in accordance with the expected pharmacokinetics is possible for individual patients. This is expected to reduce toxicity by avoiding over-dosing those patients with slow clearance, and to increase efficacy by avoiding under-dosing those with better-than-average renal function.

Both drugs may be given intraperitoneally and there has been much interest in this route for the treatment of low-bulk ovarian cancer confined to the peritoneal cavity. Intraperitoneal infusion of cisplatin achieves an AUC some 12 times higher in the peritoneal cavity than in the plasma and it is possible to combine this with intravenous infusion of sodium thiosulphate, which partially inactivates cisplatin as it escapes from the peritoneum (Howell, 1982). The usefulness of intraperitoneal therapy is limited by the penetration of the drug into solid tumours by simple diffusion. High concentrations of platinum are achieved only within 2 mm of the peritoneal surface of tumours (Los, 1990). This is borne out by the clinical experience of lasting responses to intraperitoneal therapy only in patients with very small or 'miliary' peritoneal tumours (Howell, 1987b; Markman, 1989).

Cisplatin is notoriously emetogenic and maximum antiemetic therapy with a combination of conventional agents including high-dose metoclopramide and dexamethasone is expected to prevent vomiting in only around 50% of patients. Acute vomiting lasts 12–24 hours, but delayed vomiting is common. In one study patients were asked to record nausea and vomiting at home during the week after therapy: while high-dose metoclopramide successfully prevented vomiting in 62% of patients during the 24 hours spent in hospital, 93% reported nausea or vomiting after discharge, with 60% vomiting during the period 48–72 hours post-dose (Kris, 1985).

Acute vomiting may be reduced by giving cisplatin by slow infusion over 8 hours (Jordan, 1985), or by dividing the dose over several days. There is also evidence for a diurnal variation, with vomiting reduced when cisplatin is administered in the evening rather than the morning (Hrushesky, 1986). Not surprisingly, cisplatin therapy has been the main target of research into novel anti-emetic agents. Carboplatin is moderately severely emetogenic. Persistent or late vomiting may occur but is less common than with cisplatin.

2.8 ANTI-TUMOUR ANTIBIOTICS

Several useful anti-tumour agents have been obtained from microbial fermentation, including some of the unusual nucleosides (cytosine arabinoside, 5-azacytidine) which are discussed in the section on antimetabolites.

2.8.1 ACTINOMYCIN-D

Actinomycin-D (a.k.a. dactinomycin) was originally isolated from *Streptomyces sp.* in 1940. It is used in the treatment of Wilm's tumour, Ewing's sarcoma, embryonal rhabdomyosarcoma and choriocarcinoma, working by intercalation into the DNA double helix, where it prevents transcription. It also causes single-strand DNA breaks. It enhances the effects of radiotherapy and can provoke 'radiation recall' reactions in previously irradiated tissues.

Human pharmacokinetics were studied by Tattersall *et al.* (1975) who found a rapid distribution phase followed by prolonged elimination with $t_{\frac{1}{2}}\beta$ of around 36 hr. Urinary and faecal excretion continued for seven days, though totalled only 34% of the administered dose and blood separation showed persistent intracellular sequestration of actinomycin-D in white blood cells after nine days.

There is some evidence of schedule-dependency of the anti-tumour activity of actinomycin-D in mice, with the anti-tumour effect depending on high (C_{MAX} rather than AUC (Schabel, 1974). This has not been confirmed in humans. Dactinomycin is moderately severely emetogenic and vomiting may persist for longer than 24 hours after the dose, in keeping with the drug's pharmacokinetics. One study claimed that toxicity was reduced by the use of slow infusion therapy (Blumenreich, 1985) although others point out that overall toxicity may be more acceptable with infrequent bolus dosing (Benjamin, 1976).

2.8.2 ANTHRACYCLINES

Doxorubicin (proprietory Adriamycin) is the most widely used naturally ocurring cytotoxic agent. Its cousins, daunomycin, which has similar activity and toxicity, and idarubicin, which is less toxic, are preferred in some centres for non-lymphocytic leukaemias. Epirubicin is less toxic though probably equally less potent (Miles, 1990).

Anthracyclines stimulate topoisomerase-II-dependent DNA cleavage, possibly by intercalating into DNA and interrupting the normal process of DNA breakage and repair. They can also undergo reduction to yield the semiquinone free radical, in turn generating O · free radicals and H_2O_2 which can react with each other or with ferrous ions to produce the highly destructive hydroxyl radical, OH^-. In addition, anthracyclines can chelate iron and the resulting complexes can bind to DNA and generate hydroxyl radicals in its immediate vicinity. The two basic mechanisms, DNA intercalation/topoisomerase-II-dependent cleavage and free radical formation, may contribute unequally to the toxic and useful effects of the anthracyclines. This has led to important developments in their use, incorporating pharmacodynamic manipulation and the use of chemoprotective agents.

Table 2.12 Doxorubicin

Action:	(1) intercalation into DNA and topoisomerase-II dependent breaks (2) free radical formation with or without iron
Metabolism:	hepatic: doxorubinol + aglycones
Administration:	i.v. bolus or infusion; vesicant
Distribution:	V_d around 0.4 l/kg
CSF:	poor penetration
Kinetics:	$t_{\frac{1}{2}}\alpha$ 3–10 min; $t_{\frac{1}{2}}\beta$ 1–3 hr; $t_{\frac{1}{2}}\gamma$ > 24 hr
Clearance:	biliary: 50% of dose in 5 days renal clearance insignificant
Vomiting:	moderate; latency 4–6 hr; duration > 6 hr, sometimes several days

Doxorubicin (Table 2.12) diffuses across membranes when un-ionized, although it does not penetrate the blood–brain barrier. It is bound avidly within cell nuclei. The observed pharmacokinetics reflect this, with a plasma profile conforming to a two- or three-compartment model, the final compartment representing intranuclear-bound drug. The corresponding half-lives are $t_{\frac{1}{2}}\alpha$ 3–10 min, $t_{\frac{1}{2}}\beta$ 1–3 hr and $t_{\frac{1}{2}}\gamma$ 20–30 hr (Greene, 1983; Eksborg, 1989). Of drug in the plasma, 75% is protein bound.

Drug metabolism occurs in the liver: the primary metabolite is doxorubicinol and both this and the parent drug may form 7-deoxyaglycones, although all these metabolites are less active and less abundant than the parent drug. The liver is also the main site of excretion, with 40–50% of a dose appearing in the bile over 5 days as both parent drug and metabolites (Benjamin, 1977; Riggs, 1983). It is tempting to consider whether this biliary excretion of doxorubicin may contribute to the prolonged nausea and vomiting sometimes provoked by it (section 2.1, above), but no studies have directly addressed this question.

The rate of clearance is limited by the slow release of drug from the tissues and dose reduction is not advised for mild or moderate hepatic dysfunction (Brenner, 1984); but patients with biliary obstruction have reduced plasma clearance, increased AUC and increased toxicity (Riggs, 1983).

There has been much interest in the pharmacodynamics of doxorubicin. It is likely that the anti-tumour response relates to total drug exposure (AUC) while cardiotoxicity depends more on maximum concentration (C_{MAX}) and is reduced by the use of slow infusions or small divided dose schedules (Legha, 1982; Eksborg, 1989). This may reflect the relative contributions of free radical formation and DNA intercalation, the former being more important at higher drug concentrations. Cardiac muscle is relatively deficient in catalase and is particularly vulnerable to free radical damage. The iron chelator ICRF–187 reduces the contribution of free-radical formation and is effective in preventing cardiotoxicity without abrogating the anti-tumour effect (Speyer, 1988).

Unfortunately, the other toxicities, including nausea and vomiting, do not respond as well to pharmacodynamic manipulation. Two studies comparing bolus with 96-hour infusion (Martoni, 1983) and weekly with three-weekly bolus therapy (Twelves, 1991) failed to show any significant differences in efficacy or toxicity, although one recent report claimed reduced gastro-intestinal toxicity with a 96-hour infusion regimen (Bugat, 1989). Similarly, ICRF-187 does not appear to reduce the nausea and vomiting of doxorubicin therapy (Speyer, 1988).

In the search for synthetic anthracycline analogues, a new class of compounds, anthracenediones, was synthesized in the late 1970s. The most active, mitoxantrone, is active against breast cancer, leukaemias and lymphomas. It works by intercalation into DNA, causing cross-strand links and breaks, but it does not share the anthracyclines' ability to generate free hydroxyl radicals. Plasma pharmacokinetics show a similar three-phase fall with $t_{\frac{1}{2}}\alpha$ 10 min, $t_{\frac{1}{2}}\beta$ 1.4 hr and $t_{\frac{1}{2}}\gamma$ 30 hr (Smyth, 1986). The drug persists in certain tissues for weeks after a dose. Renal clearance is insignificant but elimination may be delayed in hepatic impairment. Nausea and vomiting occur but are considerably milder than with the anthracyclines.

2.8.3 MITOMYCIN C

This drug was isolated from *Streptomyces sp.* in 1958 and has been used with effect against a wide variety of solid tumours. It is a **bioreductive** alkylating agent, that is one which requires reductive metabolism to activate it. A semiquinone radical is formed which, in anaerobic conditions, may bind directly to DNA. Similar reactions may occur at two sites in the molecule, giving sequential bivalent bonding to DNA, especially adenine and guanine residues. This produces inter-strand links. However, the semiquinone may react with O_2 to release superoxide, hydroxyl radicals or hydrogen peroxide with less specific toxicity. For this reason, mitomycin may be preferentially toxic to hypoxic cells (Francasso, 1986) and new agents are being developed which accentuate this feature.

Mitomycin C is inconsistently absorbed from the GI tract, so is given intravenously. A typical regimen is 10–15 mg/m^2 i.v. bolus every six weeks. More frequent administration leads to cumulative myelosuppression. Plasma pharmacokinetics show a bi-exponential decline of the parent drug, with $t_{\frac{1}{2}}\alpha$ 8 min; $t_{\frac{1}{2}}\beta$ 48 mins. Renal clearance accounts for only 10% of the dose, though a higher concentration is found in bile (Dorr, 1988). Neither renal nor hepatic impairment affect the disposition of the drug sufficiently to necessitate a dose reduction. Intraperitoneal and intravesical administration have been used to achieve high local concentrations with little systemic absorption (Adams, 1984; Wajsman, 1984).

Table 2.13 Bleomycin

Action:	DNA intercation then free radicals; single + double-strand DNA breaks
Metabolism:	associates spontaneously with Fe^{++}
Administration:	i.v. bolus or infusion; i.m.; intracavity
Distribution:	V_d 0.5 l/kg; slow entry into cells 50% bioavailable after intracavity use
CSF:	good penetration of brain metastases
Kinetics:	$t\frac{1}{2}\alpha$ 24 min; $t\frac{1}{2}\beta$ 4 hr
Clearance:	renal: 50% dose recovered in 24 hr
Vomiting:	mild and infrequent

Nausea and vomiting occur but are rarely a major problem with mitomycin-C therapy. Cumulative myelosuppression is usually the dose-limiting toxicity. Less common serious toxicities include a haemolytic-uraemic syndrome, interstitial pneumonitis and cardiotoxicity.

2.8.4 BLEOMYCIN

Bleomycin (Table 2.13) is a mixture of peptides obtained from a fungal culture. Some can be synthesized chemically and are currently undergoing clinical trials. The natural product is well established in combination regimens for germ cell tumours, lymphomas and head and neck cancers and is used in experimental treatments for other solid tumours, notably cervical carcinoma. Its usefulness in combination regimens stems partly from its virtual absence of myelotoxicity.

Its mode of action has some parallels with the iron-dependent free radical formation of anthracyclines. It forms a complex with ferrous iron and oxygen, then intercalates between strands of DNA. Free OH^- radicals are then generated by the bleomycin-Fe-O_2 complex and lead to cleavage of the deoxyribose ring and breakage of one or both of the DNA strands.

Pharmacokinetics after bolus i.v. injection fit a two-compartment model with $t_{\frac{1}{2}}\alpha$ 24 min; $t_{\frac{1}{2}}\beta$ 4 hr. V_d is 17.5 l/m^2 (≈0.5 l/kg), similar to

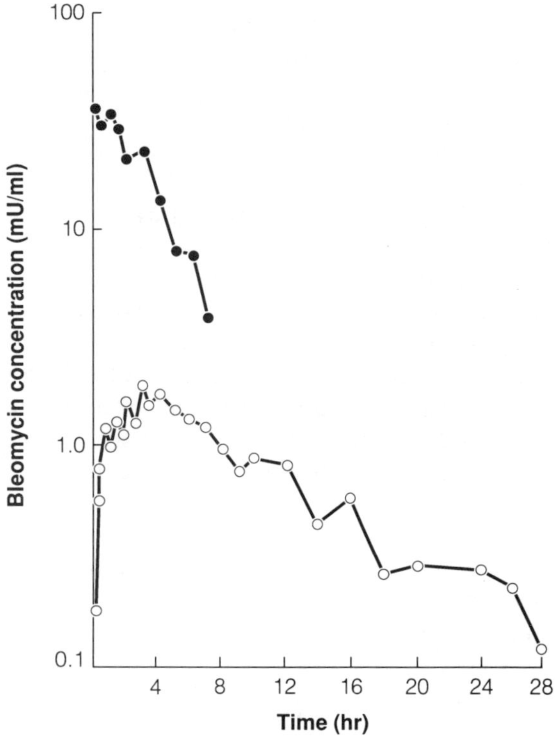

Figure 2.8 Absorption of bleomycin from the peritoneal cavity. Peritoneal (●) and plasma (○) bleomycin concentrations following i.p. instillation of 60 U/m^2 bleomycin in 2 litres saline over 1 hour (mean values for 11 patients). The plasma C_{MAX} occured at 3 hours. (Reproduced from Howell *et al.*, 1987.)

total body water. Clearance is mainly renal, with 45% of a dose appearing in the urine within 24 hours and increased $t_{\frac{1}{2}}\beta$ and toxicity have been reported in patients with impaired renal function (Alberts, 1978; McLeod, 1987). Bleomycins have a high molecular weight (~1,500) and penetrate cell membranes slowly (Roy, 1984); however, absorption from both pleural and peritoneal cavities is relatively prompt (Fig. 2.8). When plasma bleomycin levels are measured after injection of the drug into one of these cavities ('intracavity' administration), peak plasma level (C_{MAX}) occurs within 2 hr and the systemic bioavailability, assessed as the ratio of total AUC after intracavity *versus* intravenous dosing, is around 50% (Alberts, 1979; Howell, 1987a). Similarly, one study showed good uptake of radiolabelled bleomycin into brain metastases (Front, 1987).

Vomiting does occur but is rarely a problem with bleomycin therapy. Occasionally vomiting occurs for a few hours after intracavity administration, but published data suggest that this is infrequent (Ostrowski, 1986). The dose-limiting toxicity of bleomycin is interstitial pneumonitis and pulmonary fibrosis. These are related to cumulative dose, becoming common above 450 mg total. A pharmacodynamic relationship, with lower toxicity from continuous infusion than bolus therapy, has been suggested from animal experiments, but this awaits clinical validation (Jensen, 1990).

2.9 PLANT ALKALOIDS

Unlike fungi, plants have yielded up relatively few of the anti-cancer agents in current use, though much effort is currently devoted to screening chemicals extracted from the ever-disappearing flora of the tropical rainforests. The only agents currently established are the vinca alkaloids (vincristine, vinblastine and vindesine), extracted from the periwinkle, *Vinca rosea*, and the epipodophyllotoxins (etoposide [VP-16] and teniposide [VM-26]), synthetic derivatives from the mandrake, *Podophyllum peltatum*. Several new plant-derived agents are under investigation, notably navelbine, a semi-synthetic vinca alkaloid and taxol, from the western yew, *Taxus brevifolia*.

2.9.1 VINCA ALKALOIDS

These drugs work by binding to tubulin, the protein building-block of the microtubules involved in mitosis, and disrupting its polymerization. This leads to arrest of mitosis during metaphase. They are used extensively in combination chemotherapy regimens for acute leukaemia, lymphomas and a wide range of solid tumours, particularly those with a high mitotic rate such as childhood tumours, germ cell tumours and small cell lung cancer.

Vincristine (VCR), vinblastine (VBL) and vindesine (VDS) have similar pharmacokinetic properties. All are given by intravenous bolus and have a short distribution phase ($t_{\frac{1}{2}}\alpha$ 2–5 min), an intermediate phase of clearance of free drug ($t_{\frac{1}{2}}\beta$ 50–140 min) and a prolonged terminal phase representing slow release of the drug from tissues and blood cells ($t_{\frac{1}{2}}\gamma$ 24–85 hr) (Nelson, 1982). Clearance is almost exclusively hepatic, with >70% of the dose eventually excreted in faeces, although no firm policy is established for dose-reduction in hepatic impairment. CSF penetration is poor (Jackson, 1981).

The major toxicity of VCR is neuropathy, related to the disruption of microtubular function in neuronal axons. This is less frequent with VDS and much less so with VBL, the dose of which is limited by myelosuppression.

Table 2.14 Etoposide

Action:	topoisomerase-II-dependent DNA cleavage
Administration:	i.v. infusion; oral
Binding:	95% protein-bound in plasma
Distribution:	V_d 0.4 l/kg; oral bioavailability ≈ 50%
CSF/brain:	CSF 0.3–10% plasma levels; higher in some brain tumours
Kinetics:	$t_{\frac{1}{2}}\alpha$ 90 min.; $t_{\frac{1}{2}}\beta$ 6 hr
Clearance:	30% excreted unchanged in urine; remainder cleared by liver
Vomiting:	mild-to-moderate

2.9.2 ETOPOSIDE

Etoposide (Table 2.14) (and its analogue teniposide), like the vinca alkaloids, binds to tubulin. However, its anti-tumour activity stems not from this but from its ability to arrest cells in S or G_2 phase by causing DNA strand breaks. It does this in association with topoisomerase-II, a nuclear enzyme which breaks DNA as part of the normal process of repair. It is used in combination regimens for lymphomas and germ cell tumours and is the most effective single agent for the treatment of small cell lung cancer.

Etoposide may be given orally, though its bioavailability by this route is variable (Harvey, 1985). Intravenously, it is given by short infusion, since bolus injections cause hypotension. It is 95% protein bound in plasma (Allen, 1982). Pharmacokinetics conform to a two-compartment model with $t_{\frac{1}{2}}\alpha \approx 90$ min; $t_{\frac{1}{2}}\beta \approx 6$ hr (D'Incalci, 1982). Renal clearance is about one third of the total plasma clearance and only 30% of the dose is recovered unchanged in the urine, with 20% recovered as metabolites and the rest being excreted in bile or lost to the tissues. CSF levels are <10% of plasma levels, but this is partly accounted for by the different protein concentrations in the two fluids.

Etoposide is **phase-specific**, that is it affects cells only at certain stages of the mitotic cycle. This, along with its lack of a prolonged terminal elimination phase, may account for its schedule-dependency and the pharmacodynamic features discussed in section 2.3, above.

Vomiting is not a major problem with etoposide therapy. The mild emesis provoked by short intravenous infusions is usually easily controlled with simple anti-emetics. More recently, low-dose oral etoposide, given for prolonged courses, has proven useful in the treatment of advanced small cell lung cancer (Clark, 1990). A proportion of patients treated in this way complain of nausea and occasional vomiting.

2.10 ANTI-METABOLITES

This rather unhelpful term is applied to a diverse group of drugs which act by interfering with the synthesis of purine and pyrimidine bases, their linkage to a sugar to form nucleosides, or their subsequent phosphorylation to nucleotides, the building-blocks of the nucleic acids DNA and RNA. They rely for their anti-tumour activity on the increased demand for nucleic acid synthesis in malignant cells and, in some cases, their relative lack of precursors. In addition, some agents act as **false nucleotides**, becoming incorporated into DNA or RNA in place of the normal purine and pyrimidine nucleotides, and thereafter disturbing their function.

Most anti-metabolites are analogues of the naturally ocurring bases or nucleosides. A further compound, methotrexate, interferes with folic acid metabolism, so depleting the supply of one-carbon groups required for the *de novo* synthesis of purines and thymidylate.

Table 2.15 Cytosine arabinoside

Action:	analogue of deoxycytidine
Metabolism:	converted to araCTP in target cell
Administration:	wide dose range; i.v., i.t., s.c.
Distribution:	body water; active transport into cells
CSF:	moderate: around 30% of plasma
Kinetics:	$t_{\frac{1}{2}}\alpha$ 12–25 min; $t_{\frac{1}{2}}\beta$ 2–20 hr
Clearance:	catabolite araU excreted renally, accounting for 70–80% of the dose
Vomiting:	severe and early after high-doses; latency up to 12 hr at lower doses

2.10.1 CYTOSINE ARABINOSIDE

Cytosine arabinoside (a.k.a. arabinosylcytosine; 1β-D-arabinofuranosylcytosine; araC) (Table 2.15) is an isomer of deoxycytidine, differing only in the orientation of a hydroxyl group on the sugar ring. In human cells it is phosphorylated in the same way as its natural counterpart to form the nucleotide ara-cytosine triphosphate (araCTP), but this 'false nucleotide' can both inhibit DNA polymerase and, after incorporation into DNA, terminate DNA chain elongation. It is most frequently used in combinations for remission induction or consolidation treatment for acute non-lymphocytic leukaemia and has been used in certain high-grade lymphomas, but has little activity in solid tumours.

AraC is hydrophilic and crosses cell membranes by a nucleoside active transport mechanism which results in its rapid distribution in total body water. It is metabolized rapidly, with either the generation of the active nucleotide araCTP or deamination to the inactive uridine analogues, ara-uridine monophosphate (araUMP) and ara-uridine (araU), which is the major urinary excretion product. Thus its clinical activity depends on the activity of transport mechanisms and the balance between activation and deamination within malignant cells.

There is rapid disappearance from the plasma after a bolus injection, fitting a two-compartment pharmacokinetic model with $t_{\frac{1}{2}}\alpha$ 12–25 min and $t_{\frac{1}{2}}\beta$ 2–20 hr (Kreis, 1985; Avramis, 1989; Liliemark, 1985). Very little araC appears in the urine (Kreis, 1985), but the main plasma catabolite, araU, is excreted renally with $t_{\frac{1}{2}}$ 3–6 hr and 70–80% of the dose appears in the urine in this form. Serum protein binding is negligible (Slevin, 1983a). CSF penetration is relatively brisk for a hydrophilic drug and although the CSF: plasma concentration ratio did not exceed 22% during a 3-hour infusion of high dose araC, the CSF clearance was slower, leading to a CSF concentration higher than the simultaneous plasma level three hours (Slevin, 1983b).

AraC is given in a wide range of doses and its main toxicities are severe myelotoxicity and gastro-intestinal mucositis. At low or medium dose (e.g. 20–200 $mg/m^2/day$) it causes mild-to-moderate nausea and vomiting, but vomiting may be severe with the high dose regimens (up to 3 g/m^2 12 hourly). Vomiting generally starts during or shortly after a 3-hour infusion and lasts somewhat longer than 12 hours.

2.10.2 5-AZACYTIDINE

This is an analogue of cytidine rather than deoxycytidine, but like araC its most useful activity is against acute non-lymphocytic leukaemia. It differs from cytidine in having nitrogen at the 5-position of its heterocyclic ring, making it unstable in solution. Like araC, it enters cells via a nucleoside transport mechanism. It is then phosphorylated to azacytidine triphosphate (azaCTP) which competes with native CTP for incorporation into RNA and disrupts RNA function in several ways. It may also be incorporated to some extent into DNA and may inhibit the methylation of DNA cytidine residues. Cytidine methylation is a normal mechanism of gene inactivation, thus 5-azacytidine may lead to alterations in gene expression and cellular differentiation (Jones, 1983).

The pharmacokinetics of 5-azacytidine are poorly understood because of its lability and the lack of a specific assay method. Isotope tracer studies show rapid distribution of radioactivity in total body water, minimal protein binding, poor CSF penetration and a plasma $t_{\frac{1}{2}}$ of around $3\frac{1}{2}$ hours, but little of the measured radioactivity represents parent drug (Israili, 1976).

Bolus intravenous 5-azacytidine is potently emetogenic and this effect, though not the anti-mitotic effect, is strongly schedule-dependent. When the same dose is administered by continuous intravenous infusion, nausea and vomiting are not a problem, although myelosuppression and anti-leukaemic activity are the same (Vogler, 1976).

2.10.3 5-FLUOROURACIL

5-Fluorouracil (5-FU) was one of the first drugs to be rationally designed and synthesized to achieve a specific biochemical action (Heidelberger, 1957). It has a wide spectrum of activity and forms an important part of current treatments for cancers of the breast and gastro-intestinal tract. It differs from uracil only in the substitution of fluorine for hydrogen at the 5-position of its heterocyclic ring. Its cytotoxicity may relate in part to the substitution of fluorinated uridine triphosphate residues into RNA, but it may interfere with pyrimidine metabolism in other ways. It can inhibit thymidylate synthetase, the enzyme responsible for *de novo* synthesis of thymidylate, which normally involves the addition of a methyl group at the 5-position of deoxyuridine monophosphate. As well as depleting the cell's supply of thymidylate required for DNA synthesis, it has recently been shown that inhibitors of thymidylate synthetase may lead to a build up of deoxy-uridine nucleotides, which become wrongly incorporated into DNA (Curtin, 1991).

5-FU is usually given by intravenous bolus injection or infusion. Oral bioavailability is extremely unreliable (Finch, 1979) and oral 5-FU is no longer used, although a newer compound, ftorafur, which acts partly as a pro-drug for 5-FU, is suitable for oral use. 5-FU is distributed in the extracellular fluid space (V_d around 0.2 l/kg) and transported into cells by an active transport mechanism. It is rapidly metabolized, forming either active fluoro-nucleotides or inactive catabolites (mainly fluoro-β-alanine). Catabolism occurs preferentially in the liver, where clearance may equal hepatic blood flow.

Plasma pharmacokinetics have been matched to a variety of classical and physiological models. $T_{\frac{1}{2}}$ is reported to be in the order of 10–20 minutes; however, there is evidence of non-linear kinetics, with saturation of metabolic clearance at high concentration (McDermott, 1982). Intracellular 5-FU and metabolites persist for much longer and it is possible that incorporation of fluoro-UTP into RNA creates a pool of fluoro-nucleotide which is released slowly as the RNA is subsequently broken down. Distribution into CSF is good, but may be reduced with infusional therapy as evidence in monkeys suggests that BBB penetration depends on achieving a high C_{MAX} in the plasma (Kerr, 1984).

The story of 5-FU's saturable metabolism becomes more complicated with the observation of a circadian variability to the metabolic clearance. Harris *et al.* (1990) measured the activity of the rate-limiting catabolic enzyme, dihydroprimidine dehydrogenase (DPD) in serial white blood cell samples from patients on chronic 5-FU infusions. They found a sinusoidal circadian variability in its activity, inversely matched by variations in the plasma 5-FU concentration (Fig. 2.1, above). Another phenomenon has been reported by Findlay *et al.* (1991), who were able to monitor 5-FU's metabolism within tumour tissue using magnetic resonance spectroscopy. They found wide variability in the tumours' ability to anabolise or catabolise the drug, and noted that concurrent administration of interferon-α tended to favour the anabolic pathway.

There has been much interest in 5-FU's pharmacodynamics: like several other anti-metabolites it combines a short plasma half-life with cell-cycle phase specificity, so its effects are likely to be schedule-dependent. This is indeed the case: anti-tumour responses and patterns of toxicity vary widely according to the schedule of administration. When given by bolus injection or short infusion, myelosuppression is dose-limiting, mucositis is common and vomiting is not infrequent. Protracted infusions of the drug produce neither myelotoxicity nor vomiting and the dose-intensity (and AUC) may be increased until mucositis or a new side-effect, hand–foot dermatitis, limits the dose. Colorectal tumour responses are more frequent with infusional therapy (Hansen, 1989), suggesting that colorectal tumour cells are more sensitive to the AUC or period of exposure whilst bone marrow stem cells and the CTZ are more sensitive to C_{max}.

2.10.4 METHOTREXATE

Methotrexate is a powerful competitive inhibitor of the enzyme dihydrofolate reductase (DHFR). It is one of the best established and most widely applied cytotoxic agents and one for which vomiting is a problem only at high dose.

Inhibition of DHFR prevents the generation of reduced folate which is needed as a cofactor for several cellular processes, in particular the *de novo* synthesis of thymidylate by the enzyme thymidylate synthetase. Reduced folate is also required for purine synthesis. DHFR inhibition also leads to accumulation of dihydrofolate, which itself inhibits thymidylate synthetase.

Methotrexate is used orally, intravenously by bolus or infusion, intramuscularly, intra-arterially and intrathecally. Oral methotrexate is absorbed by an easily saturable folate transport system giving oral bioavailability of around 50% at low dose, but making this route unsuitable for medium- or high-dose therapy. Pharmacokinetics after i.v. bolus administration show more than one phase, with $t_{\frac{1}{2}}\alpha$ around 1–2 hr and $t_{\frac{1}{2}}\beta$ around 8–12 hours (Chabner, 1978; Stoller, 1975). V_d is around 0.18 l/kg for the central and 0.76 l/kg for the peripheral compartment, corresponding to extracellular fluid and total body water respectively. Plasma binding is around 95% but becomes saturated above 50 μmol/l, leading to non-linear pharmacokinetics when total plasma levels are measured (Steele, 1981).

The renal clearance of methotrexate approximates to the creatinine clearance. When high doses are used, the concentration in the urine may exceed its solubility at acid pH and intratubular precipitation may occur. For this reason it is necessary to maintain alkaline urine and adequate flow during high-dose methotrexate therapy. The terminal phase ($t_{\frac{1}{2}}\gamma$) is prolonged in patients with 'third space' fluid collections such as ascites, which act as drug reservoirs (Chabner, 1978). Several groups have used a small test dose of methotrexate to measure plasma clearance in individual patients in order to calculate the infusion rate required to produce the desired plasma level for high-dose therapy (Kerr, 1983).

Medium and high dose methotrexate regimens must include the biochemical rescue of normal tissues at an interval after the methotrexate has been given. This is usually done with calcium leukovorin (folinic acid), a reduced folate. Leukovorin is usually started 24 hours after initiating methotrexate and its dose and duration is titrated to the plasma levels of methotrexate remaining. Drug level monitoring is considered mandatory for high-dose methotrexate/leukovorin rescue regimens. Vomiting is a common side effect of methotrexate only when given at high dose.

2.11 CONCLUSIONS

Some drugs with powerful cytotoxicity cause little vomiting and vice-versa. Others that require metabolism to active species provoke vomiting only after a long 'latent' period, yet when their metabolism is studied in detail we find that the latency far exceeds the time required to generate active metabolites. In many cases vomiting does not start until long after the drug has been all but cleared from the bloodstream. We must concede that the physiologist, not the pharmacokineticist, will hold the key to the phenomenon of latency.

However, pharmacokinetics has been useful in explaining the problems that arise with certain classes of drug. Drugs with high lipid solubility, such as the nitrosoureas and methylmelamine metabolites, may persist at low levels in the CNS at a time when plasma levels have fallen. Doxorubicin may still be present in high concentration in the bile several days after a dose.

Perhaps the most important outcome of the study of pharmacokinetics has been an appreciation of the variability in drug handling by different individuals. Even those with normal measured renal or hepatic function show wide differences for certain drugs. As HPLC and other assay techniques become ever more accessible, so therapeutic drug monitoring and the tailoring of doses to individuals becomes a practical option. Our goal must be, for each patient, to optimize dosing and schedule so as to provide the best possible drug profile for a drug's beneficial effects whilst keeping toxicity within acceptable limits. Similarly, anti-emetic drug therapy should be planned to take account of the expected pharmacokinetic profile and latency within individuals.

ACKNOWLEDGEMENTS

The author gratefully acknowledges the suggestions and comments of Dr Paul Thompson, Department of Oncology, Auckland Hospital, New Zealand.

REFERENCES

Adams, S.C., Patt, Y.Z. and Rosenblum, M.G. (1984) Pharmacokinetics of mitomycin C following intraperitoneal administration. *Proc. ASCO*, **3**, 361.

Adolphe, A.B., Glasofer, E.P., Troetel, W.M. *et al.* (1975) Pharmacokinetics of streptozotocin. *Cancer Chemother. Rep.*, **59**, 547–56.

Alberts, D.S., Chen, H.S.G., Liu, R. *et al.* (1978) Bleomycin pharmacokinetics in man I: Intravenous administration. *Cancer Chemother. Pharmacol.*, **1**, 177–81.

Alberts, D.S., Chen, H.S.G., Mayersohn, M. *et al.*, (1979) Bleomycin pharmacokinetics in man II: intracavity administration. *Cancer Chemother. Pharmacol.*, **2**, 127–32.

Allen, L.M. and Creaven, P.J. (1975) Pharmacokinetics of ifosfamide. *Clin. Pharmacol. Ther.*, **17**, 492–8.

Allen, L.M., Tejada, F., Okonmah, A.D., *et al.* (1982) Combination therapy of the epipodopyllotoxin derivatives, teniposide and etoposide: a pharmacodynamic rationale. *Cancer Chemother. Pharmacol.*, **7**, 151–56.

Ames, M.M. and Powis, G. (1983) Pharmacokinetics of nitrosoureas, in *Pharmacokinetics of Anticancer Agents in Humans*, (Eds. M.M. Ames, G. Powis and J.S. Kovach) pp. 113–34, Elsevier, Amsterdam.

Arndt, C.A., Balis, F.M., McCulley, C.L. *et al.* (1988) CSF penetration of active metabolites of cyclophosphamide and ifosfamide in rhesus monkeys *Cancer Res.*, **48**, 2113–15.

Avramis, V.I., Weinberg, K.I., Sato, J.K. *et al.* (1989) Pharmacology studies of 1β-D-arabinofuranosylcytosine in paediatric patients with leukaemia and lymphoma after a biochemically optimal regimen of loading bolus plus continuous infusion of the drug. *Cancer Res.*, **49**, 241–7.

Benjamin, R.S., Hall, S.W., Burgess, M.A. *et al.* (1976) A pharmacokinetically based phase-I/II study of single-dose actinomycin D. *Cancer Treat. Rep.*, **60**, 289–91.

Benjamin, R.S., Riggs, C.E., and Bachur, N.R. (1977) Plasma pharmacokinetics of adriamycin and its metabolites in humans with normal hepatic and renal function. *Cancer Res.*, **37**, 1416–20.

Benvenuto, J.A., Stewart, D.J., Benjamin, R.S. *et al.* (1981) Pharmacology of pentamethylmelamine in humans. *Cancer Res.*, **41**, 566–9.

Blumenreich, M.S., Woodcock, T.M. and Richman, S.P. (1985) A Phase-I trial of dactinomycin IV infusion in patients with advanced malignancies. *Cancer*, **56**, 256–8.

Borison, H.L., Borison, R. and McCarthy, L.E. (1981) Phylogenic and neurologic aspects of the vomiting process *J. Clin. Pharmacol.* **21** (8–9 Suppl): 23S–29S.

Borison, H.L. (1986) Anatomy and physiology of the chemoreceptor trigger zone and area postrema; in *Nausea and Vomiting: Mechanisms and Treatment*, (Eds C.J. Davis, G.V. Lake-Bakaar, and D.G. Grahame-Smith) pp. 10–17, Springer-Verlag, Berlin.

Breithaupt, H., Dammann, A. and Aigner, K. (1982) Pharmacokinetics of DTIC and its metabolite AIC following different dose schedules. *Cancer Chemother. Pharmacol.*, **9**, 103–9.

Brenner, D.E., Wiernik, P.H., Wesley, M. *et al.* (1984) Acute doxorubicin toxicity: relationship to pretreatment liver function, response and pharmacokinetics. *Cancer*, **53**, 1042–8.

Bugat, R., Robert, J., Herrera, A. *et al.* (1989) Clinical and pharmacokinetic study of 96-hr infusions of doxorubicin in advanced cancer patients. *Eur. J. Cancer Clin. Oncol.*, **25**, 505–11.

Calvert, A.H., Newell, D.R., Gumbrell, L.A. *et al.* (1989) The clinical pharmacokinetics of carboplatin: prospective validation of a dosage formula for use in high-dose single-agent and combination studies *Proc. Am. Soc. Clin. Oncol.*, **8**, 70.

Casimir, A., Kavanagh, J., Liu, F. *et al.* (1983) Phase-I trial of IV procarbazine administered as a

5-day continuous infusion *Proc. Am. Assoc. Cancer Res.*, **24**, 144.

Chabner, B.A., Sponzo, R., Hubbard, S. *et al.* (1973) High dose intermittent IV infusion of procarbazine. *Cancer Chemother. Rep.* **57**, 361–3.

Chabner, B.A., Stoller, R.G., Hande, K.R. *et al.* (1978) Methotrexate disposition in humans. *Drug Metab. Rev.*, **8**, 107–17.

Chen, H.S.G. and Gross, J.F. (1979) Physiologically based pharmacokinetic models for anticancer drugs. *Cancer Chemother. Pharmacol.*, **2**, 85–94.

Clark, P.I., Cottier, B., Joel, S.P. *et al.* (1990) Prolonged administration of single-agent oral etoposide in patients with untreated small cell lung cancer *Proc. ASCO*, **9**, 226.

Cohen, J.L., Jao, J.Y. and Jusko, W.J. (1971) Pharmacokinetics of cyclophosphamide in man. *Br. J. Pharmacol.*, **43**, 677–80.

Connors, T.A., Cox, P.J., Farmer, P.B. *et al.* (1974) Some studies of the active intermediates formed in the microsomal metabolism of cyclophosphamide and ifosfamide. *Biochem. Pharmac.*, **23**, 115–29.

Corden, B.J., Fine, R.L., Ozols, R.F. and Collins, J.M. (1985) Clinical pharmacology of high-dose cisplatin. *Cancer Chemother. Pharmacol.* **14**, 38–41.

Cornwell, G.G., Pajak, T.P., McIntyre, O.R. *et al.* (1982) Influence of renal failure on myelosuppressive effects of melphalan. *Cancer Treat. Rep.*, **66**, 475–81.

Cowan, D.H. and Bergsagel, D.E. (1971) Intermittent treatment for metastatic malignant melanoma with high-dose 5(3,3-dimethyl-l-triazeno) imidazole- 4-carboxamide. *Cancer Chemother. Rep.*, **55**, 178–81.

Curtin, N.J., Harris, A.L. and Aherne, G.W. (1991) Mechanism of cell death following thymidylate synthase inhibition: 2′-deoxyuridine-5′-triphosphate accumulation, DNA damage, and growth inhibition following exposure to CB3717 and dipyridamole. *Cancer Res.*, **51**, 2346–52.

D'Incalci, M., Bolis, G., Mangioni, C. *et al.* (1978) Variable oral absorption of HMM in man. *Cancer Treat. Rep.*, **62**, 2117–9.

D'Incalci, M., Bolis, G., Facchinetti, T. *et al.* (1979) Decreased half life of cyclophosphamide in patients under continual treatment. *Eur. J. Cancer*, **15**, 7–10.

D'Incalci, M., Farina, P., Sessa, C. *et al.* (1982) Pharmacokinetics of VP-16-213 given by different administration methods. *Cancer Chemother. Pharmacol.*, **7**, 141–5.

Dorr, R.T. (1988) New findings in the pharmacokinetic, metabolic and drug-resistance aspects of mitomycin C. *Semin. Oncol.*, **15**(Suppl.4), 32–41.

Egorin, M.J., Forrest, A., Belani, C.P. *et al.* (1987–9) A limited sampling strategy for cyclophosphamide pharmacokinetics. *Cancer Res.*, **49**, 3129–33.

Ehrsson, H., Eksborg, S., Osterborg, A. *et al.* (1989) Oral melphalan pharmacokinetics: relation to dose in patients with multiple myeloma. *Med. Oncol. Tumour Pharmacother.*, **6**, 151–4.

Ehrsson, H., Eksborg, S., Wallin, I. *et al.* (1990) Oral melphalan pharmacokinetics: influence of interferon-induced fever. *Clin. Pharmacol. Ther.*, **47**, 86–90.

Einhorn, L.H., Pennington, K. and McClean, J. (1990) Phase-II trial of daily oral VP–16 in refractory small cell lung cancer. *Semin. Oncol.*, **17**(Suppl.2), 32–35.

Eksborg, S. (1989) Pharmacokinetics of anthracyclines. *Acta. Oncol.*, **28**, 873–6.

El-Yazigi, A. and Martin, C.R. (1988) Capillary gas chromatography and thermionic NP-specific detection of BCNU or CCNU in stability and pharmacokinetic studies. *Pharm. Res.*, **5**, 220–5.

Fetting, J.H., Grochow, L.B., Folstein, M.F. *et al.* (1982) The course of nausea and vomiting after high dose cyclophosphamide. *Cancer Treat. Rep.*, **66**, 1487–93.

Fichtinger-Schepman, A.M.J., van Oosterom, V.T., Lohman, P.H.M. *et al.* (1987) Cisplatin-induced DNA adducts in peripheral leukocytes from seven cancer patients. *Cancer Res.*, **47**, 3000– 4.

Finch, R.E., Bending, M.R. and Lant, A.F. (1979) Plasma levels of 5FU after oral and intravenous administration in cancer patients. *Br. J. Clin. Pharmacol.*, **7**, 613–7.

Findlay, M., Mansi, J.L., Hill, A. *et al.* (1991) Modulation of continuous low-dose 5FU with alpha-interferon in colo-rectal cancer – clinical results and metabolic monitoring of 5FU using $_{19}$F MRI. Spectroscopy. *Eur. J. Cancer*, **27** (Suppl. 2), S83.

Foster, B.J., Harding, B.J., Leyland-Jones, B. *et al.* (1986) Hexamethylmelamine: a critical review of an active drug. *Cancer Treat. Rev.*, **13**, 195–202.

Fracasso, P.M. and Sartorelli, A.C. (1986) Cytotoxicity and DNA lesions produced by Mitomycin C and porfiromycin in hypoxic and aerobic EMT6 and CHO cells. *Cancer Res.*, **46**, 3939–44.

Freireich, E.A., Gehan, E.A., Rall, D.P. *et al.* (1966) Cross-species comparisons of drug dosage using body surface area. *Cancer Chemother. Rep.*, **50**, 219–44.

Front, D., Even-Sapir, E., Iosilevsky, G., *et al.* (1987) Monitoring of ^{57}Co-Bleomycin delivery to brain metastases and their tumours of origin. *J. Neurosurg.*, **67**, 506–10.

Goren, M.P., Wright, R.K., Pratt C.B. *et al.* (1986) Dechloroethylation of ifosfamide and neuro-toxicity [letter]. *Lancet* Nov **22**, 1219–20.

Gormley, P.E., Gangji, D., Wood, J.H. and Poplack, D.G. (1981) Pharmacokinetic study of CSF penetration of cis-DDP(II). *Cancer Chemother. Pharmacol.*, **5**, 257–60.

Gouyette, A., Hartmann, O. and Pico, J.L. (1986) Pharmacokinetics of high-dose melphalan in children and adults. *Cancer Chemother. Phamacol.*, **16**, 84–9.

Greene, R.F., Collins, J.M., Jenkins, J.F. *et al.* (1983) Plasma pharmacokinetics of adriamycin and adriamycinol: implications for the design of in vitro experiments and treatment protocols *Cancer Res.*, **43**, 3417–21.

Hansen, R.M., Quebberman, E. and Anderson, T. (1989) 5-Flurouracil by protracted venous infusion. *Oncology*, **46**, 245–50.

Harland, S.J., Newell, D.R., Siddik, Z.H. *et al.* (1984) Pharmacokinetics of cis-diammine-1, 1-cyclobutane dicarboxylate platinum(II) [carboplatin] in patients with normal and impaired renal function. *Cancer Res.*, **44**, 1693–7.

Harris, A.L. and Cantwell, B.M.J. (1986) Mechanisms and treatment of cytotoxic-induced nausea and vomiting, in *Nausea and vomiting: mechanisms and treatment* (eds. C.J. Davis, G.V. Lake-Bakaar and D.G. Grahame-Smith) pp. 78–93, Springer-Verlag, Berlin.

Harris, B.E., Song, R., Soong, S.J. and Diasio, R.B. (1990) Relationship between dihydropyrimidine dehydrogenase activity and plasma 5-Flurouracil levels with evidence for circadian variation of enzyme activity and plasma drug levels in cancer patients receiving 5-Fluorouracil by protracted continuous infusion. *Cancer Res.*, **50**, 197–201.

Harvey, V.J., Slevin, M.L., Joel, S.P. *et al.* (1985) Variable bioavailability following repeated oral doses of etoposide. *Eur. J. Cancer Clin. Oncol.*, **21**, 1315–9.

Heidelberger, C., Chaudhuari, N.K., Danenberg, P. *et al.* (1957) Fluorinated pyrimidines: a new class of tumour inhibitory compounds. *Nature*, **179**, 663–66.

Howell, S.B., Schiefer, M., Andrews, P.A. *et al.* (1987, i) The pharmacology of intraperitoneally administered bleomycin. *J. Clin. Oncol.*, **5**, 2009–16.

Howell, S.B., Zimm, S., Markman, M. *et al.* (1987, ii) Long-term survival of advanced refractory ovarian carcinoma patients with small-volume disease treated with intraperitoneal chemotherapy. *J. Clin. Oncol.*, **5**, 1607–12.

Howell, S.B., Pfeifle, C.E., Wung, W. *et al.* (1982) Intraperitoneal cisplatin with systemic thiosulphate protection. *Ann. Int. Med.*, **97**, 845–51.

Hrushesky, W.J. and von Roemeling, R. (1986) Chemotherapy-induced vomiting: circadian drug timing as a source of predictable within-patient variability. *Cancer Treat. Rep.*, **70**, 1347–8.

Israili, Z.H., Vogler, W.R., Mingioli, E.S. *et al.* (1976) The disposition and pharmacokinetics in humans of 5-azacytidine administered intravenously as a bolus or by continuous infusion. *Cancer Res.*, **36**, 1453–61.

Jackson, D.V., Sethi, V.S., Spurr, C.L. *et al.* (1981) Pharmacokinetics of vincristine in the cerebrospinal fluid of humans. *Cancer Res.*, **41**, 1466–8.

Jensen, J.L., Goel, R. and Venner, P.M. (1990) The effect of corticosteroid administration on bleomycin lung toxicity. *Cancer*, **65**, 1291–7.

Jodrell, D., Zuhowski, E., Egorin, M. *et al.* (1991) Intermittent bolus dosing with suramin: the use of adaptive control with feedback. *Proc. Am. Soc. Clin. Oncol.*, **10**, 92.

Jones, P.A., Taylor, S.M. and Wilson, V. (1983) DNA modification, differentiation and transformation *J. Exp. Zool.*, **228**, 287–95.

Jordan, N.S., Schauer, P.K., Schauer, A. *et al.* (1985) The effect of administration rate on cisplatin-induced emesis. *J. Clin. Oncol.*, **3**, 559–61.

Juma, F.D., Rogers, H.J. and Trounce, J.R. (1980) The pharmacokinetics of cyclophosphamide, phosphoramide mustard and nor-nitrogen mustard studied by gas chromatography in patients receiving cyclphosphamide therapy. *Br. J. Clin. Pharmacol.*, **10**, 327–35.

Juma, F.D. (1984) Effect of liver failure on the pharmacokinetics of cyclophosphamide. *Eur. J. Clin. Pharmacol.*, **26**, 591–3.

Kerr, I.G., Jolivet, J., Collins, J.M. *et al.* (1983) Test dose for predicting high dose methotrexate infusions. *Clin. Pharmacol. Ther.*, **33**, 44–51.

Kerr, I.G., Zimm, S., Collins, U.M. *et al.* (1984) Effect of intravenous dose and schedule on CSF pharmacokinetics of 5FU in the monkey. *Cancer Res.*, **44**, 4929–32.

Kleinerman, E.S., Zwelling, L.A. and Muchmore, A.V. (1980) Enhancement of naturally occurring human spontaneous monocyte cytotoxicity by *cis*-diamminedichloroplatinum(II). *Cancer Res.*, **40**, 3099–102.

Koriech, O.H. and Shukla, V.S. (1981) Dacarbazine in malignant melanoma: reduced toxicity with protection from light. *Clin. Radiol.*, **32**, 53–55.

Kreis, W. Chaudhri, F., Chan, K. *et al.* (1985) Pharmacokinetics of low-dose 1β-D-arabinofuranosylcytosine given by continuous intravenous infusion over 21 days. *Cancer Res.*, **45**, 6498–501.

Kris, M.G., Gralla, R.U., Clark, R.A. *et al.* (1985) Incidence, course and severity of delayed nausea and vomiting following the administration of high-dose cisplatin. *J. Clin. Oncol.*, **3**, 1379–84.

Lazarus, H.M., Herzig, R.H. *et al.* (1983) Intensive melphalan chemotherapy and cryopreserved autologous bonemarrow transplantation for the treatment of refractory cancer. *J. Clin. Oncol.*, **1**, 359–67.

Legha, S.S., Benjamin, R.S., MacKay, B. *et al.* (1982) Reduction of doxorubicin toxicity by prolonged continuous intravenous infusion. *Ann. Intern. Med.*, **96**, 133–9.

LeRoy, A.F., Lutz, R.J., Dedrick, R.L. *et al.* (1979) Pharmacokinetic study of cisplatin in the beagle dog: thermodynamic and kinetic behaviour of DDP in a biologic milieu. *Cancer Treat. Rep.*, **63**, 59–71.

Liliemark, J.O., Plunkett, W. and Dixon, D.O. (1985) Relationship of 1β-D-arabinofuranosylcytosine (araC) in plasma to araC-triphosphate levels in leukaemic cells during treatment with high-dose araC. *Cancer Res.*, **45**, 5952–7.

Lindley, C.M., Bernard, S. and Fields, S.M. (1989) Incidence and duration of chemotherapy-induced nausea and vomiting in the outpatient oncology population. *J. Clin. Oncol.*, **7**, 1142–9.

Litterst, C.L., Gram, T.E., Dedrick, R. *et al.* (1976) Distribution and disposition of platinum following intravenous administration of *cis*-DDP(II) to dogs. *Cancer Res.*, **36**, 2340–4.

Loo, T.L., Luce, J.K., Jardin, J.H. *et al.* (1968) Pharmacologic studies of the antitumour agent DTIC. *Cancer Res.*, **28**, 2448–53.

Los, G., Mutsaers, P.H., Lenglet, W.J. *et al.* (1990) Platinum distribution in intraperitoneal tumours after intraperitoneal cisplatin treatment. *Cancer Chemother. Pharmacol.*, **25**, 389–94.

Luce, J.K., Thurman, W.G., Issacs, B.L. and Talley, R.W. (1970) Clinical trials with the antitumour agent 5-(3,3-dimethyl-l-triazeno) imidazole-4-carboxamide [DTIC]. *Cancer Chemother. Rep.*, **54**, 119–24.

Markman, M., Reichman, B., Hakes, T. *et al.* (1989) Intraperitoneal chemotherapy as treatment for ovarian carcinoma and gastrointestinal malignancies: the Memorial Sloan-Kettering experience. *Acta Med. Austriaca.*, **16**, 65–7.

Martoni, A., DiMarco, A.R., Campaggi, C.M. *et al.* (1983) Doxorubicin and epirubicin: clinical experience and pharmacokinetics. *Drugs Exptl. Clin. Res.*, **9**, 767–74.

Mbidde, E.K., Selby, P.J., Perren, T.J. *et al.* (1988) High-dose BCNU chemotherapy with autologous bone marrow transplantation and full dose radiotherapy for grade IV astrocytoma. *Br. J. Cancer*, **58**, 779–82.

McDermott, B.J., van der Berg, H.W. and Murphy, R.F. (1982) Nonlinear pharmacokinetics for the elimination of 5-fluorouracil after intravenous administration in cancer patients. *Cancer Chemother. Pharmacol.*, **9**, 173–8.

McLeod, B.F., Lawrence, H.J., Smith, D.W. *et al.* (1987) Fatal bleomycin toxicity from a low cumulative dose in a patient with renal insufficiency. *Cancer*, **660**, 2617–20.

Meulemans, A. Giroux, B., Hannoun, P. *et al.* (1989) Permeability of two nitrosoureas, carmustine and fotemustine, in rat cortex. *Chemotherapy*, **35**, 313–9.

Miles, D.W., Richards, M.A., Rubens, R.D. *et al.* (1990) High-dose epirubicin as primary therapy in advanced breast carcinoma: a phase-II study. *Proc. Br. Assoc. Cancer Res./Assoc. Cancer Physicians*, **31/5**, 94.

Miller, J.C. and Einhorn, L.H. (1990) Phase-II study of daily oral etoposide in refractory germm cell tumours. *Semin. Oncol.*, **17** (Suppl 2): 36–39.

Nadkarni, M.V., Trams, E.G. and Smith, P.K. *et al.* (1956) Observations on the rapid disappearance of radioactivity from blood after intravenous triethylene melamine-C^{14}. *Proc AACR*, **2**, 136.

Nelson, R.L., Allen, L.M. and Creaven, P.J. (1976) Pharmacokinetics of divided-dose ifosfamide. *Clin. Pharmacol. Ther.*, **19**, 365–70.

Nelson, R.L. (1982) The comparative clinical pharmacology and pharmacokinetics of vindesine, vincristine and vinblastine in human patients with cancer. *Med. Paed. Oncol.*, **10**, 115–27.

Nowakowska-Dulawa, E. (1990) Circadian rhythm of 5-fluorouracil pharmacokinetics and tolerance. *Chronobiologia*, **17**, 27–35.

Oliverio, V.T., Denham, C., deVita, V.T. *et al.* (1964) Some pharmacologic properties of a new antitumour agent, N-isopropyl-α-(2-methylhydrazino)-p-toluamide HCl [procarbazine]. *Cancer Chemother. Rep.*, **42**, 1–7.

Onsrud, M., Bosnes, V. and Grahm, I. (1986) Cisplatinum as adjunct to surgery in early stage ovarian carcinoma: effects on lymphocyte cell populations. *Gynaecol. Oncol.*, **23**, 323–28.

Ostrowski, M.J. (1986) An assessment of the long-term results of controlling the reaccumulation of malignant effusions using intracavity bleomycin. *Cancer*, **57**, 721–7.

Patton, T.F., Repta, A.J. and Sternson, L.A. (1983) Clinical pharmacology of cisplatin, in *Pharmacokinetics of anticancer agents in humans* (eds M.M. Ames, G. Powis and Kovach) pp. 155–86, Amsterdam, Elsevier.

Peters, W.P., Stuart, A., Klotman, M. *et al.* (1989) High-dose combination cyclophosphamide, cisplatin and melphalan with autologous bone-marrow support. A clinical and pharmacologic study. *Cancer Chemother. Pharmacol.*, **23**, 377–83.

Reece, P.A., Stafford, I., Russell, J., and Hill, P.G. (1985) Non-linear renal clearance of ultrafilterable platinum in patients treated with *cis*-DDP. *Cancer Chemother. Pharmac.*, **15**, 295–9.

Reece, P.A., Hill, H.S., Green, R.M. *et al.* (1988) Renal clearance and protein binding of melphalan in patients with cancer. *Cancer Chemother. Pharmacol.*, **22**, 348–52.

Riggs, C.E. and Bachur, N.R. (1983) Clinical pharmacokinetics of anthracycline antibiotics, in *Pharmacokinetics of anticancer agents in humans*, (eds. M.M. Ames, G. Powis and J.S. Kovach) pp. 229–78, Elsevier, Amsterdam.

Rosenberg, B., van Camp, L. Trosko, J.E. *et al.* (1969) Platinum compounds: a new class of potent antitumour agents. *Nature*, **222**, 385–6.

Rosenberg, B. (1985) Fundamental studies with cisplatin. *Cancer*, **54**, 2303–16.

Roy, S.N. and Horowitz, S.B. (1984) Characterization of the association of radiolabelled bleomycin A_2 with HeLa cells. *Cancer Res.*, **44**, 1541–6.

Rutty, C.J., Abel, G. and Harrap, K.R. (1979) *In vitro* cytotoxicity of hexamethylmelamine and its analogues. *Br. J. Cancer*, **40**, 317–8.

Schabel, F.M. (1974) New experimental drug combinations with potential clinical utility. *Biochem. Pharmacol.*, **2** (Suppl), 163–76.

Schwartz, D.E., Bollag, W. and Obrecht, P. (1967) Distribution and excretion studies of procarbazine in animals and man. *Arzneimittel-Forsch*, **17**, 1389–93.

Shiba, D.A. and Weinkam, R.J. (1982) Quantitative analysis of procarbazine, procarbazine metabolites and chemical degradation products with application to pharmacokinetic studies. *J. Chromatogr.*, **229**, 397–407.

Shiba, D.A. and Weinkam, R.U. (1983) The *in vivo* cytotoxic activity of procarbazine and procarbazine metabolites against L1210 cells in CDF_1 mice and the effects of pretreatment with procarbazine, phenobarbital, diphenylhydantoin and methylprednisolone upon *in vivo* procarbazine activity. *Cancer Chemother. Pharmacol.*, **11**, 124–29.

Skibba, U.L., Ramirez, G. *et al.* (1969) Preliminary clinical trial and the physiologic disposition of DTIC in man. *Cancer Res.*, **29**, 1944–51.

Sladek, N.E., Priest, I., Doeden, D. *et al.* (1980) Plasma half-life and urinary excretion of cyclophosphamide in children. *Cancer Treat. Rep.*, **64**, 1061–66.

Slevin, M.L., Woolard, R.C., Lister, T.A. *et al.* (1983a) Relationship between protein binding and extravascular drug concentrations of a water-soluble drug, cytosine arabinoside. *J. Royal Soc. Med.*, **76**, 365–8.

Slevin, M.L., Piall, E.M., Aherne, G.W. *et al.* (1983b) Effect of dose and schedule on pharmacokinetics of high-dose cytosine arabinoside in plasma and cerebrospinal fluid. *J. Clin. Oncol.*, **1**, 546–51.

Slevin, M.L., Clark, P.I., Joel, S.P. *et al.* (1989) A randomised trial to evaluate the effect of schedule on the activity of etoposide in small-cell lung cancer. *J. Clin. Oncol.*, **7**, 1333–40.

Smyth, J.F., Macpherson, J.S., Warrington, P.S. *et al.* (1986) The clinical pharmacology of mitoxantrone. *Cancer Chemother. Pharmacol.*, **17**, 149–52.

Speyer, J.L., Green, M.D., Kramer, E. *et al.* (1988) Protective effect of the bis-piperazinedione, ICRF-187 against doxorubicin-induced cardiac toxicity in women with advanced breast cancer. *New Eng. J. Med.*, **319**, 745–52.

Sponzo, R.W., De Vita, V.T. and Oliverio, V.T. (1973) Physiologic disposition of CCNU and methyl-CCNU in man. *Cancer*, **31**, 1154–9.

Steele, W.H., Lawrence, J.R., Stuart, J.F.B. and McNeil, C.A. (1981) The protein binding of methotrexate in the serum of patients with neoplastic disease. *Cancer Chemother. Pharmacol.*, **7**, 61–4.

Stoller, R.G., Jacobs, S.A., Drake, J.C. *et al.* (1975) Pharmacokinetics of high-dose methotrexate. *Cancer Chemother. Rep.*, **6**, 19–24.

Tattersall, M.H.N., Sodergren, S.K., Sengupta, D.H. *et al.* (1975) Pharmacokinetics of actinomycin D in patients with malignant melanoma. *Clin. Pharmacol. Ther.*, **17**, 701–18.

Thatcher, N., Sharma, H., Harrison, R. *et al.* (1982) Blood clearance of three radioactively labelled platinum complexes. *Cancer Chemother. Pharmacol.*, **9**, 13–16.

Tranchand, B., Ploin, Y.D. and Minuit, M.P. (1989) High dose melphalan dosage adjustment: possibility of using a test-dose. *Cancer Chemother. Pharmacol.*, **23**, 95–100.

Twelves, C.J., Dobbs, N.A., Aldhous, M. *et al.* (1991) Comparative pharmacokinetics of doxorubicin given by three different schedules with equal dose intensity in patients with breast cancer. *Cancer Chemother. Pharmacol.*, **28**, 302–307.

Vogler, W.R., Miller, D.S. and Keller, J.W. (1976) 5-Azacytidine (NSC-102816): a new drug for the treatment of myeloblastic leukaemia. *Blood*, **48**, 331–7.

Voisin, E.M., Ruthsatz, M. Collins, J.M. and Hoyle, P.C. (1991) Extrapolation of animal toxicity to humans: interspecies comparisons in drug development. *Regul. Toxicol. Pharmacol.*, **12**(2), 107–16.

Wajsman, Z., Dhafir, R.A., Pfeffer, M. *et al.* (1984) Studies of mitomycin C absorption after intravesical treatment of superficial bladder tumours, *J. Urol.*, **132**, 30–3.

Wharton, J.T., Rutledge, F., Smith, J.P. *et al.* (1979) Hexamethylmelamine: an evaluation of its role in the treatment of ovarian cancer. *Am. J. Obstet. Gynaecol.*, **133**, 833–44.

Worzalla, J.F., Johnson, B.M., Ramirez, G. *et al.* (1973) N-demethylation of the antineoplastic agent hexamethylmelamine in rats and man. *Cancer Res.*, **33**, 2810–15.

Zucchetti, M., D'Incalci, M., Willems, Y. *et al.* (1988) Lack of effect of cisplatin on iv L-PAM plasma pharmacokinetics in ovarian cancer patients. *Cancer Chemother. Pharmacol.*, **22**, 87–89.

3

Toxicology of chemotherapeutic agents

I.R. JUDSON

3.1 INTRODUCTION

The majority of cancer chemotherapeutic agents have an effect on nucleic acid synthesis and consequently exert their anti-tumour effects through the inhibition of cell growth and division. There has been an enormous increase in the understanding of how cancer cells differ from normal cells in relation to control mechanisms, but as yet this knowledge has not led to the development of selective agents which are capable of targeting specific control processes. In general, anti-proliferative agents exhibit poor selectivity – hence the more rapidly proliferating tissues in the body, such as the bone marrow, are also affected. Chemotherapeutic drugs are usually administered at or near to the maximum tolerated dose in order to optimize their anti-tumour effect. Other side effects which are unrelated to the anti-proliferative effect vary much more widely between different agents and may be amenable to symptomatic treatment. The commonest side effects are summarized in Table 3.1. Differences in the likely severity of toxicities between different agents, which depend in part on patient susceptibility, dosage, and schedule of administration, are not included here. However, it should be noted that certain drugs – cisplatin, for example – are far more prone to cause a variety of severe toxicities than a drug such as chlorambucil for which myelosuppression is the only significant acute side effect.

3.1.1 IMPACT OF SIDE EFFECTS ON QUALITY OF LIFE AND COMPLIANCE

The frequency and severity of chemotherapy-related side effects may have an important impact on both the quality of life of cancer patients and their compliance with treatment. While not all cytotoxic agents produce the same adverse effects, the common lay picture of cancer treatment causing vomiting and hair loss emphasizes the fear which these toxicities provoke. In a study of patients' perceptions of cancer chemotherapy side effects, in which physical and psychological problems were ranked according to severity, vomiting, nausea and hair loss were considered the most serious problem (Coates *et al.*, 1983). Apprehension about injections, concern about the effects of treatment on work and family, tiredness and sleeping difficulties were also highlighted. In a separate study relating side effects to compliance, hair loss, nausea and loss of appetite were reported most commonly and correlated with poor attendance at

Emesis in Anti-cancer Therapy
Mechanisms and treatment
Published in 1993 by Chapman & Hall, London
ISBN 0 412 37250 9

Table 3.1 Principal side effects of chemotherapeutic agents

	Myelosuppression	Alopecia	Gastro-intestinal mucosa	Nausea and vomiting	Kidney	Bladder	Heart	Peripheral nervous system	CNS	Lung	Liver	Skin
Actinomycin D	+	+	+	+	–	–	–	–	–	–	–	+
Bleomycin	–	+	+	–	–	–	–	–	–	+	–	+
Busulphan	+	(+)	–	+	–	–	–	–	–	+	(+)	+
Carboplatin	+	–	–	+	+/–	–	–	–	(+)	–	(+)	–
Carmustine (BCNU)	+	–	+	+	–	–	–	–	–	+	+/–	–
Chlorambucil	+	–	–	+	–	–	–	–	–	–	–	–
Cisplatin	+	–	–	+	+	–	–	+	–	–	–	–
Cyclophosphamide	+	+	–	+	–	+	(+)	–	–	–	–	–
Cytosine arabinoside	+	–	+	–	–	–	–	+/–	(+)	–	+	–
Dacarbazine (DTIC)	+	+	–	+	–	–	–	–	–	–	+	–
Daunorubicin	+	+	+	+	–	–	+	–	–	–	–	–
Doxorubicin	+	+	+	+	–	–	+	–	–	–	–	–
Epirubicin	+	+	+	+	–	–	+	–	–	–	–	–
Etoposide	+	+	+	–	–	–	–	–	–	–	–	–
5-Fluorouracil	+	+/–	+	+	–	–	+	+/–	+	–	–	–
Hexamethylmelamine	+/–	–	–	+	–	–	–	+	–	–	–	–
Hydroxyruea	+	–	+	–	–	–	–	–	–	–	–	–
Ifosfamide	+	+	–	+	+	+	–	–	+	–	–	–
Lomustine (CCNU)	+	–	–	+	–	–	–	–	–	–	+/–	–
Melphalan	+	+	+	+	–	–	–	–	–	–	–	–
6-Mercaptopurine	+	–	+	–	–	–	–	–	–	–	+	–
Methotrexate	+	–	+	+/–	(+)	–	–	–	–	–	–	+
Mitoxantrone	+	+/–	–	+	–	–	+	–	–	–	–	–
Mitomycin C	+	+/–	+	+	+	–	–	–	–	–	–	–
Mustine	+	+	+	+	–	–	–	–	–	–	–	–
Procarbazine	+	–	–	+	–	–	–	+	+	–	–	–
Streptozotocin	+	–	+	+	+	–	–	–	–	–	+/–	–
Teniposide	+	+	+	+	–	–	–	–	–	–	–	–
6-Thioguanine	+	–	+	+	–	–	–	–	–	–	–	–
Thiotepa	+	+	(+)	+	–	–	–	–	(+)	–	–	–
Treosulphan	+	–	–	–	–	–	–	–	–	+/–	–	–
Vinblastine	+	+	+	+	–	–	–	+	–	–	–	–
Vincristine	+	+	–	–	–	–	–	+	–	–	–	–
Vindesine	+	+	–	+/–	–	–	–	+	–	–	–	–

+: present, –: absent, +/–: occasional or minor, (+): important in high dose therapy chemotherapy clinics, particularly among younger patients (Richardson *et al.*, 1988). Preparing patients for these problems is an important part of helping them to cope (Goodman *et al.*, 1989).

3.1.2 FACTORS AFFECTING THE SEVERITY OF SIDE EFFECTS

The severity of chemotherapy-related side effects is influenced by the overall physical condition of the patient, as well as age, prior therapy and nutritional status. Extensive prior chemotherapy predisposes to myelosuppression, as does radiotherapy to large areas of bone marrow. Prior or simultaneous radiotherapy may increase the likelihood of mucositis or skin necrosis. Poor performance status, hepatomegaly, low albumin, elevated blood urea and alkaline phosphatase have all been identified as risk factors for fatal toxicity in small cell lung cancer patients (Morittu *et al.*, 1989). Factors which are known to increase the likely toxicity of chemotherapy need to be taken into account when deciding on the timing and dosage of such treatment.

3.2 ANTI-PROLIFERATIVE SIDE EFFECTS

3.2.1 MYELOSUPPRESSION

The commonest and potentially most serious side effect of cytotoxic drugs is that of bone marrow suppression; this may take the form of leukopenia, mainly granulocytopenia, thrombocytopenia and anaemia. The bone marrow is one of the most rapidly dividing tissues in the body, hence its susceptibility to anti-proliferative agents.

3.2.1.1 Leukopenia

Leukopenia is more likely to occur than thrombocytopenia or anaemia due to the short half-life of granulocytes (6–12 h) compared with that of platelets or erythrocytes. Granulocytes are essential for maintaining body defences against bacteria, fungi and viruses. Bacterial infection usually involves the patient's endogenous flora. The risk of serious, life-threatening infection increases with the severity and duration of granulocytopenia. A granulocyte count of $<0.5 \times 10^9/l$ is assoicated with a significant incidence of major infection, particularly if it remains below this level for more than seven days. Mucositis is usually associated with leukopenia indicating that damage to buccal mucosal cells and increased susceptibility to infection are both involved.

The pattern of myelosuppression varies according to the potential for damaging bone marrow stem cells. Anti-metabolites which only affect dividing cells are least likely to cause lasting damage. Conversely, alkylating agents which kill non-cycling cells, including early precursors, may cause severe, sometimes cumulative, bone marrow suppression. This difference is well illustrated by differences in the requirement for bone marrow autotransplantation as an adjunct to high dose chemotherapy with a variety of agents. In the case of those drugs which spare bone marrow stem cells, autologous bone marrow rescue does not shorten the duration of leukopenia, see Table 3.2.

Table 3.2 Requirement for adjunctive bone marrow autotransplantation in chemotherapy

Drug	Autograft required	Limiting toxicity ± BMT
Melphalan	+	Gut
Busulphan	+	Lung, liver
BCNU	+	Lung, liver
Thiotepa	+	Neurotoxicity
Carboplatin	±	Kidney, liver, CNS
Cyclophosphamide	–	Heart, bladder
Etoposide	–	Mucositis
Cytosine arabinoside	–	Eyes, gut, skin

In the majority of cases, duration of leukopenia is short and recovery is predictable. Since cytotoxic agents have a small therapeutic index and are given at maximally tolerated doses, the white blood cell count (WBC) nadir may be used as a guide to the correct dose in individual patients. However, it has to be remembered that neutropenic fever demands prompt administration of intravenous broad spectrum antibiotics. Intensive high dose chemotherapy may result in prolonged neutropenia requiring the use of prophylactic antibiotics, including anti-fungal agents. The duration of neutropenia, but not thrombocytopenia, may be shortened by the use of autologous bone marrow transplantation (Table 3.2, above). In the future it may prove possible to virtually eliminate the problem of myelosuppression due to conventional dose chemotherapy by the use of haemopoietic growth factors. At present it is possible to shorten the duration and severity of granulocytopenia by the use of G-CSF or GM-CSF but the effects on platelet recovery are limited. It has proved possible to use these agents to allow safe dose escalations to be performed with agents such as doxorubicin (Bronchud *et al.*, 1989). Their use in high dose chemotherapy and bone marrow transplantation is currently being investigated as is the possible role of combinations such as IL-3 + GM-CSF and erythropoietin + GM-CSF.

A small number of drugs are marrow sparing, including vincristine, bleomycin, low-dose methotrexate and moderate-dose cisplatin. Such agents can be used together with more myelosuppressive agents to produce combinations with an improved therapeutic index.

3.2.1.2 Thrombocytopenia

Thrombocytopenia is rarely dose limiting for drugs in conventional dosage, exceptions being the nitrosoureas such as CCNU (lomustine) and BCNU (carmustine), mitomycin C and carboplatin. When it occurs, thrombocytopenia may be cumulative and prolonged: recovery, for example, may take up to six weeks following carmustine. Serious complications are rare with a platelet count of $>50 \times 10^9/l$ but bleeding from the gut mucosa, gums and genito-urinary tract may occur below this level. More serious is the risk of cerebral haemorrhage. Platelet transfusions may be given in the case of active bleeding or prophylactically when the platelet count is $<20 \times 10^9/l$. Petechial haemorrhages in the skin are a useful indication of inadequate platelet number and function.

3.2.1.3 Anaemia

Anaemia secondary to cancer chemotherapy is rarely acute but may result from prolonged treatment, particularly in patients with reduced bone marrow reserve or poor nutrition. Cisplatin is a well recognized cause of anaemia. Fortunately, treatment by blood transfusion is simple and effective.

3.2.2 ALOPECIA

The hair follicle is particularly vulnerable to cytotoxic drugs since up to 90% of follicles are in active cell division at any one time. Head and body hair may be affected and although the loss is temporary, hair may regrow with an altered texture and colour. Hair loss is a side effect of most major drug classes including anthracyclines, epipodophyllotoxins and nitrogen mustards. Severity is related to dose and route of administration – for example, cyclophosphamide given orally does not produce significant alopecia but this does occur with larger doses given i.v. Similarly, low doses of doxorubicin given weekly are less likely to cause severe alopecia than a standard 3-weekly bolus injection. Etoposide, however, produces severe alopecia regardless of route or dose schedule.

The importance of this side effect lies in the psychological impact of the associated change in body image. This is particularly important in younger patients. Wigs or hair pieces can be used to disguise the problem and, with certain drugs including doxorubicin and to a lesser extent cyclophosphamide, scalp cooling may be used to limit the degree of hair loss (Giaccone *et al.*, 1988; Parker, 1987). Scalp cooling to 22–24°C reduces the blood flow to the hair follicles, hence the delivery of cytotoxic agent, and reduces the metabolism of follicle cells. Cooling needs to be maintained until plasma drug levels have fallen below a certain threshold, hence this technique is only applicable to drugs which are administrated by i.v. bolus and have a relatively short plasma half-life. When the half-life is prolonged, for example, by liver impairment in the case of doxorubicin, scalp cooling is likely to be ineffective.

3.2.3 GASTRO-INTESTINAL TOXICITY

3.2.3.1 Upper gastro-intestinal tract

Oral mucositis or stomatitis is caused by a combination of damage to the oral mucosa and granulocytopenia. The cells lining the oral cavity, as elsewhere in the gut, are rapidly dividing with a cycle time of 12–24 hours and are therefore susceptible to anti-proliferative drugs. Severe inflammation and ulceration of the oral or oesophageal mucosa may prevent the patient from eating or even drinking. Loss of taste acuity associated with damage to taste buds may further exacerbate existing eating difficulties associated with poor appetite and chemotherapy-induced nausea. Specific infections may be identified, for example, *Candida albicans*, *Herpes simplex*, but often normal mouth flora only will be isolated.

Concomitant local radiotherapy, poor dental hygiene and dental prostheses all predispose to mucositis. The drugs particularly associated with this toxicity include 5-fluorouracil (5-FU), methotrexate, doxorubicin, vincristine and cytosine arabinoside, but high-dose chemotherapy and total body radiation may also result in severe stomatitis and oesophagitis. The risk of mucositis may be ameliorated by alterations in schedule of administration, for example, 5-FU may be given in larger dosage by continuous infusion before dose-limiting mucositis occurs.

Mouth care, involving attention to dental hygiene, prevention of fungal infection, and avoidance of trauma may help to limit the incidence of mucositis. It has been claimed that allopurinol mouthwashes may ameliorate 5-FU-induced stomatitis, but this has not been substantiated in a number of randomized trials (Loprinzi *et al.*, 1990). Continuous infusions of opiates may be helpful in controlling the pain due to stomatitis and oesophagitis. Local symptomatic measures, such as the use of analgesic gels and local anaesthetic sprays, have only a limited role.

3.2.3.2 Lower gastro-intestinal tract

Cytosine arabinoside, 5-FU and methotrexate may cause diarrhoea secondary to damage to the gastro-intestinal mucosa. In the case of 5-FU + folinic acid this may be dose limiting and may occasionally lead to fatal dehydration. Anti-diarrhoeal agents have little effect and recovery may be slow. High dose chemotherapy and total body irradiation may also cause severe damage to the gut lining leading to diarrhoea, blood loss and poor absorption. This becomes the dose limiting toxicity for high dose melphalan when autologous bone marrow transplantation is used to allow further dose escalation. Management may require the use of parenteral nutrition in addition to careful replacement of fluid and electrolyte losses.

3.3 ACUTE NON ANTI-PROLIFERATIVE TOXICITIES

Cancer chemotherapy may cause a variety of non-specific acute toxicities which are unrelated to the anti-proliferative effects. Anorexia, lethargy, depression, altered taste sensation, impaired sexual activity, nausea and vomiting have all been described. Emesis is undoubtedly the most important of these and perhaps the easiest to quantify. However, other toxicities should not be underestimated in terms of their potential impact on quality of life. For example, altered taste sensation may destroy the patient's enjoyment of food which is then also likely to exacerbate pre-existing anorexia, whether caused by the disease or the chemotherapy. This is a relatively common side effect of cytotoxic drugs which has received little attention. Depression and lethargy are not uncommon and may be so severe as to be dose limiting for certain drugs. The causes are uncertain although hepatotoxicity and central nerve system toxicity may sometimes be responsible. The use of quality of life assessments during treatment is becoming more common and will probably lead to a better understanding of such problems and an improved awareness of their impact on the acceptability of treatment.

3.3.1 NAUSEA AND VOMITING

A detailed description of the mechanism of cancer chemotherapy-induced nausea and vomiting may be found in Chapter 7. There is no doubt that this is one of the most important side effects from the point of view of patients' quality of life while receiving chemotherapy. There is no direct relationship between the cytotoxic potency of a particular drug, that is the dose causing significant antitumour effects, and its emetic potential. Certain drug classes are generally more emetic but chemotherapeutic agents vary substantially in this regard. Undoubtedly, the most emetic drug is cisplatin followed by mustine, DTIC, actinomycin D, doxorubicin, carboplatin and cyclophosphamide. Bleomycin, methotrexate and the vinca alkaloids rarely cause significant nausea.

Some less toxic analogues, such as carboplatin and epirubicin, are significantly less emetic than their respective parent compounds cisplatin and doxorubicin but there remains a need for the development of more effective anti-emetic therapy.

Clearly, the 5-HT_3 receptor antagonists represent an important advance although they are not completely effective in abolishing emesis associated with cisplatin, high dose chemotherapy or the anticipation of chemotherapy. Delayed emesis may stem from entirely different processes such as damage to gastro-intestinal mucosa and is much less amenable to treatment with current 5-HT_3 receptor antagonists. Recent evidence suggests that dexamethasone is more effective than ondansetron in the treatment of delayed emesis (Jones *et al.*, 1991). Nevertheless, the success of the 5-HT_3 receptor antagonists approach does clearly demonstrate the value of an improved understanding of this complex problem, one which led to the development of these agents.

3.4 SPECIFIC ORGAN TOXICITIES

In addition to anti-proliferative and general effects, many cytotoxic agents produce specific organ toxicities, some of which are cumulative and may be dose limiting. Problems such as renal impairment, which may not be reversible, become particularly important when treating children or young adults for diseases which are potentially curable. Long-term sequelae need to be considered very carefully in these situations.

3.4.1 KIDNEY

A number of chemotherapeutic agents – the most important being cisplatin – may directly cause renal damage. Cisplatin causes irreversible cumulative tubular damage resulting in a progressive fall in glomerular filtration rate, ideally measured by ^{51}Cr-EDTA clearance (Daugaard *et al.*, 1988). Proteinuria and magnesium deficiency also result. Magnesium replacement therapy may be used to prevent symptoms such as tetany. Saline hydration does partly ameliorate the problem and there is some evidence that smaller individual doses may be less harmful (Daugaard *et al.*, 1988). A number of agents have been used in an attempt to prevent cisplatin nephrotoxicity including sodium thiosulphate, diethyldithiocarbamate and selenium but none have entered routine clinical practice owing to poor tolerability or concern about the potential for reversing anti-tumour activity. The use of intraperitoneal cisplatin in combination with i.v. thiosulphate appears to be effective (Howell *et al.*, 1983). Carboplatin, in out-patient dosage, appears to be virtually devoid of significant nephrotoxicity, but a knowledge of renal function is helpful in determining the appropriate dose (Calvert *et al.*, 1990).

Ifosfamide may produce renal tubular toxicity resulting in a fall in glomerular filtration rate. More rarely, a severe tubular leak syndrome may develop leading to hypokalaemia, hypocalcaemia and hypophosphataemia, polyuria and metabolic acidosis (Smeitink *et al.*, 1988). Mitomycin C has been associated with a haemolytic-uraemic syndrome associated with glomerular lesions. There appears to be evidence of dose dependency and the complication is more likely in patients who have received higher cumulative doses. Occasionally this may occur in association with other serious toxicities such as pulmonary oedema and other evidence of microangiopathic disease (Verweij *et al.*, 1987). High-dose methotrexate can cause renal impairment and this is thought to be due to drug precipitation in the renal tubules. This problem is usually prevented by the use of careful hydration together with urinary alkalinization, which enhances methotrexate solubility in the urine. Because a significant proportion of methotrexate is cleared by the kidney, methotrexate toxicity may be greatly enhanced in patients with impaired renal function.

Renal impairment may result from hyperuricaemia occurring due to tumour breakdown, particularly at the start of treatment for leukaemia or lymphoma. Rapid cell lysis causes release of nucleic acids which are broken down to uric acid. Owing to its limited solubility in the acid pH of the urine, uric acid may precipitate in the distal renal tubules causing obstruction. The tumour lysis syndrome is also characterized by hyperkalaemia, hyperphosphataemia and hypocalcaemia. Allopurinol inhibits the enzyme xanthine oxidase, limiting the rise in uric acid and this, together with an adequate diuresis, is usually sufficient to prevent renal toxicity associated with tumour lysis.

3.4.2 BLADDER

Cyclophosphamide and ifosfamide are metabolically activated to alkylating species. Both drugs release acrolein, a toxic metabolite which is concentrated in the urine and causes acute haemorrhagic cystitis. In addition to the immediate toxicity, there is an associated risk of secondary bladder cancer. Forced diuresis together with urethral catheterization to keep the bladder empty have been used with high-dose cyclophosphamide but the use of 2-mercapto-ethanesulphonate (mesna) is preferred. Mesna reacts with acrolein preventing its toxicity and can be coadministrated by i.v. infusion or intermittent bolus (Burkert, 1983).

3.4.3 HEART

Cardiotoxicity has been reported as a complication of treatment with anthracyclines such as doxorubicin, its 4′-epimer epirubicin, daunorubicin, and the related compound mitoxantrone, as well as by cyclophosphamide, actinomycin D, 5-FU, mitomycin C and busulphan. Cardiotoxicity due to anthracyclines may be acute or chronic. The acute syndrome comprises supraventricular and ventricular arrhythmias, heart block and a fall in ejection fraction which can lead to left ventricular failure. The chronic cardiotoxicity is irreversible and cumulative – for doxorubicin, for example, the recommended maximum cumulative dose is 550 mg/m^2, at which dose the risk of cardiac failure remains less than 5%. Substantial damage may occur before the onset of symptoms which may, in fact, not develop until after treatment has been completed. For example, the increased cardiac work load imposed by pregnancy may unmask cardiac damage in a woman previously treated with doxorubicin.

Patients with chronic cardiac impairment usually complain of increased breathlessness but may present in acute left ventricular failure. There are rare cases of successful cardiac transplantion having been performed in patients who have been cured of cancer at the expense of chronic left ventricular failure. However, this is unusual and in the majority of cases the decline in left ventricular function is measurable, using isotope ventriculography or echocardiography, but does not cause symptoms. It is advisable to carefully monitor patients receiving these agents in order to avert serious toxicity by stopping treatment before the damage becomes too severe. Special care needs to be taken in patients with pre-existing cardiac disease or those who have received mediastinal irradiation since these factors predispose to cardiac damage (Schwartz *et al.*, 1987). This risk has always to be weighed against the need to deliver effective chemotherapy which should not be compromised unnecessarily.

Weekly administration of lower doses and continuous infusion therapy have both been shown to reduce the cardiotoxicity of doxorubicin and a number of free radical scavengers have been tested on the premise that the cardiotoxicity due to anthracyclines is related to free radical generation in the myocardium. One such study in man has demonstrated that the bispiperazinedione ICRF-187 can protect the myocardium from the effects of doxorubicin without affecting other toxicities or diminishing the anti-tumour activity of the drug (Speyer *et al.*, 1990). The mechanism of this protection is unclear but may be due to iron chelation preventing the generation of free radicals by the doxorubicin-iron complex. The other approach to the problem is the development of less cardiotoxic analogues. The anthrapyrazoles appear to be a very promising group of compounds from this point of view. They appear to combine a reduced ability to form free radicals with lower toxicity with respect to nausea and vomiting, mucositis and alopecia compared with doxorubicin. Early experience with CI-941 (now DuP-941) in breast cancer suggests that this has been achieved without any loss of anti-tumour activity (Judson, 1991).

5-fluorouracil has been reported to cause coronary spasm, chest pain and arrhythmias and, rarely, may lead to left ventricular failure following an acute toxic cardiomyopathy. The mechanism or cardiotoxicity remains obscure but the drug should probably be avoided in patients with ischaemic heart disease or a history of dysrrhythmias (Ensley *et al.*, 1989). Acute myocardial necrosis may also occur as a complication of high-dose cyclophosphamide.

3.4.4 NERVOUS SYSTEM

Peripheral and central nervous system toxicities may complicate chemotherapy with a variety of drugs. Central nervous system toxicity is associated with drugs or their metabolites which are capable of crossing the blood–brain barrier but the mechanisms are ill understood. The drugs most commonly associated with peripheral neuropathy, the vinca alkaloids, affect neurotubular function in a similar way to their effect on the mitotic spindle through which they exert their anti-tumour activity. Other drugs which may cause peripheral toxicity include cisplatin, 5-FU, procarbazine, hexamethylmelamine, and cytosine arabinoside.

3.4.4.1 Peripheral neuropathy

There are some differences between cytotoxic agents in the type of peripheral toxicity observed but the commonest problem is a 'glove and stocking' loss of sensation, usually associated with unpleasant paraesthesiae. Relatively minor degrees of objective sensory impairment may prove disabling, making the performance of simple tasks such as dressing or writing very difficult. Loss of pain sensation may lead to burns or other trauma and this is particularly important in the elderly who may already have an impaired peripheral circulation leading to poor healing – for example, in the feet. Loss of vibration sense can be used to monitor the progression of neurotoxicity. Toxicity is generally dose-related and cumulative.

In the case of the vinca alkaloids, motor weakness may be a relatively early feature, sometimes in association with muscle pain. If severe weakness occurs recovery may take many months. On the other hand, cisplatin produces a predominantly sensory lesion which may nevertheless affect gait due to lack of proprioception. The damage caused by cisplatin may not be entirely reversible.

Walking difficulties may be caused by a combination of sensory ataxia and weakness due to motor involvement. Weakness may progress from slight difficultly in rising from a chair or boarding a bus to total paraplegia. Progression of neuropathy may sometimes occur after cessation of treatment hence it is not always possible to prevent such extreme toxicity. Loss of tendon reflexes is extremely common in patients treated with vincristine or cisplatin and precedes the development of weakness. Although a useful indicator of toxicity, loss of tendon reflexes in itself is not an indication for stopping treatment, and there is no substitute for careful monitoring of sensory function.

Recovery of peripheral nerve injury in experimental models has been accelerated by the use of ACTH or melanocyte-stimulating hormone-like peptides. An analogue of ACTH has been shown to ameliorate the neurotoxicity of cisplatin in patients with ovarian cancer without affecting the anti-tumour activity of the drug (Gerrittsen *et al.*, 1990). Some benefit has also been reported with ethiophos (WR-2721) (Mollman *et al.*, 1988). The non-neurotoxic analogue carboplatin is now available as an alternative treatment to cisplatin for many indications.

3.4.4.2 Ototoxicity

Another major toxicity of cisplatin therapy is high tone deafness and vestibular disturbances leading to difficulties with balance. Tinnitus may occur, in association with hearing loss, or in isolation. Ototoxicity is more likely to occur in older patients and in those with impaired renal function. Rapid administration of cisplatin increases the risk of toxicity, perhaps indicating the importance of peak plasma concentration, as does the co-administration of frusemide, which is also contra-indicated from the point of view of nephrotoxicity. Recovery, if it occurs at all, is usually incomplete. Monitoring patients by regular audiometry is vital to provide an early warning of impending serious hearing loss. The cisplatin analogue carboplatin does not appear to be ototoxic and should be substituted where serious toxicity is anticipated.

3.4.4.3 Autonomic neuropathy

Toxicity to the autonomic nervous system may cause paralytic ileus, loss of bladder tone, impotence and hypotension. Vincristine is particularly prone to cause paralytic ileus which may mimic an acute intestinal obstruction with peritonitis. This complication is said to be more likely in patients with impaired hepatic function leading to reduced vincristine clearance. Treatment of constipation may help to prevent the development of ileus and awareness of concomitant medication such as opiate analgesia is clearly important.

3.4.4.4 Central nervous system

Encephalopathy has been reported with a number of drugs, presenting as ataxia, drowsiness, changes in mood, confusion, psychosis or even coma. This is a major problem with ifosfamide, which may produce central nervous system (CNS) toxicity in up to 30% of patients. Risk factors include impaired renal function, low albumin, prior CNS disease, pelvic tumour and short infusion time (Meanwell *et al.*, 1986). Somnolence, ataxia and weakness may complicate 5-FU treatment; ataxia and confusion are also a complication of high-dose cytosine arabinoside, and procarbazine may cause confusion and psychosis. High-dose corticosteroids, used in the treatment of haemopoietic malignancies, may result in steroid psychosis which is characterized by confusion and paranoid delusions. This usually reverses rapidly following withdrawal of the drug.

Intrathecal chemotherapy is used as prophylaxis against meningeal recurrence in acute lymphoblastic leukaemia and certain types of non Hodgkin's lymphoma and for the treatment of carcinomatous meningitis. Methotrexate is used routinely, sometimes together with hydrocortisone and cytosine arabinoside. In the case of prophylactic or adjuvant treatment cranial irradiation may also be employed. The two modalities have additive toxic effects on cerebral function leading to memory difficulties, impairment of concentration, and a decline in intellectual capacity (Bleyer *et al.*, 1981). The severity correlates with the dose of radiation given. In addition, prolonged use of intrathecal methotrexate for treatment of established meningeal disease may lead to leukoencephalopathy which may cause severe neurological dysfunction, sometimes mimicking the symptoms of meningeal disease itself. Careful monitoring should enable the drug to be stopped before serious irreversible damage has occurred (Wasserstrom *et al.*, 1982).

3.4.5 LUNG

A particularly distressing problem associated with certain chemotherapy agents is that of pulmonary toxicity which has been linked with the administration of bleomycin, carmustine (BCNU) and busulphan, also, more rarely, with mitomycin C, cyclophosphamide, chlorambucil, melphalan, cytosine arabinoside, procarbazine and methotrexate. The clinical picture varies, but, in general, toxicity is dose related and may develop several weeks to months following completion of therapy.

At this time, an inflammatory infiltrate can be observed, associated with histological changes in alveolar walls and blood vessels, which may progress to severe pulmonary fibrosis. Diagnosis may be difficult owing to the paucity of physical signs which may be confined to fine basal crepitations. A chest X-ray may be unhelpful initially and there is dispute as to the value of the carbon monoxide transfer factor (McKeage *et al.*, 1990). Symptomatically the patient is likely to complain of shortness of breath and a dry cough but may become progressively limited with the development of dyspnoea and tachypnoea at rest.

A number of early cases respond to treatment with high-dose corticosteroids and withdrawal of the offending drug. However, the presence of dyspnoea at rest and a low pO_2 together with frank consolidation on the chest radiograph implies a grave prognosis and such patients frequently progress to fatal respiratory failure.

Predisposing factors include pulmonary radiotherapy, especially total body irradiation prior to bone marrow transplantation, pre-existing pulmonary disease, age, cigarette smoking and, particularly in the case of bleomycin, exposure to high oxygen concentrations. Drug toxicity needs to be distinguished from pneumonitis due to opportunistic infections such as cytomegalovirus, *Pneumocystis carinii*, aspergillosis and mycoplasma. It may be appropriate to treat empirically for the commoner of these organisms while awaiting the results of microbiological investigations. Bronchial lavage is a useful technique for obtaining samples from which to identify infective organisms and may avoid the performance of an open lung biopsy.

Bleomycin-induced pulmonary fibrosis may occur following a relatively short period of exposure but is more likely to develop in patients who have received >500 units of the drug. The mechanism appears to involve the production of free radicals, hence the detrimental effect of high oxygen concentrations. There is also evidence that macrophages are involved, both from histological studies and, for example, from the observation that protection may be conferred by antibodies against tumour necrosis factor (TNF). Although corticosteroids may have a limited role in treatment of these cases, there is no effective therapy for severe cases. In addition, there does not seem to be a reliable test for early diagnosis of this potentially devastating problem.

Clearly, prevention would be preferable and in addition to the potential role for anti-FNC antibodies there is experimental evidence in favour of a variety of preventive measures. These include the use of chelating agents and antioxidants to limit free radical formation, and glucocorticoids and antifibrotic drugs such as penicillamine to limit the inflammatory response and subsequent fibrosis. Also of benefit may be dietary manipulations such as the use of fish oil derivatives. However, all of these approaches have yet to be proven in man (Scheulen, 1987). In the case of bleomycin, there is some evidence in favour of prolonged infusion as a means of reducing pulmonary toxicity.

Unlike bleomycin-induced toxicity, pulmonary fibrosis following carmustine (BCNU) may take years to develop and appears to affect the upper lobes preferentially. The chest radiograph may remain normal and the problem may be much more common than previously recognized (O'Driscoll *et al.*, 1990).

3.4.6 LIVER

Given the central role of the liver in the metabolism of many drugs, it is not surprising that a large number of agents may produce abnormalities as measured by liver function tests. It is also important to remember that drugs which are largely cleared by this route may give rise to increased toxicity in the presence of liver impairment such as that due to metastatic disease.

The list of drugs which may cause liver toxicity is a long one. Hepatotoxicity may vary from reversible abnormalities in liver function tests to the development of hepatic fibrosis and cirrhosis. The drugs most likely to cause serious liver injury are methotrexate, cytosine arabinoside and 6-mercaptopurine (6-MP) but nitrosoureas and asparaginase commonly cause reversible abnormalities of liver function tests and other drugs which occasionally cause hepatotoxicity include interferon, chlorambucil, busulphan, hydroxyurea, DTIC and cisplatin.

Dose-related hepatotoxicity may occur with 6-MP and may mimic obstructive liver disease. Pre-existing liver disease may preclude the use of certain agents and care needs to be taken to monitor liver function tests during therapy. In the case of methotrexate given regularly over a period of years for chronic non-malignant conditions such as psoriasis or rheumatoid arthritis, it has been claimed that the incidence of hepatic fibrosis may be as high as 25% with a proportion of patients progressing to cirrhosis. It is now routine to monitor such patients regularly by percutaneous liver biopsy to provide an early warning of the development of cirrhosis but a recent large study suggests that the risk of fibrotic liver disease has been exaggerated (Shergy *et al.*, 1988).

3.4.6 Skin

A number of drugs may cause an allergic rash but more serious skin toxicities do occur. Bleomycin causes skin pigmentation, particularly in skin creases and at the sites of scratching. On the hands and over peripheral joints, the skin may become thickened and red and may eventually peel and blister. A similar toxicity to feet and hands has been observed in patients receiving 5-FU by prolonged continuous infusion; this is said to respond to pyridoxine. The rash associated with methotrexate may take the form of a radiation recall reaction. Conjunctivitis has also been described as a complication of methotrexate and 5-FU therapy. In the latter case this may be complicated by tear duct stenosis.

Extravasation of certain vesicant drugs such as doxorubicin and vincristine during intravenous administration may result in skin necrosis. Particular care is required during prolonged infusions which, in consequence, need to be given via a central venous catheter. This property of anti-tumour agents also correlates with an increased risk of thrombophlebitis in the blood vessels used for administration.

3.5 LATE SIDE EFFECTS

There are now a number of cancers which may be cured by intensive combination chemotherapy and the late sequelae of such therapy need to be considered very carefully. In addition to specific organ toxicities which can present some time after the completion of treatment – as in the case of BCNU-induced pulmonary fibrosis – chemotherapy may also affect the gonads, leading to infertility and hormone changes. Another major concern is the mutagenicity of many cytotoxic agents which can lead to the development of second tumours. The need to eliminate these problems is well recognized and is currently an important feature of research into the treatment of Hodgkin's disease and certain paediatric tumours.

3.5.1 ENDOCRINE EFFECTS

3.5.1.1 Ovaries

Age is the major risk factor for chemotherapy-induced ovarian failure which is much less common in women <30 years of age and still less common following treatment before puberty. Additional factors include the drugs used as well as dosage and duration of treatment. Alkylating agents such as cyclophosphamide, chlorambucil, melphalan, mustine and busulphan are particularly prone to cause ovarian dysfunction. In the case of cyclophosphamide, the cumulative dose likely to cause amenorrhea has been determined in relation to age: for example, 9.3 g in 30–39 year old women, 20.4 g in 20–29 year olds (Hobbie *et al.*, 1989). This risk is exacerbated by pelvic radiotherapy. Cranial radiation may occasionally cause secondary ovarian failure due to damage to the hypothalamic–pituitary axis.

Attempts have been made to protect the ovaries from chemotherapy – for example, by the use of oral contraceptives. The results of clinical studies, however, are inconclusive and any benefit seems unlikely by this route. Hormonal replacement therapy in ovarian failure may be required if the symptoms of oestrogen withdrawal such as hot flushes, loss of libido and vaginal dryness, are severe. In younger women with ovarian failure there are the additional concerns of osteoporosis and increased risk of cardiovascular disease. Caution is required in the case of breast cancer where the tumour may be oestrogen-sensitive. In the case of prepubertal ovarian failure, hormonal replacement may be required to promote the development of secondary sexual characteristics.

3.5.1.2 Testes

Infertility is much more likely to occur in young men treated with alkylating agents, although the effects are similarly related to cumulative dose and the duration of treatment. An approximate threshold for azoospermia with cyclophosphamide appears to be a cumulative dose of 11 g. The majority of patients treated for Hodgkin's disease with ≥5 courses of MOPP (mustine, vincristine, procarbazine and prednisolone) or ChlVPP (chlorambucil and vinblastine replacing the first two drugs) will develop azoospermia.

Testosterone may be required during puberty in the case of prepubertal damage and occasionally for the treatment of loss of libido and impotence in adults with testicular failure. However, recovery of function may sometimes occur up to several years after the completion of therapy. The most important consideration is the possibility of sperm banking prior to chemotherapy, providing the sperm count is adequate, in order to give the patient the option of fathering children by artificial insemination in the future.

3.5.2 SECOND MALIGNANCIES

A number of alkylating agents have been implicated as a cause of second malignancies following apparently successful chemotherapy in patients with lymphomas, a variety of solid tumours, and childhood cancers. The drugs which have been proven to be carcinogenic in man include melphalan, chlorambucil, treosulphan, cyclophosphamide and busulphan. The MOPP combination is clearly carcinogenic and both mustine and procarbazine, the latter being particularly carcinogenic in animals, have been implicated (Fraser *et al.*, 1989). The concomitant use of radiotherapy increases the risk. There is also some evidence that the nitrosoureas are carcinogenic. A number of other agents are also known to be mutagenic, such as doxorubicin, but the link with second tumours is less clearcut.

The second malignancy associated with prior chemotherapy is acute myeloid leukaemia (AML). Unfortunately the chemotherapy-induced disease appears to behave differently in that it tends to take a much more aggressive course and is generally refractory to treatment. The risk of inducing AML appears to be related both to the individual drug and to duration of treatment. For example, melphalan has been reported to be more leukaemogenic than cyclophosphamide. There appear to be cumulative dose thresholds below which the risk is low in a similar way to the effects on reproductive function.

Patients receiving radiotherapy have an increased incidence of other tumours: breast cancer and sarcomas, for example, often occur at the edge of the radiotherapy field. The risk of second malignancy is enhanced by combined modality treatment, that is chemotherapy + radiotherapy.

In the case of Hodgkin's disease, where the greatest experience has been acquired, there is a cumulative risk of developing AML of 0.3 to 1% per year starting 1 to 2 years after treatment and peaking at about 8 years before declining after 10 years (Zarrabi *et al.*, 1989). There have been suggestions that patients with Hodgkin's disease may have an inherent tendency to develop malignancies, but this is unproven, unlike children with hereditary retinoblastoma who do carry a significant risk of further malignancies due to the heterozygous lack of a tumour suppressor gene.

Current trials are addressing this issue by attempting to define the minimum duration of treatment in a number of disease types, eliminating certain agents where possible. The combination of adriamycin, bleomycin, vinblastine and DTIC (ABVD) appears to have a lower potential for causing AML in Hodgkin's patients, while maintaining good activity (Santoro *et al.*, 1987). Similarly, treatment for testicular cancer, usually with cisplatin, vinblastine and bleomycin, does not appear to cause AML. However, a recent report suggests that the replacement of vinblastine by etoposide does lead to an increased risk of leukaemia (Pedersen-Bjergaard *et al.*, 1991). Although so far there is no evidence for a significant increase in the incidence of leukaemia (Valagussa *et al.*, 1987), reports of secondary AML following adjuvant chemotherapy in breast cancer are a cause for concern, particulary if primary chemotherapy becomes more widely employed (Geller *et al.*, 1989). Conversely, some authors claim to have shown that adjuvant chemotherapy might have a protective effect against the development of new primary tumours (Arriagada and Rutqvist, 1991).

3.6 CONCLUSIONS

Because of the poor therapeutic index of most anti-cancer agents – which, of necessity, are used at their maximum tolerated dose – serious side effects are unfortunately common. Some acute toxicities are completely reversible and have their major impact on patients' quality of life during treatment. Others may occur many years later with potentially devastating, even fatal consequences. It is vital that research continues into the development of less toxic schedules of administration – shorter duration, less toxic analogues of existing agents and new drugs with a more favourable toxicity profile, for example. However, it must be remembered that current cancer chemotherapy is capable of curing or significantly palliating more than a quarter of all cancers and concern over toxicity should not be allowed to obscure this success.

REFERENCES

Arriagada, R. and Rutqvist, L.E. (1991) Adjuvant chemotherapy in early breast cancer and incidence of new primary malignancies. *Lancet*, **338**, 535–38.

Bleyer, W. (1981) Neurologic sequelae of methotrexate and ionizing radiation: A new classification. *Cancer Treat. Rep.*, **65**, 89–98.

Bronchud, M.H. *et al.* (1989) The use of granulocyte colony-stimulating factor to increase the intensity of treatment with doxorubicin in patients with advanced breast and ovarian cancer. *Br. J. Cancer*, **60**, 121–25.

Burkert, H. (1983) Clinical overview of mesna. *Cancer Treat. Rev.*, **10**, 175–81.

Calvert, A.H. *et al.* (1990) Carboplatin dosage: Prospective evaluation of a simple formula based on renal function. *J. Clin. Oncol.*, **7**, 1748–56.

Coates, A. *et al.* (1983) On the receiving end – Patient perception of the side-effects of cancer chemotherapy. *Eur. J. Cancer*, **19**, 203–9.

Daugaard, G., Rossing, N. and Rørth, M. (1988) Effects of cisplatin on different measures of glomerular function in the human kidney with special emphasis on high-dose. *Cancer Chemother. Pharmacol.*, **21**, 163–67.

Ensley, J.F. *et al.* (1989) The clinical syndrome of 5-fluorouracil cardiotoxicity. *Invest. New Drugs*, **7**, 101–9.

Fraser, M.C. and Tucker, M.A. (1989) Second malignancies following cancer therapy. *Seminars in Oncol. Nursing*, **5**, 43–55.

Geller, R.B. *et al.* (1989) Secondary acute myelocytic leukemia after adjuvant therapy for early-stage breast carcinoma. *Cancer*, **64**, 629–34.

Gerrittsen van der Hoop, R. *et al.* (1990) Prevention of cisplatin neurotoxicity with an ACTH(4–9) analogue in patients with ovarian cancer. *New Engl. J. Med.*, **322**, 89–94.

Goodman, M. (1989) Managing the side effects of chemotherapy. *Seminars in Oncol. Nursing*, **5**(2, suppl 1), 29–51.

Giaccone, M.D. *et al.* (1988) Scalp hypothermia in the prevention of doxorubicin-induced hair loss. *Cancer Nursing*, **11**, 170–73.

Hobbie, W.L. and Schwartz, C.L. (1989) Endocrine late effects among suvivors of cancer. *Seminar in Oncol. Nursing*, **5**, 14–21.

Howell, S.B. *et al.* (1983) Intraperitoneal *cis*-diamminedichloroplatinum with systemic thiosulfate protection. *Cancer Res.*, **43**, 1426–31.

Jones, A.L. *et al.* (1991) Comparison of dexamethasone and ondansetron in the prophylaxis of emesis induced by moderately emetogenic chemotherapy. *Lancet*, **338**, 483–87.

Judson, I.R. (1991) Anthrapyrazoles: true successor to the anthracyclines? *Anti-Cancer Drugs*, **2**, 223–31.

Loprinzi, C.L. *et al.* (1990) A controlled evaluation of an allopurinol mouthwash as prophylaxis against 5-fluorouracil-induced stomatitis. *Cancer*, **65**, 1879–82.

McKeage, M.J. *et al.* (1990) Carbon monoxide diffusing capacity is a poor predictor of clinically significant bleomycin lung. *J. Clin. Oncol.*, **8**, 779–83.

Meanwell, C.A. *et al.* (1986) Prediction of ifosfamide/mesna associated encephalopathy. *Eur. J. Cancer*, **22**, 815–19.

Mollman, J.E. *et al.* (1988) Cisplatin neuropathy: risk factors, prognosis and protection by WR-2721. *Cancer*, **61**, 2192–95.

Morittu, L. *et al.* (1989) Patients at risk of chemotherapy-associated toxicity in small cell lung cancer. *Br. J. Cancer*, **59**, 801–4.

O'Driscoll, B.R. *et al.* (1990) Active lung fibrosis up to 17 years after chemotherapy with carmustine (BCNU) in childhood. *New Engl. Med.*, **323**, 378–82.

Parker, R. (1987) The effectiveness of scalp hypothermia in preventing cyclophosphamide-induced alopecia. *Oncol. Nurs. Forum*, **14**, 49–53.

Pedersen-Bjergaard, J. *et al.* (1991) Increased risk of myelodysplasia and leukaemia after etoposide, cisplatin, and bleomycin for germ-cell tumours. *Lancet*, **338**, 359–63.

Richardson, J.L., Marks, G. and Levine, A. (1988) The influence of symptoms of disease and side effects of treatment on compliance with cancer therapy. *J. Clin. Oncol.*, **6**, 1746–52.

Santoro, A. *et al.* (1987) Long-term results of combined chemotherapy-radiotherapy approach in Hodgkin's disease: Superiority of ABVD plus radiotherapy versus MOPP plus radiotherapy. *J. Clin. Oncol.*, **5**, 27–37.

Scheulen, M.E. (1987) Reduction of pulmonary toxicity. *Cancer Treat. Rev.*, **14**, 231–43.

Smeitink, J. *et al.* (1988) Nephrotoxicity associated with ifosfamide. *Eur. J. Pediatr.*, **148**, 164–66.

Schwartz, R.G. *et al.* (1987) Congestive heart failure and left ventricular dysfunction complicating doxorubicin therapy. *Am. J. Med.*, **82**, 1109–17.

Shergy, W.J. *et al.* (1988) Methotrexate-associated hepatotoxicity: Retrospective analysis of 210 patients with rheumatoid arthritis. *Am. J. Med.*, **85**, 771–74.

Speyer, J.L. *et al.* (1990) Protective effect of the bispiperazinedione ICRF-187 against doxorubicin-induced cardiac toxicity in women with advanced breast cancer. *New Engl. J. Med.*, **319**, 745–51.

Valagussa, P., Tancini, G. and Bonadonna, G. (1987) Second malignancies after CMF for resectable breast cancer. *J. Clin. Oncol.*, **5**, 1138–42.

Verweij, J., van der Burg, M.E.L. and Pinedo, H.M. (1987) Mitomycin C-induced hemolytic uremic syndrome. Six case reports and review of the literature on renal, pulmonary and cardiac side effects of the drug. *Radiotherapy and Oncol.*, **8**, 33–41.

Wasserstrom, W.R., Class, J.P. and Posner, J.B. (1982) Diagnosis and treatment of leptomeningeal metastases from solid tumours. *Cancer*, **49**, 759–72.

Zarrabi, M.H. and Rosner, F. (1989) Second neoplasms in Hodgkin's disease: current controversies. *Haematol. Oncol. Clinics of N. America*, **3**, 303–18.

4

Nausea in anti-cancer therapy: Measurement and mechanisms

M. TONATO, F. ROILA and A. DEL FAVERO

4.1 INTRODUCTION

Nausea is an unpleasant sensation of discomfort referred to the upper gut; it is associated with the awareness of the urge to vomit. Nausea can result from a wide variety of organic and psychogenic disorders and, in cancer patients receiving chemotherapy, is perceived as the most distressing side effect of anti-neoplastic treatment (Coates *et al.*, 1983).

In a recent study, the frequency of nausea was evaluated during the last six months of life in 342 Norwegian cancer patients. Nausea was a symptom in 44% of patients and only 2% of them obtained complete relief from symptoms despite anti-emetic treatment. There was a close connection between opiate or cytostatic treatment and nausea. The highest frequency was found among patients with gastro-intestinal and ovarian cancer, whilst the lowest frequency was found in the prostate cancer group (Gran *et al.*, 1990).

In contrast to vomiting, very little is known about the physiology of nausea. The manifestation of nausea is accompanied by a loss of gastric tone and a decrease in peristaltic activity along with contraction of the duodenum and a reflux of intestinal contents into the stomach. Frequently, nausea is accompanied by sweating, pallor, salivation, dizziness, lightheadedness and tachycardia, all of which are mediated by the autonomic nervous system.

Although nausea, vomiting and retching are often considered to be part of the same process and to have identical underlying mechanisms, this assumption may be incorrect. Nausea, for example, may occur without vomiting, and vice versa. Nevertheless, as nausea usually precedes vomiting, and sub-emetic doses of emetic agents can evoke nausea alone, it has been suggested that nausea represents low level activation of the vomiting pathway (Andrews *et al.*, 1988).

Accurate measurement of nausea is an essential part of evaluation of side effects caused by cancer chemotherapy and of the efficacy of any anti-emetic treatments. Assessment methodology, however, is far from being standardized and, as this chapter suggests, needs careful consideration.

In discussing the measurement of nausea we will focus our attention on four main topics: what is to be measured; who should measure what; the various methods available, and how to select and use these.

4.2 DEFINING THE PARAMETERS TO BE MEASURED

Nausea can be the essential component in four distinct emetic syndromes in patients

Emesis in Anti-cancer Therapy
Mechanisms and treatment
Published in 1993 by Chapman & Hall, London
ISBN 0 412 37250 9

receiving chemotherapy (Gralla *et al.*, 1984): acute chemotherapy-induced emesis; persistent or delayed emesis; anticipatory emesis, and emesis not related to chemotherapy received.

The physiological mechanisms of each of these syndromes have not yet been fully elucidated: we do not really know, for example, if substantial differences exist. However, what is certain is that different methods of assessment may be needed when evaluating the various syndromes. They need, therefore, to be clearly defined and differentiated in evaluating any anti-emetic treatment.

Being a subjective phenomenon, nausea assessment, by definition, is difficult and relies almost entirely on reports by the patient. In measuring nausea, it is therefore important that the patients have a clear understanding of the phenomenon to be assessed. They must understand the exact meaning of the word nausea, be aware of its various dimensions and of the ways in which nausea evaluation is performed. It should be considered that even the patient's interpretation of the word nausea might be a special problem. In fact, this word was not understood by two-thirds of the patients participating in a study on nausea measurement and the term 'sick stomach' was the most common patient description of the term (Rhodes *et al.*, 1984). Nausea must be assessed separately from vomiting. Even when evaluating the efficacy of anti-emetic therapy, during which nausea and vomiting can be assembled together in a common score, the two components need a separate assessment. Thus, these symptoms can occur independently, can be influenced in a different way by anti-emetic therapy or by environmental factors, and, most important, are measured by different methods (Del Favero *et al.*, 1990). A separate evaluation of nausea and vomiting was indeed the finding in 91% of 384 papers dealing with anti-emetic treatment evaluation that have been published since January 1983

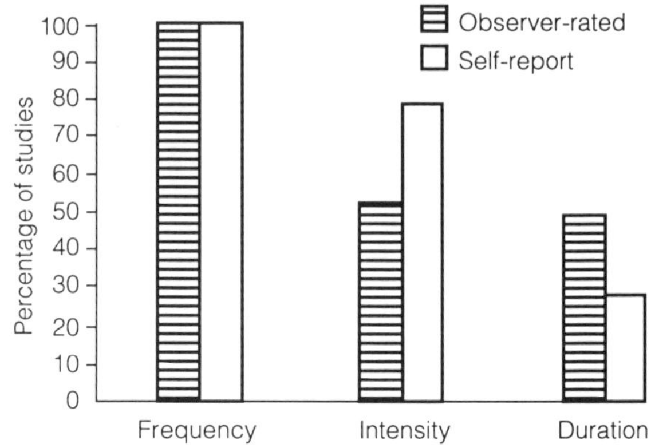

Figure 4.1 Percentage of studies using observer-rated or self-report methodology to measure dimensions of nausea.

and it therefore now appears to be a widely accepted procedure.

Nausea is characterized by three distinct and relatively independent characteristics: frequency, intensity and duration. All these elements must be taken into consideration when measuring nausea since they give rise to different clinical concerns and may call for different therapeutic approaches. They can be measured in a relatively precise way and represent the elementary quantitative dimensions of nausea. Moreover, they can be used to construct more complex composite dimensions of nausea (see below) in an attempt to objectively quantify the global, entirely subjective experience of nausea which is in itself a multidimensional phenomenon.

Unfortunately, apart from frequency, the above-mentioned dimensions of nausea are not always measured in clinical trials (Fig. 4.1). The duration of nausea is measured considerably less often than are its frequency and intensity, despite the fact that duration is likely to be just as much of a concern to the patient as the other dimensions.

A satisfactory assessment of nausea requires the evaluation of the qualitative as well as the quantitative aspects of the experience.

Qualitative measurement presents a much more difficult task, but in spite of this, the measurement of how 'unpleasant' or 'severe' nausea is for the patient must remain an essential part of nausea assessment.

In addition to the above-mentioned direct measurements of nausea a variety of indirect measurements have been suggested (e.g. change in appetite, general well being, patient's preference amongst anti-emetic treatments, etc.) (Cotanch *et al.*, 1983). Such measurements, however, have not been widely employed, have not been validated, and many factors can bias the results. It remains to be demonstrated if such measurements can provide useful additional information to that of the direct measurements of nausea.

More intriguing is the interpretation of the data provided by studies which are aimed at obtaining an indirect assessment of nausea. These measure some of the physiological parameters which may correlate with the patients' report of nausea.

In one of these studies, using a biomedical instrumentation developed by NASA for evaluating space adaptation sickness, physiological parameters were monitored continuously for 12 hours in 8 patients after chemotherapy administration (Morrow *et al.*, 1987). Patients' reports of nausea were accompanied by a replicable physiological pattern: increase of pallor, decrease of temperature, blood volume, pulse and heart rate. Furthermore, a correlation between these physiological measures and patient-report intensity of nausea was shown, confirming the results of previous reports (Cotanch *et al.*, 1983; Burish *et al.*, 1981; Burish *et al.*, 1987; Cotanch *et al.*, 1987; Lyles *et al.*, 1982).

In other studies, however, no modification occurred in physiological measures such as heart rate (Ahles *et al.*, 1984; Levitt *et al.*, 1981), blood pressure, respiratory rate, vital capacity and temperature (Levitt *et al.*, 1981) in patients referring pre or postchemotherapy nausea. In patients with anticipatory nausea and vomiting an increase of heart rate was shown; this was not shown in patients who exhibited only anticipatory nausea (Ahles *et al.*, 1984).

It seems clear that the modification of these physiological measures of nausea are difficult to interpret: both because of the contrasting data available, and because they can be influenced by many other factors which may not be related to nausea. More data are therefore needed before a better understanding of the role of physiological measures in the assessment of nausea can be achieved.

More interesting, although limited, are the data derived from studies aimed at finding humoral markers of nausea. Some studies in man have reported marked increase in plasma arginine–vasopressin levels, with no significant change in plasma osmolarity or blood pressure, after administration of various nausea-causing stimuli (apomorphine, ethanol infusion, etc.) (Shelton *et al.*, 1977; Rowe *et al.*, 1979). This phenomenon was confirmed in two small studies conducted in cancer patients undergoing chemotherapy (Fisher *et al.*, 1982; Edwards *et al.*, 1989).

In the Fisher study arginine–vasopressin levels increased 0–40 min before nausea and vomiting and peaked at 28–115 min after their occurrence. In the Edwards study, relative increases in arginine–vasopressin levels were significantly greater in patients who vomited and in those who experienced moderate or severe nausea compared to those who either did not exhibit emesis or had mild or no nausea.

From these studies it is impossible to distinguish the effects of arginine–vasopressin on either the nausea or the vomiting. It is also difficult to understand if arginine–vasopressin has a mediating role in the pathogenesis of chemotherapy-induced emesis, or instead if its increase represents a response to nausea.

A recent study (Nussey *et al.*, 1988) tested the plasma response of arginine–vasopressin

Table 4.1 Measurement of nausea: Review of the literature 1983–1990

What has been measured (%)	Frequency 100	Intensity 70	Duration 34	
Who measures (%)	Patient's report 35	Observer report 21	Both 6	NS 38
Scales employed (%)	VAS 29	Score 49	Both 4	NS 18

384/478 published reports evaluable for nausea assessment: 50% full papers; 46% abstracts; 4% short reports or letters.
NS = not specified.

and oxytocin to apomorphine, and ipecacuanha-induced nausea and vomiting in normal volunteers and patients with idiopathic diabetes insipidus. Apomorphine-induced nausea was followed by marked increases in plasma arginine–vasopressin in normal subjects, but not in patients with idiopathic diabetes insipidus. Therefore, the role of arginine–vasopressin does not seem essential in the emetic response in humans, and its increase could be an effect of nausea and not a cause.

Some humoral agents, when exogenously administered, have been shown to induce vomiting in animal models: angiotensin II, neurotensin, leu- and met-enkephalin, cholecystokinin, insulin, gastrin, bombesin, peptide YY and thyrotropin-releasing hormone. However, these emetogenic doses are often high and do not reflect blood levels which may possibly be reached naturally in various emetic syndromes or conditions (Kucharczyk *et al.*, 1990). No correlation of these humoral agents with nausea has yet been demonstrated.

A close correspondence between tachygastria (evaluated through an electrogastrogram) and nausea occurring in motion sickness syndrome has recently been shown (Stern *et al.*, 1987). The neurohumoral mechanisms that mediate tachygastria are unknown, but a stress-mediated catecholamine release that temporarily suppresses gastric vagal imput and precipitates tachygastria has been suggested. Here again it is impossible to know if tachygastria is the cause or the effect of nausea; it cannot therefore be used as a marker of nausea, particularly in chemotherapy-treated patients where this phenomenon has not yet been demonstrated. Again, more studies are needed to investigate possible humoral mediators of nausea.

4.3 THE CLINICAL MEASUREMENT OF NAUSEA

Nausea does not constitute an observable phenomenon since it is a purely subjective experience. It is unlikely that an external observer can be aware that a patient is nauseated unless that patient tells him. Thus, it is always the patient who allows nausea to be measured. This can be done by the patient him- or herself using a self-report scale or through an interview with the patient by an external observer who subsequently scores the patient's nausea using one of the available methods.

It should be added that the patient's self report can in itself be biased. Anti-emetic drugs or behavioural interventions can impair the patients' state of consciousness or alter their perception of distress.

Table 4.1 shows the percentage of studies which have used observer-rated or self-report methodology to record various dimensions of nausea. Not unexpectedly, observer-rated nausea is used rather less than self-report methodology. Nevertheless, a physician, or alternatively a nurse with particular training in nausea assessment, could be employed as an external rater and in studies on children an observer parent could be used.

If observer-rated measurements are employed it is suggested that two independent raters be used whenever possible; averaging two independent ratings increases their reliability. Appropriate training of the observer also seems to be useful in order to increase inter-rater agreement.

4.3.1 MEASUREMENT METHODS

Much instrumentation is available to measure the quantitative and qualitative aspects of nausea. However, in contrast to the consensus reached on the criteria for the assessment of vomiting, ways to measure nausea have not yet been adequately validated and standardized.

There follows a concise review of the advantages and limitations of the most widely used scales in the measurement of different dimensions of nausea.

4.3.1.1 Frequency of nausea

The degree of protection from nausea (as well as from vomiting) remains the main efficacy parameter with which to assess the validity of any new anti-emetic treatment. Any study of this requires that the frequency of nausea be reported. The measurement can be a simple one, based on a yes/no answer to a specific question by the patient on the presence of nausea; alternatively, it can be based on a four-or-more-point scale. Overall, 100% of published studies report complete protection from nausea (Table 4.1, above).

4.3.1.2 Intensity of nausea

Intensity is another frequently used dimension of nausea (see also Table 4.1). Two types of scales have been employed: visual analogue scales (VAS) and descriptive ordinal scales (DS).

A VAS scale is usually a 100 mm long vertical line with the extremes marked as 'no nausea' (bottom) and the 'worst nausea I have ever felt' (top), with no intermediate divisions or descriptive terms. A score from 0–100 is determined by measuring the distance from the bottom to the mark placed by the patient along the line.

Investigators who have used VAS with children have incorporated the scale in a sketch of a thermometer and the children colour in their degree of nausea. Some minor variations of this type of VAS have also been used such as scales with a horizontal or semicircular line. In some cases the VAS is incorporated in the line-intermediate divisions and/or in discrete descriptive terms (i.e. nausea slight; mild; severe). These types of scales, however, do not seem to offer any advantage: even worse, they could introduce some bias in the measurement provided by the more usual VAS.

Another type of analogue scale used to evaluate intensity of nausea is the analogue continuous chromatic scale (ACCS) (Del Favero *et al.*, 1990).

This scale consists of a coloured horizontal strip, 100 mm long and 25 mm wide, containing no marking except for the anchor points at each end, the extremes being 'no nausea' (left) and 'worst nausea I have ever felt' (right); these words are on a white background at the two extremities of the coloured strip. The colour is graduated from left to right from pale pink to dark red. The coloured strip lies on one face of a double-sided device, the patient evaluates the intensity of the nausea by positioning a transparent slider containing a narrow black line perpendicular to the coloured strip. The opposite side of the ruler contains a 0–100 mm scale, which fits exactly the ACCS on the other face. This is not visible to the patient. This allows the observer to immediately record the nausea score. The position of the slider is fixed by a stopper fitted inside the device.

Many types of descriptive scales have been employed that use three or more points along with various verbal ratings (Morrow *et al.*, 1984). A scale rating 0, no nausea; 1, slight nausea; 2, moderate nausea; and 3, severe nausea, is one of the simplest and most widely used.

Few studies have assessed the reliability and validity of VAS scales in measuring intensity of nausea. Reliability of VAS has been evaluated in a group of 18 cancer patients who had filled out VAS twice, 10–15 minutes apart. The coefficient of correlation was high (0.83), showing a good reliability. Validity of the VAS was established showing either a significant correlation between each patient's score and that of a clinical observer who was unaware of the patient's self-report of nausea (Fetting *et al.*, 1982) or (in a double-blind crossover study) showing a strong correlation of VAS with the patient preference expressed for the control of nausea achieved by treatment after two cycles of chemotherapy (Pater *et al.*, 1985).

In children under nine years old the use of VAS for evaluating nausea has been found to be a difficult procedure (Redd *et al.*, 1987). A rating scale with verbal descriptions as signposts along the scale (including faces above the numbers in the scale in children younger than 10 years) has therefore been used (Zeltzer *et al.*, 1984; LeBaron *et al.*, 1984). The validity of this method was initially suggested by an 80% agreement betwen the ratings of parents and children when they were assessed independently (Zeltzer *et al.*, 1984). Subsequently, validity was confirmed in a study in 161 healthy school children and 64 children with cancer who were asked to rate nausea and vomiting from a series of vignettes. Even five-year-old children were found to respond in a manner similar to adult raters (Zeltzer *et al.*, 1988).

Only a few studies have simultaneously assessed nausea using different scales and only two have evaluated the agreement of these scales (Del Favero *et al.*, 1990; Havsteen *et al.*, 1986). In both studies there was a high correlation between a four-point descriptive scale (DS) and the VAS for nausea (correlation coefficient 0.899 and 0.68 respectively). A good correlation was also shown (r = 0.74 and r = 0.60 respectively) when the ACCS was compared with the visual analogue and descriptive scales. The ACCS had been previously evaluated to assess pain, and proved to be more sensitive than VAS, allowing a greater discrimination of grades of pain (Grossi *et al.*, 1983) but not in the case of nausea (Del Favero *et al.*, 1990).

The substantial equivalence of VAS and DS was also demonstrated by measuring their sensitivity. The comparative sensitivities of the two scales was found to be similar when assessed by their ability to demonstrate changes in the dimensions of nausea occurring in the same patient at different evaluation times and to discriminate two groups treated with different anti-emetic treatment (Del Favero *et al.*, 1990). In conclusion the analogue scale did not appear to offer a specific advantage over a simple DS.

4.3.1.3 Duration of nausea

The duration of nausea has been reported only in a low percentage (29%) of studies (see Table 1), probably because it is an intermittent phenomenon and its assessment may be difficult and require frequent evaluations. Most commonly, patients are asked, at each point of evaluation, how many minutes they have experienced nausea during the previous time period. Its measurement can be biased both by the level of recall capability of the patient and by the number and/or time intervals of evaluations. However, when one considers that duration of nausea could be equal to or more distressing than intensity, it would be useful to have it evaluated in all trials on anti-emetics.

4.3.1.4 Composite dimensions of nausea

Nausea has recently been evaluated according to other dimensions that include **maximal intensity**, defined as the highest value of the score obtained with a descriptive or analogue scale at any evaluation carried out over the observation time (Del Favero *et al.*, 1990). Other composite measures of nausea are as follows:

(1) Entity (E): defined as the sum of all the values of intensity (I) of nausea recorded with a descriptive or analogue scale at each evaluation time ($\Sigma = I$).
(2) Quantity (Q): defined as the sum of the products of the intensity multiplied by the duration (D) recorded at each evaluation time ($Q = \Sigma(I \times D)$.

A good correlation between these different dimensions has been shown irrespective of the scale employed. Furthermore, using E and most particularly Q of nausea, the power of the statistical analysis in discriminating differences between groups of patients submitted to different anti-emetic treatments increases, as does the correlation between VAS and DS. Composite measurements of nausea seem therefore to be the most sensitive way to quantify this purely subjective symptom (Del Favero *et al.*, 1990), not an unexpected finding if one takes into account the fact that nausea is a multidimensional phenomenon and is likely therefore to be better defined by a multidimensional scale.

4.3.1.5 Other scales to evaluate nausea and vomiting

Other indices have been proposed to measure the global experience of nausea and vomiting in patients receiving chemotherapy by evaluating both the quantitative as well as the qualitative aspects of the emetic experience (i.e. Duke Descriptive Scale [Cotanch *et al.*, 1983]). Two of these instruments (described below) were developed and tested some years ago (Rhodes *et al.*, 1984; Morrow *et al.*, 1984).

The Rhodex index is a 5-item (duration of nausea; frequency of nausea; distress from nausea; frequency of vomiting, and amount of vomiting), 5-point Likert-type scale.

The Morrow Assessment of Nausea and Emesis scale (MANE) is a self-report scale which assesses the following aspects: anticipatory nausea; anticipatory vomiting; post-treatment nausea, and post-treatment vomiting. Elements assessed by MANE are: frequency (4-point scale [during or after every treatment to never]); duration (hours nausea and vomiting last); severity (6-point scale [very mild to intolerable]); and time when nausea and vomiting were worse (6-point scale [during treatment to 24-hr after treatment]).

Although reliability and validity of these scales has been demonstrated, they have been used very little in anti-emetic research. Furthermore, if these scales are appropriate for subjective measurements, such as that of nausea, assessment of vomiting should be made by direct observation employing trained staff. The patient's own recall of a vomiting experience may not in fact be accurate, especially when they have taken anti-emetic drugs that induce sedation, memory loss and hallucinations.

4.4 CHOOSING THE APPROPRIATE MEASUREMENT METHOD

Any choice of the best way to measure nausea should be based on careful consideration of the type of nausea we are dealing with, the aim of the measurement in question and the relative merits of various types of measurements.

Anticipatory nausea usually requires only a yes/no assessment and can be performed by directly interviewing the patient; delayed nausea is most often evaluated by a diary card completed by the patient him- or herself; the patient also scores the intensity of the symptom by a DS.

Choice of measurement for post-chemotherapy acute nausea can be more complex. In this case both the aim of the measurement and the performance of the available scales must be considered in order to make the best choice.

Analogue scales have been proposed as the best measurement for many subjective symptoms (i.e. pain) because they offer a greater sensitivity with respect to DS (Huskisson *et al.*, 1974), but this has not been found in nausea evaluation (Del Favero *et al.*, 1990). A further advantage of VAS could be represented by the fact that the distribution of maximal intensity values obtained by it is uniform (Del Favero *et al.*, 1990) and this may be relevant according to the choice of statistical analysis method to be employed. The disadvantage of VAS is the requirement for a careful explanation of its use to the patient by a trained assistant on the first few occasions. Despite this, a small percentage of patients are still unable to complete a VAS. Another limitation of VAS, as has been said, is the fact that this tool measures mainly a quantitative single aspect (intensity) of what is a multidimensional phenomenon. To circumvent this limitation we have proposed the measurement of composite dimensions of nausea such as Q or E (Del Favero *et al.*, 1990).

Descriptive scales, despite the well known defects common to all discrete scales, appear to offer the important specific advantage of simplicity with no important drawbacks with respect to VAS. Analogue and descriptive scales probably can be usefully combined to make the evaluation process more complete and precise. In fact, the possibility that many factors (i.e. patient expectations, environment) influence the tolerance to or alter the perception of severity of nausea suggests an advantage in maintaining two different measurements of the same phenomenon.

4.5 CONCLUSIONS

Nausea is a subjective feeling and therefore cannot be measured by an objective 'gold-standard' method from which either assessment of sensitivity or specificity of various methods of measurement could be derived. Consequently, uncertainties still exist over the 'best' method of assessing chemotherapy-induced nausea in cancer patients enrolled in clinical trials on anti-emetics.

Both VAS and DS have proven to be useful. A simple DS can be adopted to quantify nausea when analogue scales are not at hand, provided that a standard way of presenting the scale is assured and that the main efficacy parameter used to assess the validity of an anti-emetic treatment is complete protection from nausea and vomiting. VAS can be combined with DS to strengthen the consistency of the results. In comparative clinical trials, measurement of more complex dimensions of nausea, such as Q or E, can add a measure of sensitivity in detecting differences.

A consensus on the best way to assess nausea so that a better comparison of the results obtained in clinical trials can be made would be welcome.

REFERENCES

Ahles, T.A., Cohen, R.E., Little, D., *et al.* (1984) Toward a behavioral assessment of anticipatory symptoms associated with cancer chemotherapy. *J. Behav. Ther. Exp. Psychiat.*, **15**, 141–45.

Andrews, P.L.R. Rapeport, W.G. and Sanger, G.J. (1988) Neuropharmacology of emesis induced by anti-cancer therapy, *Trends in Pharmacol Sci.*, **9**, 334–41.

Burish, T.G. and Lyles, J.N. (1981) Effectiveness of relaxation training in reducing adverse reactions to cancer chemotherapy. *J. Behav. Med.*, **4**, 65–78.

Burish, T.G., Carey, M.P., Krozely, M.G., *et al.* (1987) Conditioned side effects induced by cancer chemotherapy: prevention through behavioral treatment. *J. Consult. Clin. Psychol.*, **55**, 1, 42–48.

Coates, A., Abraham, S., Kaye, S.B., *et al.* (1983) On receiving end-patient perception of the side effects of cancer chemotherapy. *Eur. J. Cancer Clin. Oncol.*, **19**, 203–8.

Cotanch, P.H. (1983) Relaxation training for control of nausea and vomiting in patients receiving chemotherapy. *Cancer Nurs.*, **6**, 277–83.

Cotanch, P.H. and Strum, S. (1987) Progressive muscle relaxation as an anti-emetic therapy for cancer patients. *Oncol. Nurs. Forum*, **14**, 33–37.

Del Favero, A., Roila, F., Basurto, C. *et al.* (1990) Assessment of nausea. *Eur. J. Clin. Pharmacol.*, **38**, 115–20.

Edwards, C.M., Carmichael, J., Baylis, P.H., *et al.* (1989) Arginine vasopressin – a mediator of chemotherapy-induced emesis? *Br. J. Cancer*, **59**, 467–70.

Fetting, J.H., Grochow, L.B., Folstein, M.F. *et al.* (1982) The course of nausea and vomiting after high-dose cyclophosphamide. *Cancer Treat. Rep.*, **66**, 1487–93.

Fisher, R.D., Rentschier, R.E., Nelson, J.C. *et al.* (1982) Elevation of plasma antidiuretic hormone (ADH) associated with chemotherapy-induced emesis in man. *Cancer Treat. Rep.* **66**, 25–29.

Gralla, R.J. (1984) Response in the assessment of nausea and vomiting: Past problems, current issues, and suggestions for future research. *Cancer*, **53** (suppl), 2278–80.

Gran, L. and Borchgrevink, C.F. (1990) Nausea in cancer patients – an analysis of its frequency and an evaluation of treatment in a Norwegian population. *Tidsski Nor Laegeforen*, **110**, 63–65.

Grossi, E., Borghi, C., Cerchiari, E.L. *et al.* (1983) Analogue chromatic continuous scale (ACCS): a new method for pain assessment. *Clin. Exper. Rheumatol.*, **1**, 337–40.

Havsteen, H., Nielsen, H. and Kiaer, M. (1986) The use of visual analogue scale (VAS) in patients receiving cisplatin-containing cancer chemotherapy. *Proc. ASCO*, **5**, 263.

Heim, M., Romer, W. and Queisser, W. (1981) Clinical experience with levonantradol hydrochloride in the prevention of cancer chemotherapy-induced nausea and vomiting. *J. Clin. Pharmacol.*, **21** (Suppl.) 86–89.

Huskisson, E.C. (1974) Measurement of pain. *Lancet* II, 1127–31.

Kucharczyk, J., and Harding, R.K. (1990) Regulatory peptides and the onset of nausea and vomiting. *Cancer Physiol. Pharmacol.*, **68**, 289–93.

LeBaron, S. and Zelzter, L.K. (1984) Assessment of acute pain and anxiety in children and adolescents by self-reports, observer reports, and a behaviour checklist. *J. Consult. Clin. Psychol.*, **52**, 729–38.

Levitt, M., Wilson, A., Bowman, D., *et al.* (1981) Physiologic observations in a controlled clinical trial of the antiemetic effectiveness of 5, 10 and 15 mg of tetrahydrocannabinol in cancer chemotherapy. Ophthalmologic implications. *J. Clin. Pharmacol.* **21** (Suppl.), 103–9.

Lyles, J.N., Burish, T.G., Krozely, M.G., *et al.* (1982) Efficacy of relaxation training and guided imagery in reducing the aversiveness of cancer chemotherapy. *J. Consult. Clin. Psychol.*, **50**, 509–24.

Morrow, G.R. (1984) The assessment of nausea and vomiting. Past problems, current issues, and suggestions for future research. *Cancer*, **53** (suppl), 2267–78.

Morrow, G.R. (1987) Physiologic measures of chemotherapy induced nausea and vomiting. *Proc. ASCO*, **6**, 266.

Nussey, S.S., Hawthorn, J., Page, S.R. *et al.* (1988) Responses of plasma oxytocin and arginine vasopressin to nausea induced by apomorphine and ipecacuanha. *Clin. Endocrinol.*, **28**, 297–304.

Pater, J.L., Willan, A.R., Erlichman, C., *et al.* (1985) A validation of self-reported measures of nausea (N) and vomiting (V). *Proc. ASCO*, **4**, 265.

Redd, W.H., Jacobsen, P.B., Die-Trill, M., *et al.* (1987) Cognitive/attentional distraction in the control of conditioned nausea in pediatric cancer patients receiving chemotherapy. *J. Consult. Clin. Psychol.*, **55**, 391–95.

Rhodes, V.A., Watson, P.M. and Johnson, M.H. (1984) Development of reliable and valid measures of nausea and vomiting. *Cancer Nurs.*, **7**, 33–41.

Rowe, J.W., Shelton, R.L., Helderman, J.H., *et al.* (1979) Influence of the reflex on vasopressin release in man. *Kidney Int.*, **16**, 729–35.

Shelton, R.L., Kinney, R.M. and Robertson, G.L. (1977) Emesis, a species specific stimulus for vasopressin release. *Clin. Res.*, **25**, 301A.

Stern, R.M., Koch, K.L., Stewart, W.R. *et al.* (1987) Spectral analysis of tachygastria recorded during motion sickness. *Gastroenterol.*, **92**, 92–97.

Zeltzer, L.K., LeBaron, S. and Zeltzer, P.M. (1984) A prospective assessment of chemotherapy-related nausea and vomiting in children with cancer. *Amer. J. Pediatr. Hematol. Oncol.*, **6**, 5–16.

Zeltzer, L.K., LeBaron, S. and Zeltzer, P.M. (1984) The effectiveness of behavioral intervention for reducing nausea and vomiting in children and adolescents receiving chemotherapy. *J. Clin. Oncol.*, **2**, 683–90.

Zeltzer, L.K., LeBaron, S., Richie, D.M., *et al.* (1988) Can children understand and use a rating-scale to quantify somatic symptoms? Assessment of nausea and vomiting as a model. *J. Consult. Clin. Psychol.*, **56**, 567–72.

5

Changes in gastro-intestinal motility associated with vomiting and nausea

H.I.M. DAVIDSON and M.-A. PILOT

5.1 INTRODUCTION

In this chapter the gastro-intestinal motility changes which occur immediately before, during and after cytotoxic drug-induced nausea and vomiting will be discussed. The mechanisms of these changes, including some aspects of their pharmacology, will also be discussed using data from animal experiments and where possible man. In order to assess the contribution which these gastro-intestinal motility changes may make to the emetic reflex a number of emetic substances have been included which are not normally used in chemotherapy but have been used clinically for antibacterial therapy (e.g. erythromycin) or to produce emesis in an experimental situation (e.g. apomorphine).

Although the central integration of emetic stimuli has a common site in the brainstem, there are thought to be two basic mechanisms for the production of emesis. Firstly, the direct activation of the area postrema (chemoreceptor trigger zone) such as occurs with apomorphine and other centrally acting emetics which initiate emesis after entering the circulation, and secondly, the activation of visceral afferents by substances such as copper sulphate which initiate vomiting at the level of the gastro-intestinal tract (see Chapter 7). The activation of the gastro-intestinal motor correlates of vomiting occur irrespective of the mechanism of action of the emetic stimulus and so centrally and peripherally acting emetics will be reviewed together.

This chapter will also attempt to ascribe a physiological function to the gastro-intestinal motor changes which occur during vomiting and discuss the effects on motility of substances which not only induce emesis but have additional actions on the gastro-intestinal tract (e.g. diarrhoea). The gastro-intestinal changes which occur in association with the subjective feeling of nausea and the possible causal relationship between these motility changes and nausea are discussed separately.

5.2 NORMAL MOTILITY PATTERNS OF THE UPPER GASTRO-INTESTINAL TRACT

To recognize the changes in gastro-intestinal motility associated with emesis it is important to appreciate the sequence of events which

Emesis in Anti-cancer Therapy
Mechanisms and treatment
Published in 1993 by Chapman & Hall, London
ISBN 0 412 37250 9

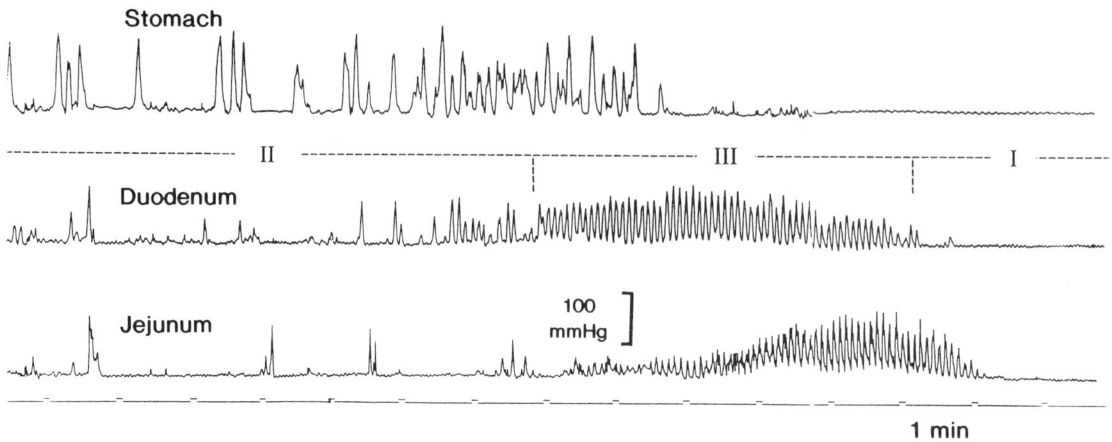

Figure 5.1 Migrating motor complex (MMC) in the human gastro-intestinal tract recorded using luminal pressure transducers. During the high contractile phase (phase 3) shown here lasting approximately 5 minutes and migrating in an aboral direction, the gut contracts at its maximum frequency. The frequency of contraction depends on the gut region – note the slower frequency of contraction in the stomach. I, II and III represent the quiescent, irregular contractile and high contractile phases of the MMC respectively.

occur during digestion. This section gives a short outline of the motility patterns recognized in the fed and fasted states.

The arrival of food in the digestive tract gives rise to an integrated and co-ordinated pattern of motor activity to facilitate the passage of nutrients to sites where they can be digested and absorbed. The presence of a bolus of food in the oesophagus triggers a peristaltic wave which travels the length of the oesophagus and terminates in the relaxation of the lower oesophageal sphincter, thus allowing the food to enter the stomach. The proximal stomach exhibits a reflex phenomenon called receptive relaxation which allows this part of the stomach to act as a reservoir for the meal. When the food has been mechanically degraded by the powerful muscular action of the antrum into particles small enough to pass through the pylorus, it is expelled progressively into the duodenum. This occurs through a finely integrated mechanism whereby single waves of contraction start in the distal stomach and migrate distally into the small bowel. The gastric emptying of liquids is exponential and is more rapid than that of solids which follows a linear pattern.

Antroduodenal co-ordination is a complex feature essential for the process of gastric emptying (Schuurkes and Van Nueten, 1990). Co-ordination of contractile activity also occurs in all parts of the small bowel, seemingly in a random fashion. Although numerous contractions can be seen to occur postprandially, single waves travelling through short segments of bowel have been observed; these are thought to be responsible for the passage of nutrients in an aboral direction (Schemann and Erhlein, 1986).

In all mammals studied to date, either by means of intraluminal pressure tubes or sensors implanted on the surface of the bowel (in animals only), highly organized pattern of motor activity also occurs in fasting, when there are little or no nutrients in the upper regions of the digestive tract (Fig. 5.1). Discrete bursts of contractile activity are observed in a proximal segment of the bowel, and travel

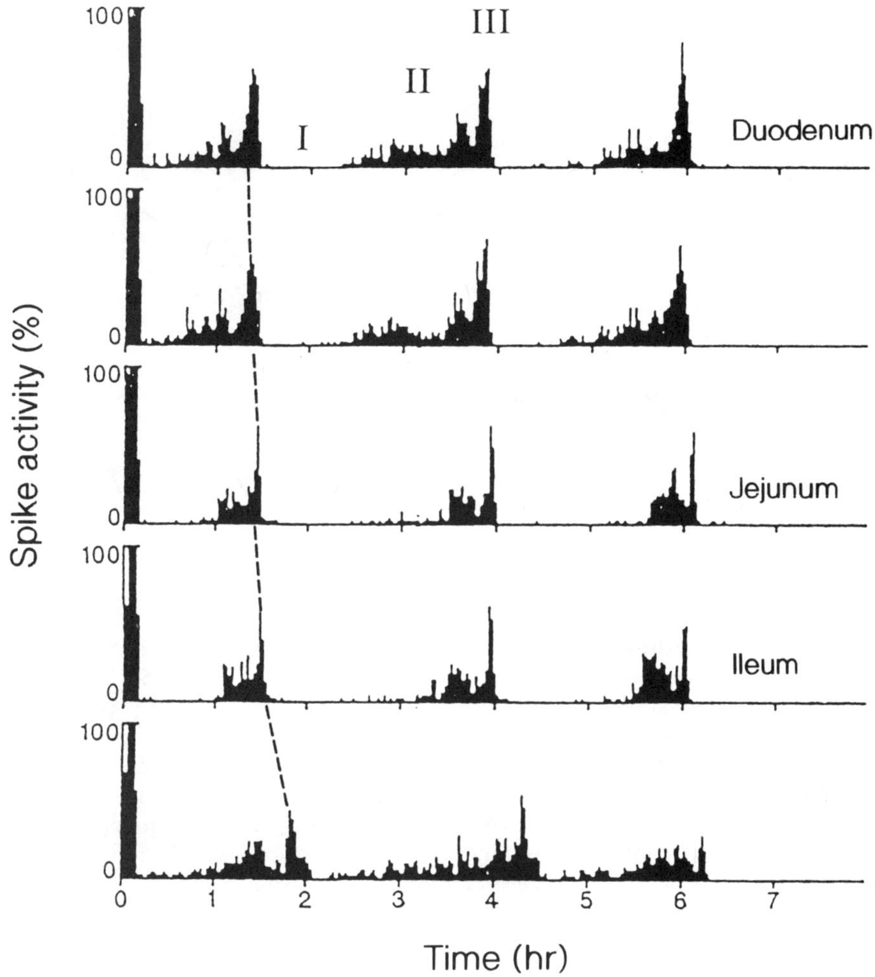

Figure 5.2 Migrating myoelectric complexes (MMC) in the canine small bowel as recorded by electrodes implanted at five sites on the duodenum, jejunum and ileum. The number of spikes have been normalized for each tracing. The first ten minutes are a calibration of 120 spikes per minute. I, II and III represent the phases of the MMC as defined above. Note that the speed of propagation is faster in the proximal bowel than distally, as indicated by the dashed line.

aborally slowly along the length of the small bowel to the distal ileum (see also Fig. 5.1). Because of the migratory nature of this type of activity it has been named the migrating motor complex, or MMC (reviewed in Wingate, 1981; Sarna, 1985). In fasted man, such complexes are observed to occur at intervals of approximately 90 minutes. This cyclical pattern of activity occurs during fasting and the arrival of food in the lumen of the intestine immediately disrupts the MMC pattern, which is then replaced by continuous contractile activity (Fig. 5.2).

In common with striated and cardiac muscle, contraction of gastro-intestinal smooth muscle is always preceded by an

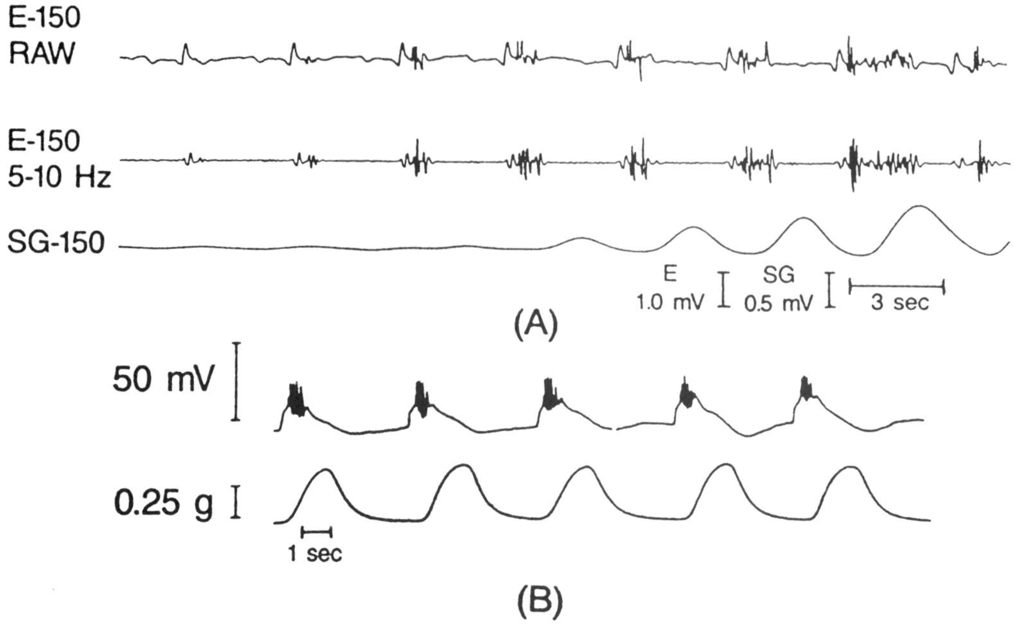

Figure 5.3 (A) *In vivo* recording of activity from an electrode (E) and strain gauge (SG) transducer implanted on small bowel serosa 150 cm from the pylorus (E-150 and SG-150 respectively). The top tracing is the raw EMG signal showing both the slow wave and accompanying spikes. Middle tracing: same signal with band pass filtering of 5–10 Hz to enhance the spike activity. The bottom tracing shows the corresponding movement of the bowel wall. Detectable movement of the gut occurs when a number of spikes accompany the slow wave. (B) *In vitro* recording showing the relationship between electrical (top trace) and contractile (bottom trace) activity. The slow wave sets the frequency of contraction and the spikes determine whether contraction occurs or not. (Reproduced with permission from Sarna and Otterson, *Gastroenterology Clinics of North America* 1989: 18, 305–375.)

electrical event. In the gut, each contraction is the result of the firing of 'spike' potentials, which can be recorded by serosal or mucosal electrodes and are therefore considered to be the myo-electrical correlates of contractile activity (Fig. 5.3). Contractions of the muscular coat of the bowel are only seen in association with spike potentials. Another type of electrical depolarization, the slow wave (also called pacesetter potential, basal electical rhythm [BER] or electrial control activity [ECA]), is also recorded in the stomach or intestine and is the result of constant and regular depolarizations (see also Fig. 5.3). The slow wave is not associated with contraction, although the rate of depolarization limits the rate at which contractions can occur at any site in the stomach or intestine. During the most intense phase of activity of the MMC (phase III), the viscus contracts at the maximum frequency for that particular site, as set by the slow wave. In humans, this rate is approximately three per minute in the stomach, and twelve per minute in the first part of the duodenum. In both the stomach and duodenum, the slow wave originates in a specialized pacesetter region but, unlike cardiac tissue, each slow wave is not accompanied by spikes and does not result in contraction.

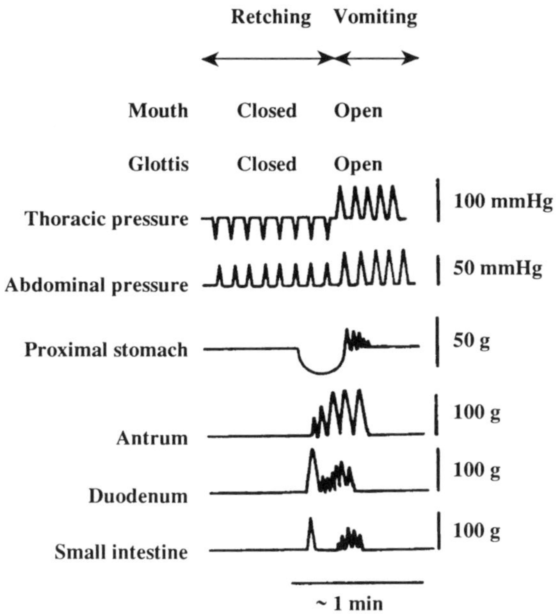

Figure 5.4 Schematic representation of the somatic and gastro-intestinal events occurring during retching and vomiting.

5.3 MOTILITY CHANGES OBSERVED IN THE GASTRO-INTESTINAL TRACT DURING EMESIS

It has been known for a number of years that during the emetic reflex respiratory and abdominal muscles play an important part in expulsion of gastro-intestinal contents (Gold and Hatcher, 1926; Miller, 1990). The characteristically powerful retching movements that occur prior to vomiting are a result of rhythmic contractions of the abdominal muscles. Synchronous with these abdominal muscle contractions, there are characteristic rhythmic contractions of the external intercostal muscles and diaphragm (Fig. 5.4). Throughout these movements the glottis is closed causing large negative changes in intrathoracic pressure and large positive changes in intra-abdominal pressure. In addition, there are accompanying autonomic and somatic events which include salivation, sweating (autonomic) and licking (somatic) which are the prodromata of vomiting. Characteristic gastro-intestinal motility events can be seen during this phase of the emetic reflex irrespective of the emetic stimulus.

Changes in gastro-intestinal motility which occur during nausea and vomiting were described as early as 1898 when Cannon used X-ray fluoroscopy in one of the first studies of stomach movements during vomiting. Subsequently, Alvarez described the reverse peristalsis that occurred in the intestine during the emetic act (Alvarez, 1917; Alvarez, 1925). However, the precise motor changes which occur along the length of the gastro-intestinal tract have only recently been quantified and described in any detail (Lang *et al.*, 1986). Since the development of equipment that allows recording at multiple points on the muscle or serosa of the bowel we know now that motility changes are not merely confined to the stomach and small intestine but that the motility patterns of the large intestine and gall bladder may also be altered during nausea and vomiting (Lang and Sarna, 1988). The section below synthesizes results from a number of studies in several species to present an overview of the changes which occur immediately prior to emesis.

5.3.1 MOTILITY CHANGES PRIOR TO EMESIS

Changes in gastric motility immediately prior to the act of vomiting have been most extensively studied and are seen initially as a relaxation of the proximal stomach (or abolition of electrical activity) (Abrahamsson *et al.*, 1973; De Ponti *et al.*, 1990). Lang and colleagues (1986) provided an excellent description of the gastro-intestinal motor correlates of vomiting in the dog using serosal strain gauges. Initially there is an inhibition of spontaneous motility in the proximal duodenum and jejunum and also an inhibition of motility in the very distal small intestine from where a single retrograde

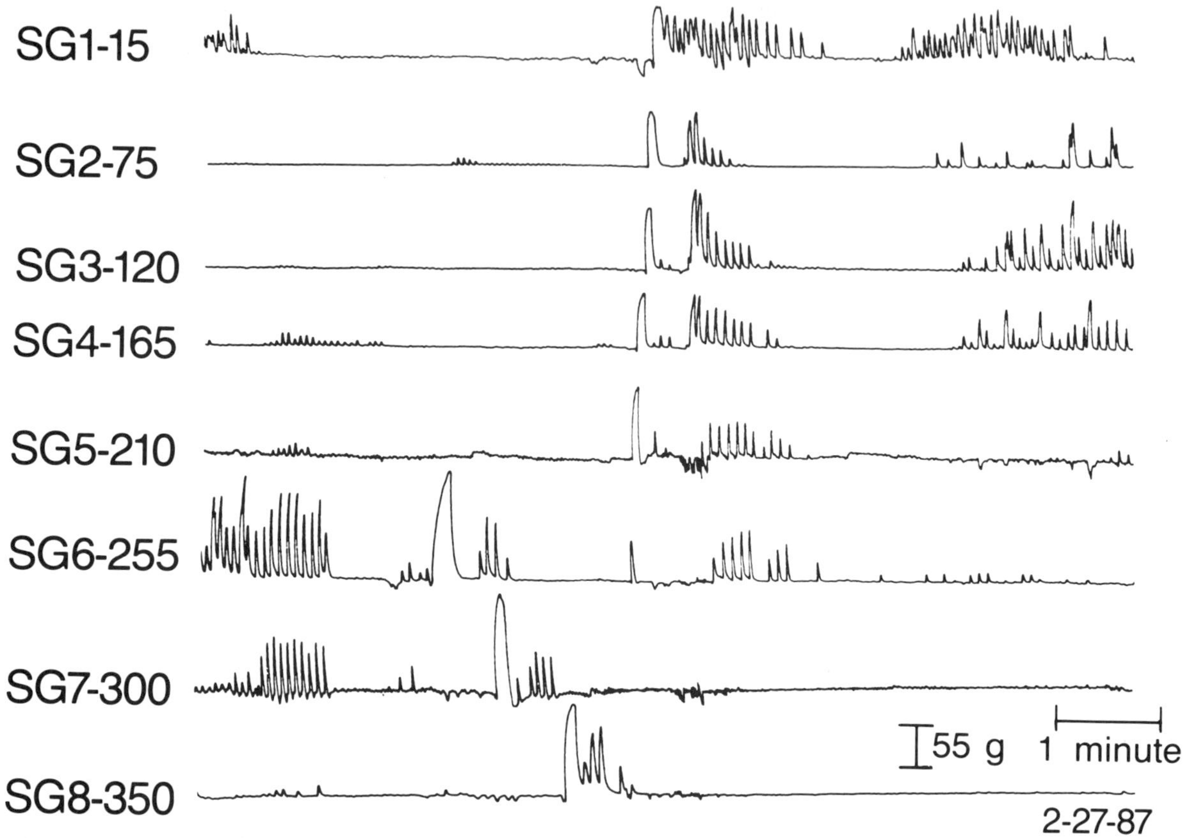

Figure 5.5 Canine intestinal contractile activity following X-radiation. A retrograde giant contraction (RGC) originating 255 cm from the pylorus (SG5) migrates orally to the duodenum. A giant migrating contraction (GMC) can also be seen originating at SG6 and passing anally. The numbers on the left-hand side indicate the distance (in cm) of the strain gauges (SG1-SG8) from the pylorus. (Reproduced with permission from Otterson *et al.*, 1988.)

giant contraction (RGC) is initiated, usually at a site in the distal jejunum (Fig. 5.5). This contraction travels proximally along the gastro-intestinal tract and appears most obvious and sustained in the duodenum.

Three features of the retroperistaltic wave are of particular interest. Firstly, the contraction is usually one to one and a half times the size of the contractions recorded in phase III of the MMC. Secondly, the rate of propagation from the origin to the duodenum is similar in different studies, with different stimuli and using either mechanical or electrical recording; in the dog the following values have been reported (mean ± se cm/sec) apomorphine 11.4 ± 0.4; spontaneous vomit 11.2 ± 1; dopamine 12.1 ± 1.3; copper sulphate 9.3 ± 1.0; gastric distension 7.8 ± 0.4 (Lang *et al.*, 1986; Lee *et al.*, 1985; Azpiroz and Malagelada, 1984). Other studies in the dog have reported lower values but the range of values were similar for the different stimuli used (Aizawa *et al.*, 1984). Interestingly, in the cat, the rate of propagation is slower, being between 2–3 cm/sec (Stewart *et al.*, 1977). Studies in which the rate of propagation was measured from the point of origin to the stomach show that the contraction travels more slowly over the duodenum and stomach than over the intestine – this contrasts with the aboral propagation of phase III of the MMC which is faster over the upper region of the gut than the lower. This observation would imply that the velocity of propagation of the contraction is not only a property of the muscle in the different regions but depends upon the way in which the muscle is activated. Finally, the region of the intestine from which the retroperistaltic contraction originates is remarkably consistent with different emetic stimuli at least in the dog: spontaneous vomiting 168 ± 22 cm apomorphine 170 ± 20 – 182 ± 18 cm from the pylorus; intestinal obstruction and intra–gastric copper sulphate 170 cm distal to the ligament of Treitz (Aizawa *et al.*, 1984; Lang *et al.*, 1986). These observations indicate that this region is somehow specialized in its musculature or innervation and this is supported by studies demonstrating that it is over this jejuno–ileal junctional region that the phase III of the MMC considerably decreases its rate of aboral propagation (Code and Marlett, 1975).

Following the oral propagation of the RGC, a burst of phasic contractions occurs which is seen along the length of the small bowel. When the RGC reaches the stomach both corpus (proximal stomach) and antrum (distal stomach) regions respond with a burst of high frequency contractions. The lower oesophagus accommodates gastric contents prior to ejection by dilating and almost acting as a funnel to provide a more efficient emptying of gastric contents (Smith and Brizzee, 1961).

5.3.2 MOTILITY AFTER EJECTION OF GASTRIC CONTENTS

Immediately following ejection of vomitus from the mouth a series of simultaneous non-propagating phasic contractions occurs in the stomach and duodenum which have been described as being 'phase III-like'. In the upper small intestine at the level of the jejunum there is a period of inhibition where no contractile activity is recorded and this lasts for approximately one minute (Lang and Sarna, 1989). In the small intestine at the level of the lower jejunum there is no cessation of contractile activity but instead a continuous series of phasic contractions is observed.

Some studies recording the electrical activity of the gut muscle have reported a prolonged (30 min) period of reduction of slow wave frequency following emesis (Akwari, 1983; Stewart, 1983). The time taken for gastro-intestinal motility and associated functions to return to normal after emesis has not been studied in detail. It is likely that with only a few minutes separating episodes of retching, and stimuli inducing emesis lasting several hours, normal motility may not be restored until prolonged periods have elapsed. One question pertinent to this relates to the 'reset time' of the motility correlates of emesis: that is, is the entire motor pattern repeated prior to each burst of retching and vomiting in a series or does it only occur with the first bout? In the cat, Stewart and Stewart *et al.* (1977; 1983), using electrical recording of muscle activity, reported that the full intestinal response was only observed prior to the first one or two episodes of vomiting prior to the first one or two episodes of vomiting in a series, although the electrical activity was disorganized prior to subsequent episodes. In these studies, the inter-episode interval required for repetition of the complete gut motor pattern was not investigated.

5.4 MECHANISMS OF GASTRO-INTESTINAL CHANGES OCCURRING DURING EMESIS

The pathways which can initiate the gastro-intestinal motor changes during vomiting can be activated by a number of substances. The activation of this motor system is produced by both cytotoxic drugs (cisplatinum), which induce emesis, and by cholecystokinin octapeptide (CCK-8) which, acting at a site within the gut wall, evokes a motility pattern almost identical to that in emesis but without evoking emesis (Lang and Marvig, 1989; Lang, 1990). In the section below the pharmacology of the motor correlates of vomiting induced by substances other than irradiation and cytotoxic drugs will also be discussed in order to provide a more comprehensive insight into mechanisms.

5.4.1 GASTRIC RELAXATION

As well as being one of the prodromata of vomiting, the phenomenon of gastric relaxation performs the physiological function of receptive relaxation during gastric filling following a meal. The control of this reflex is vagal and mediated via an inhibitory non-adrenergic, non-cholinergic (NANC) transmitter proposed to be vasoactive intestinal peptides (VIP) in vomiting carnivores such as the ferret (Andrews and Lawes, 1985). A similar mechanism is probably involved in the relaxation of the lower oesophagus seen by Smith and Brizzee (1961) prior to emesis in the cat, although the transmitter involved may not be the same.

5.4.2 SUPPRESSION OF GASTRO-INTESTINAL ELECTRICAL ACTIVITY

Both slow wave and spiking activity are reduced in the stomach and the majority of the small intestine in the pre-ejection and possibly in the early post-ejection phase of emesis (Akwari, 1983; Stewart *et al.*, 1977). The most likely candidate for this effect is once again vagal activation of NANC inhibitory neurons to the gut. In the presence of atropine, guanethidine and/or adrenergic receptor antagonists, vagal efferent stimulation either produces a relaxation or an inhibition of rhythmic contractile activity in the gastric antrum, duodenum, and small intestine of the ferret (unpublished observations). Recordings of gastric slow wave activity (ECA) in the cat reveal that the frequency can be reduced from four cycles/min to one cycle/min by vagal activation of the NANC neurons (Abrahamsson, 1986).

While the vagus could be responsible for the production of the observed activity described above, extensive direct evidence is lacking and attention has focused on paracrine or endocrine agents. In the dog, bradygastria (reduction in frequency of electrical activity) can be induced by close intra-arterial injection of adrenaline, met-enkephalin, prostaglandin E_2 and glucagon (Kim *et al.*, 1986); the latter can also produce bradygastria in man (Abell and Malagelada, 1985). The effect of adrenaline can be blocked by phentolamine and that of met-enkephalin by naloxone (Kim *et al.*, 1986). Additionally, the response to both agents was blocked by indomethacin which led to the conclusion that a prostaglandin was the final mediator of the response. The effect of glucagon was not blocked by these treatments. These observations are of particular interest in radiation-induced vomiting where increases in plasma immunoreactive β-endorphin and gastric juice (but not plasma) PGE_2 have been demonstrated to occur (Dorval *et al.*, 1985; Dubois *et al.*, 1987).

At present it is not possible to make a definitive statement about the mechanism of suppression of gut electrical activity in the pre- and post-ejection phases; however, the vagus could produce the effects via the NANC inhibitory neurons possibly using enkephalin as a neurotransmitter or even by the systemic release of glucagon from the pancreas. Additionally, the sympathetic system could be involved either directly or indirectly by the release of adrenaline from the adrenal medulla. When one considers that the inhibition of activity is rapid in onset, appears simultaneously in several gut regions and is *immediately* followed by a period of intense activity, it is more probable that it is neurally mediated whereas the delayed return of normal activity in the post-ejection phase may be humorally mediated. These aspects of the response require considerably more investigation.

5.4.3 INTESTINAL RETROPERISTALSIS

Studies in the dog have demonstrated that the retroperistaltic giant contraction (RGC) is not observed in vagotomized dogs, providing a clear indication for an involvement of the vagus (Lang *et al.*, 1986). Further pharmacological studies failed to block the response with either α or β adrenergic receptor antagonists (phentolamine, propranolol) and opiate (naloxone) or dopamine (domperidone, phenoxybenzamine) receptor antagonists (Miolan *et al.*, 1984). Using strain gauge recording (Lang *et al.*, 1986) showed that the single large retroperistaltic contraction was abolished by atropine methyl nitrate (100 μg/kg i.v.) and this, taken together with the above observations, implicates the vagal efferent activation of intramural cholinergic neurons in a number of gut regions in the production of the retro-peristaltic response. The intestine is usually functionally polarized to ensure that the peristaltic contractions produced by cholinergic and serotonergic intramural neurons propagate aborally but clearly the extrinsic nerves can somehow override this mechanism, probably by a combination of suppression of ongoing pacemaker activity and sequential activation of the vagal efferent fibres supplying successive intestinal regions (Lang and Sarna, 1989; Grundy, Andrews and Blackshaw, 1991).

Although the RGC is blocked by atropine, the post RGC phasic contractions are still present. As these are abolished by vagotomy, it is likely that they are produced by vagal activation of intramural NANC excitatory neurons. This hypothesis is supported by the observation that hexamethonium blocks all the motor correlates in the small bowel. However, some resistant component exists in the stomach. The nature of the transmitter is not known but 5-HT has been implicated in the duodenum of the dog (Miolan *et al.*, 1984); in addition, in the antrum of the ferret 5-HT can to some extent mimic the response to vagal activation of the NANC intramural neurons (Bingham, personal communication).

With the recent development of 5-HT_3 receptor antagonists as effective anti-emetics against cytotoxic drug-induced emesis in both animals and man (Chapter 9) it would be of interest to see the effect of these agents on the gastro-intestinal motor correlates of vomiting. Administered alone, this class of agents appears to have little effect on normal stomach or small bowel myoelectric activity in the dog (Davidson, Pilot and Thompson, 1990). However, this may not be the case following an emetic stimulus.

5.4.4 GIANT MIGRATING CONTRACTION (GMC)

The giant migrating contraction (GMC – not to be confused with the RGC, section 5.4.3) is an anally migrating single contraction which may be a feature of normal small and large bowel motility and occurs spontaneously. However, it is more prevalent following noxious stimuli such as vinegar instillation in to the stomach (Sarna, 1987). Although the spontaneous and initiated GMCs appear to be identical, those induced by noxious stimuli originate at more proximal sites in the intestine (Lang and Marvig, 1989). The incidence of this powerful caudally migrating contraction can be increased following emetic stimuli like radiation (Fig. 5.5, above) (Otterson *et al.*, 1988) when compared to the RGC (10 cm/sec). The propagation rate of these contractions is slow (60 cm/min) (Sarna, 1989). They are extremely efficient in propelling gastro-intestinal contents caudally and because of their strength and high incidence during fractionated doses of irradiation (Otterson *et al.* 1988) and during cramping in irritable bowel patients (Kellow and Philips, 1987), are believed to be causative of abdominal pain and radiation-associated diarrhoea. As yet, the pharmacological characteristics of this phenomenon have not been investigated. It is possible that 5-HT_3 receptors may be involved as antagonists can induce mild constipation in animals and man (Sanger *et al.*, 1991) and reduce the incidence of de-faecation following radiation in the ferret (Andrews *et al.*, unpublished observations).

5.5 THE FUNCTIONS OF THE MOTILITY CHANGES IN EMESIS

Vagotomy abolishes the gastric relaxation and retroperistalsis (RGC) preceding vomiting but not the ejection event. Since the emetic reflex does not require the motor correlates it can be deduced that the changes in motility are not responsible for triggering emesis. Hence the phenomena of vomiting and motor changes are not universally linked. Nevertheless these changes appear to be present and to form an integral part of the reflex so what is their function?

Some invertebrates and non-mammalian species (e.g. starfish, dogfish and frogs) expel unwanted material uniquely by retroperistalsis (Hatcher, 1924). In these animals this may well be the only way of expelling gut contents. The force required to expel gastric contents in these animals can easily be provided by gastric contractions alone. The 'vestigial' patterns of activity may well remain as adjuvants to the more powerful mammalian striated muscles used in the process of vomiting.

In man, in the normal course of digestion, retroperistalsis does occur, but over much shorter segments of bowel, and it is associated with the mixing of food and intestinal secretions. In vomiting, the initial gastric relaxation and reduction in emptying will prevent any form of transit from the stomach into the small bowel. Among other gastro-intestinal changes in motility, there is a single retroperistaltic wave (RGC) which begins very low down the intestine in the distal jejunum or even lower in the proximal ileum. This contraction is very powerful and tends to occlude the lumen of the gut. This pattern of activity would suggest that all gastro-intestinal contents would be swept back into the stomach for expulsion. This would seem sensible for upper gastro-intestinal contents but rather illogical for gut contents in the lower jejunum and ileum as arguably it would be more efficient to increase transit and expel them anally, a phenomenon that might require emesis and diarrhoea to occur simultaneously. The RGC provides a rapid and efficient emptying of the small intestine and oral propagation of the intestinal contents into the stomach. The GMC is equally efficient in producing an anally moving flow of contents of the large bowel. The migration of this contraction is up to ten times slower than RGC. It is recognized that the RGC is the motor correlate of vomiting in that it precedes expulsion and efficiently empties the small intestine. The GMC is perhaps the motor correlate of radiation-induced diarrhoea and associated abdominal cramping. The different time courses of the propagation of the RGC and GMC may ensure that the most recently ingested contents are expelled first by vomiting and the contents further down the gut are expelled later, in bouts of diarrhoea caused by increased incidence of GMCs and of the contents being continually propelled to the proximal colon. This guards against vomiting and diarrhoea occurring simultaneously.

Nevertheless, the gastro-intestinal correlates of vomiting are also produced when a centrally acting stimulus is administered. This appears to render the gastro-intestinal motor correlates redundant (and incidentally the somatic components as well) as the toxin has already reached the bloodstream. Although the gastro-intestinal motility disturbances which occur during vomiting appear logical, they are nevertheless not critical for expulsion of vomitus and unless they remain merely as phylogenically redundant motility patterns, their function remains uncertain.

5.6 MOTILITY CHANGES IN THE GASTRO-INTESTINAL TRACT ASSOCIATED WITH NAUSEA

Studies using provocative stimulation of the gut either with distention or luminal chemicals leave little doubt that appropriate activation of gut afferents can evoke the sensation of nausea, although this may be contributed to by the release of endogenous agents from the gut or absorbed toxins both acting on the area postrema. However, the major issue is whether the gut motor patterns observed prior to emesis are responsible for, or contribute in any way to, the genesis of nausea. It is most probable that primarily they only represent components of the motor response which readies the gut for the expulsive act of vomiting (section 5.3). Whether a toxin is acting at the level of the gut or the area postrema, the body can take no protective action until it is recognized as hazardous. The detectors (gut afferents or area postrema; see Chapter 7) that recognize it as a hazard can activate the central pathways believed to be involved in nausea. It might be argued that as the main initial function of nausea is to inhibit further ingestion and that this should be the first action taken after recognition of a hazard. The motor patterns seen in the gut are themselves produced as a reflex consequence of activation of these detectors.

Is there any direct evidence that the motor patterns observed prior to emesis can induce a sensation of nausea? Proximal gastric relaxation occurs as part of normal digestion without producing nausea, although this does tend to occur slowly as the stomach fills rather than rapidly as probably occurs prior to vomiting. In man, a decrease in gastric motility was observed by Wolf (1965) using stimuli such as caloric vestibular stimulation or motion (swinging) but the motor changes occurred both with and without nausea being induced.

The duodenal contraction which occurs immediately prior to vomiting is one of the more obvious changes from normal motility and as such was one of the first motor correlates of emesis to be described in any detail (Ingelfinger and Moss, 1942; Abbot *et al.*, 1952). In studies where duodenal contraction was found to occur with a number of different nauseogenic stimuli, namely caloric vestibular stimulation (irrigation of the inner ear), oral administration of ipecacuanha and other noxious stimuli such as cold stress, the motility effects observed were not always associated with concomitant nausea. Likewise, when nausea was present a sustained duodenal contraction was not always observed. These studies provided the first pieces of evidence to suggest that nausea and changes in gastrointestinal motility do not necessarily have a cause and effect relationship. In addition, retroperistalsis of the small intestine tends to occur as a discrete event just prior to retching and vomiting and it is difficult to see how this in isolation could account for nausea of lasting duration.

Antral tachygastria on the other hand appears a more likely candidate as it is a more continuous event and, because of its association with disordered antral motor function, it could produce sustained abnormal visceral afferent discharge patterns. There is limited evidence for a relationship between the degree of tachygastria and symptom intensity, although the relationship between onset of tachygastria (3–12 min with illusory self motion) and onset of symptoms (1–8 min) has been found to be poor (Stern *et al.*, 1987). Although this may appear to be a possible case of cause and effect, one might expect the intensity of visceral changes to reflect the degree of stimulation, as it is the stimulus that is driving both responses. Would a similar correlation be found for other events associated with nausea such as salivation or skin blood flow? A study of salivary secretion during seasickness has shown that in contrast to the expected effect there was a decrease in spontaneous and evoked secretion. This decrease was significantly correlated with the intensity of the sickness (Gordon *et al.*, 1989).

From the above arguments it appears unlikely that the gastro-intestinal motor events seen prior to retching or vomiting are the main source of the sensation of nausea, although during the period that these events occur they may well reinforce the sensation, possibly contributing to the 'wave-like' nature of the nausea and the increase in intensity, a phenomenon which is often described as vomiting becomes imminent.

5.7 GASTRO-INTESTINAL MOTILITY EFFECTS OF CHEMOTHERAPEUTIC AGENTS AND X-RADIATION

The section that follows deals with the general motility effects of cytotoxic drugs and X-radiation and reviews some of the motility changes which occur in the time domain outside the immediate events associated with emesis. Those changes seen may be due to direct effects of these stimuli on the gut or as a reflex consequence of activation of the emetic mechanism. The clinical impact of these events is also discussed.

5.7.1 EFFECT OF X-RADIATION

Radiation has wide-ranging effects on the gastro-intestinal tract: these include increased mucosal permeability, complex changes in blood flow, reduction in gastric secretion and emptying, increased mucus secretion in the lower bowel and reduction in cell division (reviewed in Dubois and Walker, 1988). The magnitude and extent of the effects depend upon the species, the dose and type of radiation, the site exposed, and the time after exposure that function is studied. In general, total body exposure to ionizing radiation at low doses (1.5 Gy) induces nausea, vomiting and reduced gastric function. At doses above 6 Gy the above, prodromal syndrome is more intense and is followed 2–5 days later by a sub-acute syndrome with diarrhoea and haematochezia superimposed upon the characteristic myelosuppression. If untreated, death may ensue due to anaemia, infection and dehydration (Dubois and Walker, 1988). This section focuses on the motility effects of radiation, although they will be influenced by the functional and later structural changes induced by the radiation.

One of the earliest studies on the effects of radiation on intestinal motility was that performed by Swann (1924), and like many of his successors he showed that exposure to X-rays caused an increase in tone of the intestine. He suggested that the mechanism responsible could be a sensitization of the autonomic nerves supplying the gut, an interesting conclusion in the light of more recent evidence suggesting a similar mechanism for induction of emesis (Andrews *et al.*, 1988). In addition to increases in tone, increases in spontaneous contraction amplitude following irradiation have been reported (Quastel, 1968) with corresponding decreases in sensitivity to 5-HT. Although more recent studies have reported an increased sensitivity to both 5-HT and acetylcholine (Gisanrin *et al.* , 1992). The latter observation is of considerable interest as it indicates that radiation may modify 5-HT receptor mechanisms in the gut, a fact that is of particular relevance because of the use of 5-HT_3 receptor antagonists as anti-emetics in radiotherapy patients. Jejunal segments of rat intestine showed similar results with respect to contraction amplitude but at very high doses of exposure (1500 rads) (Kagnoff, 1970).

More recent studies have been performed in other animals possessed of a vomiting reflex and, with multiple site recordings, changes in gastro-intestinal motility have been easier to observe. Summers *et al.* (1987) studied myoelectric activity of the proximal jejunum in conscious dogs following exposure to 938 cGy total body irradiation. In fasted animals the normal regular cyclic activity, described as the migrating myoelectric complex, was interrupted and replaced by an irregular pattern consisting of spike bursts which propagated in either direction, suggesting the initiation of contractile events which propagate in both an oral and aboral direction. This description of intestinal electrical changes after irradiation contrasts with a more recent report where irradiation of conscious dogs fitted with serosal strain gauge transducers using fractionated doses of X-rays (250 cGy, 3 times/wk for 3 wks) produced rather more subtle changes in intestinal motility (Otterson *et al.*, 1988). Normal cyclical activity recorded during fasting showed the presence of the migrating motor complex and only occasional giant caudally migrating contractions (GMCs). However, after irradiation began, a significant increase in giant migrating contractions was observed which originated from a site more proximal in the intestine than spontaneous GMCs (spontaneous 55 ± 16 cm from ileocolonic junction; radiation-induced 158 ± 7 cm). These giant migrating contractions were associated with episodes of vomiting with a highly significant correlation (Fig. 5.5, above), although, functionally, the GMC itself has a role in defaecation (Sarna, 1987).

Migrating motor complexes (MMC) showed a decrease in migration time after radiation and the pattern of the high frequency contractile phase (phase III) itself was changed to fused contractions rather than the discrete contractions seen normally. Postprandial disruption of the cycle also appeared to be increased after irradiation, that is the normal irregular contractile activity seen throughout the bowel shortly after feeding was increased in duration.

5.7.2 GASTRO-INTESTINAL MOTILITY EFFECTS OF CHEMOTHERAPEUTIC AGENTS

One of the first detailed descriptions of gastro-intestinal motility changes associated with cytotoxic drug administration was that of Akwari (1983). In this report he detailed the changes in gastro-intestinal myoelectric activity in dogs given emetic doses of cisplatin and suggested that the expulsion of vomitus could be predicted from the changes observed. It must be emphasized that this study recorded the electrical correlates of motility and not motility itself. In a more recent study by Chey *et al.* (1988), cisplatin administered to dogs produced abnormal gastro-intestinal motility in the form of orally migrating bursts of spiking activity which were shown to be highly correlated with the emetic episodes induced by this cytotoxic drug. This study showed changes in myoelectric activity recorded from serosal implanted eletrodes which were similar to those described earlier. However, in addition, motility changes occurred which were not just confined to the emetic episodes. Abnormal spike bursts in the duodenum and jejunum and oral migration of spike bursts also occurred which were not followed by emesis.

In addition to cytotoxic chemotherapeutic agents, some drugs used for antimicrobial chemotherapy such as erythromycin produce similar side effects (Klika and Goodman, 1982). Here, both gastric and intestinal motility changes have been described in man (Zara *et al.*, 1991). Within minutes of the start of an intravenous infusion there was an increase in the frequency and amplitude of gastric contractions, whereas the small bowel appear to be inhibited, although in some cases there was a transient increase in contraction frequency for approximately 15 minutes. A retroperistaltic wave was sometimes seen, accompanied by a feeling of nausea (Fig. 5.6).

In studies using the ferret (an animal which has become increasingly used as a model for the study of emesis and the efficacy of anti-emetics) cisplatin causes immediate changes in gastro-intestinal motility. Post-

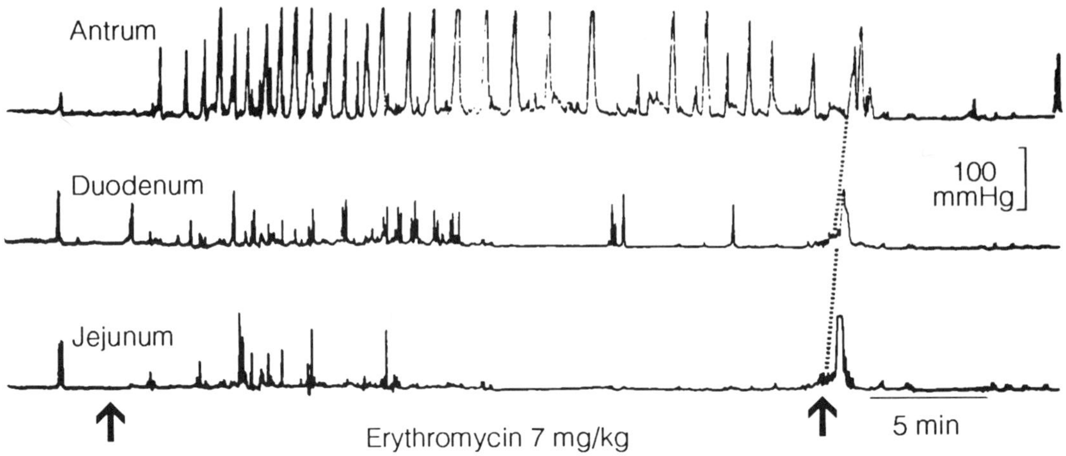

Figure 5.6 Retroperistaltic contraction in human GI tract induced by erythromycin (EM). EM (7 mg/kg) was given for 30 mins (shown by the arrows). During the infusion high amplitude contractions occurred in the stomach while the small bowel appeared to be quiescent. The retroperistalsis occurring at the end of the EM infusion was accompanied by nausea.

administration there is an increase in gastric body tone and antral and duodenal contractions which is not associated with the emetic reflex and is unaffected by pretreatment with ondansetron (proprietary name Zofran Davidson and Andrews, 1988). In addition, the motility is not dependent upon a vagal innervation (Fig. 5.7). This study suggests that cisplatin may have direct effects on enteric neurons, a conclusion supported by the studies of Racke and Schwörer (1991) on the guinea-pig duodenum.

5.7.3 WHAT ARE THE FUNCTIONAL IMPLICATIONS OF THESE MOTOR CHANGES?

Changes in motility alone suggest that alterations in gastric and intestinal function should occur following exposure to irradiation. Tests performed to assess gastric function following exposure to X-rays or cytotoxic drugs have mainly consisted of measurements of gastric emptying. Many reports have indicated a prolonged suppression in gastric emptying following irradiation or administration of cisplatinum in species which are able to vomit, e.g. monkey and dog (Dubois *et al.*, 1984; Dorval *et al.*, 1985) and those which do not have the reflex, e.g. the rat (Goodman *et al.*, 1951; Roos, Fairlie and Whitehouse, 1981; Eeckhout, 1990). It appears that the delay in gastric emptying is more pronounced when it is the abdomen itself which is exposed to irradiation (Hulse, 1966).

The effects of irradiation on small intestinal transit appear to be less pronounced than on gastric emptying. Jones and Kimeldorf (1959) and Goodman *et al.* (1951) both reported no change in pylorus to ileocecum transit time following X-radiation. One reported functional change, occurring after both irradiation and chemotherapy in man and animals, is the production of diarrhoea (Summers *et al.*, 1987; Otterson, Sarna and Moulder, 1988). In normal bowel motility it is the GMC which is believed to give rise to mass movement of colonic contents and may be involved to some extent in the process of defecation (Sarna, 1989). In animal studies the increased incidence of GMCs following exposure to ionizing

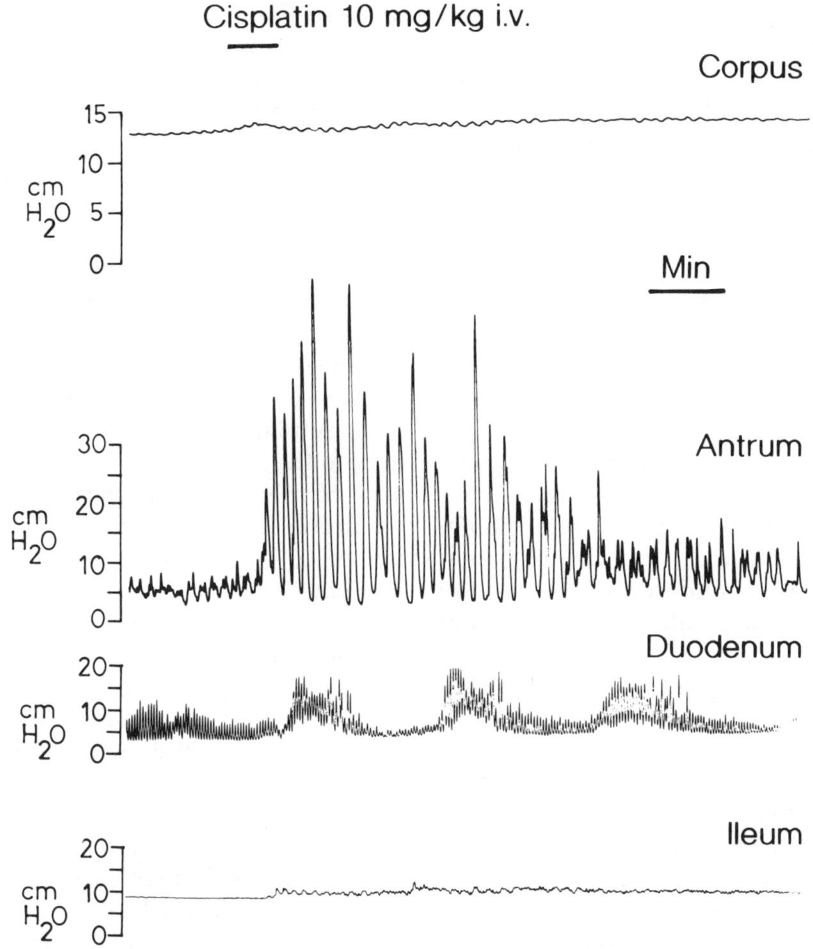

Figure 5.7 Effect of cisplatin on the gastro-intestinal contractile activity in the anaesthetized ferret. An immediate contractile response is recorded on intravenous administration of cisplatin (10 mg/kg) in the antrum and duodenum and in the proximal stomach an increase in tone occurs. This motor change does not correspond with any retching or vomiting in the animal. (Davidson and Andrews unpublished observations.)

radiation is also associated with episodes of diarrhoea (Otterson, Sarna and Moulder, 1988). The diarrhoea associated with anti-cancer therapy may therefore be a result of a selective acceleration of certain motility patterns in the lower gastro-intestinal tract.

In studies assessing the gastro-intestinal toxicity of radiation and cytotoxic administration it is evident that severe morphological changes occur in the mucosa of the intestines and these result in necrosis (Summers *et al.*, 1987) and/or haemorrhagic enterocolitis (Schaeppi *et al.*, 1973). The resultant diarrhoea is a consequence of the associated fluid and electrolyte loss that occurs when the mucosa becomes necrotic. The degree of damage to the intestine and severity of diarrhoea are related to the dose of radiation to which the animal is exposed. Dubois and Walker (1988) noted that diarrhoea appeared in dogs exposed to radiation above 6 Gy and that lower doses produced vomiting and nausea only (Chapter 8). It is apparent from these studies that diarrhoea accompanying vomiting is one of the functional changes which occurs following higher doses of radiation and may not be as common and severe in patients receiving therapeutic fractionated doses of radiation.

5.8 ARE MOTILITY CHANGES A FUNCTIONAL PART OF EMESIS?

The motor correlates of vomiting can be activated by both peripherally acting (copper sulphate) and centrally acting (apomorphine) emetic stimuli and although the proximal stomach relaxation and funnelling of the oesophagus may promote a more efficient expulsion of contents, the ejection phase of the reflex does not require the gastro-intestinal motor correlates of vomiting. This was first shown nearly 200 years ago when Magendie substituted a pig's bladder for a dog's stomach and found that it was still able to vomit (Magendie, 1824). This conclusion (confirmed in more recent studies discussed above) is further supported by experiments in the dog where administration of the α_2 receptor agonist clonidine prevents all excitatory myoelectric changes in the gut but the expulsive phase of vomiting is still evoked by its central action (Pilot *et al.*, 1986). These studies show that virtual total inhibition of gut motility will not prevent emesis. However, might it be possible to pharmacologically manipulate the gastro-intestinal disturbances associated with emesis, such as gastric stasis and retropulsion of intestinal contents, to prevent the emetic act? Some early studies claim that the effective reduction of emesis by metoclopramide in dogs given cisplatinum was due to the gastrokinetic action of increasing gastric emptying and co-ordinating the disordered motility (Alphin *et al.*, 1986). Subsequent studies revealed that metoclopramide and dazopride (both substituted benzamides) were 5-HT M-receptor (5-HT_3) antagonists (Costall *et al.*, 1987). With the advent of more specific 5-HT_3 receptor antagonists such as MDL 72222 the anti-emetic action of these compounds was attributed to blockade of neuronal 5-HT_3 receptors and not to effects on motility (Miner and Sanger, 1986). The antagonism of 5-HT_3 receptors has provided the basis for the development of highly potent anti-emetics which produce their anti-emetic action other than by prokinesis. It can be said, therefore, that it is the stimulation of specific receptors which initiate the reflex, probably on the vagal sensory terminals in the gastro-intestinal tract (Andrews and Davidson, 1990) and it is antagonism of these receptors which produces anti-emetic action and not a correction of the already initiated motor changes in the gut.

From the above brief discussion it is clear that blockade (pharmacological or surgical) of the gastro-intestinal motility changes such as gastric relaxation and intestinal retroperistalsis will not prevent the expulsive phase of emesis. However, when delayed gastric emptying is a *cause* of the emesis (e.g. in diabetes; Feldman and Smith, 1987) then prokinetic drugs that are able to overcome this delay (e.g. cisapride; Wulsche and Ehrlein, 1986) may be of benefit.

REFERENCES

Abbot, F.K., Mack, M. and Wolf, S. (1952) The relation of sustained contraction in the duodenum to nausea and vomiting. *Gastroenterology*, **20**, 238–48.

Abell, T.L. and Malagelada, J.R. (1985) Glucagon evoked dysrhythmias in humans shown by an improved electrogastrographic technique. *Gastroenterology*, **88**, 1932–40.

Abrahamsson, H., Jansson, G. and Martinson, J. (1973) Vagal relaxation of the stomach induced by apomorphine in the cat. *Acta Phys. Scand.*, **88**, 296–302.

Abrahamsson, H. (1986) Non-adrenergic non-cholinergic nervous control of gastrointestinal motility patterns. *Arch. Int. Pharmacodyn.*, **280**, Suppl., 50–61.

Aizawa, I., Negishi, K., Suzuki, T. and Itoh, Z. (1984) 'Gastrointestinal contractile activity associated with vomiting in the dog', in *Gastrointestinal Motility*, pp. 159–65 (ed C. Roman). MTP, Lancaster.

Akwari, O. (1983) The gastrointestinal tract in chemotherapy induced emesis, A final common pathway. *Drugs*, **25** (Suppl 1), 18–34.

Alphin, R.S., Proakis, A.G., Leonard C.A., Smith, W.L. *et al.* (1986) Antagonism of cisplatin-induced emesis by metoclopramide and dazopride through enhancement of gastric motility. *Dig. Dis. Sci.*, **31**, 525–29.

Alvarez, W.C. (1917) The syndrome of mild reverse peristalsis. *JAMA*, **69**, 2018–25.

Alvarez, W.C. (1925). Reverse peristalsis in the bowel: a precursor of vomiting. *JAMA*, **85**, 1051–55.

Andrews P.L.R. and Davidson, H.I.M. (1990) Activation of vagal afferent terminals by 5-hydroxytryptamine is mediated by 5-HT_3 receptors in the anaesthetized ferret. *J. Physiol.*, **422**, 920.

Andrews, P.L.R., Rapeport, W.G. and Sanger, G.J. (1988) Neuropharmacology of Emesis Induced by Anti-Cancer Therapy. *Trends Pharmacol. Sci.*, **9**, 334–341.

Davidson, H.I.M. and Andrews, P.L.R. (1988) Immediate stimulation of gastrointestinal motility by emetic doses of cisplatin in the ferret. Nausea and vomiting: A multidisciplinary perspective, symposium procedings, p. 28. Ottawa, Canada.

De Ponti, F., Malagelada, J.R., Azpiroz, F. *et al.*, (1990) Variations in gastric tone associated with duodenal motor events after activation of central emetic mechanisms in the dog. *J. Gastrointest. Motil.*, **2**, 1–11.

Dorval, E., Meuller, G.P., Eng, R. *et al.* (1985) 'Involvement of endogenous opiates in radiation-induced suppression of gastric emptying', in *Gastrointestinal Motility*, pp. 237–42 (ed C. Roman) MTP, Lancaster.

Dorval, E.D., Mueller, G.P., Eng, R.R. *et al.* (1985) Effect of ionizing radiation on gastric secretion and gastric motility in monkeys. *Gastroenterology*, **89**, 374–80.

Dubois, A., Jacobus, J.P., Grissom, M.P. *et al.* (1984) Altered gastric emptying and prevention of radiation induced vomiting in dogs. *Gastroenterology*, **86**, 444–48.

Dubois, A., Dorval, E.D., Steel, L. *et al.* (1987) Effect of ionizing radiation on prostaglandins and gastric secretion in rhesus monkeys. *Rad. Res.*, **110**, 289–93.

Dubois, A. and Walker, R.I. (1988) Prospects for management of gastrointestinal injury associated with the acute radiation syndrome. *Gastroenterology*, **95**, 500–7.

Eeckhout, C. (1990) Effects of prokinetics with different mechanisms of action on cisplatin induced slowing of gastric emptying in the rat. *J. Gastroent. Motil.*, **1**, 52.

Feldman, M. and Smith, H.J. (1987) Effect of cisapride on gastric emptying of indigestible solids in patients with gastroparesis diabeticorum. *Gastroenterology*, **92**, 171–74.

Gisanrin, O., Headford, S. and Marr, H. (1992) The effects of X-irradiation on the sensitivity of guinea-pig isolated ileum to 5-hydroxytryptamine and acetylcholine mediated responses, pp. 171–172. In mechanisms and control of emesis. (Eds A.L. Bianchi, L. Grélot, A.D. Miller, G.L. King) colloque inserm, J. Libbey Eurotext, 223.

Gold, H. and Hatcher, R.A. (1926) Studies on vomiting. *J. Pharmacol. Exper. Ther.*, **28**, 209–18.

Goodman, R.D., Lewis, A.E. and Schuck, E.A. (1952). Effects of X-irradiation on gastrointestinal transit and absorption availability. *Rad. Res.*, **169**, 242–47.

Gordon, C.R., Ben-Aryeh, H., Szargel, R. *et al.* (1989) Salivary changes associated with seasickness. *J. Auton. Nerv. Syst.*, **26**, 37–42.

Grundy, D., Andrews, P.L.R. and Blackshaw, A. (1991) 'Neural correlates of the gastrointestinal motor changes in emesis', in *Brain–gut Interactions* (eds Tache and D. Wingate) pp. 325–38 CRC Press, Boca Raton, USA.

Hatcher, R.A. (1924) The mechanism of vomiting. *Phys. Rev.*, **4**, 479–504.

Hulse, E.V. (1966) Gastric emptying in rats after part-body irradiation. *Int. J. Rad. Biol.*, **10** (6), 521–32.

Ingelfinger, F. and Moss, R.E. (1942) The activity of the descending duodenum during nausea. *Am. J. Phys.*, **136**, 561–66.

Jones, D.C. and Kimeldorf, D.J. (1959) Gastrointestinal function during exposure to X-rays. *Rad. Res.*, **11**, 832–43.

Kagnoff, M. (1970) Motor activity *in vitro* of rat small intestine following whole body irradiation. *Rad. Res.*, **42**, 565–76.

Kellow, J.E. and Phillips, S.F. (1987) Altered bowel motility in irritable bowel syndrome is correlated with symptoms. *Gastroenterology*, **92**, 1885–93.

Kim, C.H., Azpiroz, F. and Malagelada, J.R. (1986) Characteristics of spontaneous and drug-induced dysrhythmias in a chronic canine model. *Gastroenterology*, **90**, 421–27.

Klika, I.J. and Goodman, J.M. (1982) Gastrointestinal tract symptoms from intravenously administered erythromycin. *JAMA*, **248**, 1309–11.

Lang, I.M. (1990) Digestive tract motor correlates of vomiting and nausea. *Can. J. Physiol. Pharmacol.*, **68**, 242–53.

Lang, I.M. and Marvig, J. (1989) Functional localisation of specific receptors mediating gastrointestinal motor correlates of vomiting. *Am. J. Phys.*, **256**, G92–G99.

Lang, I.M., Sarna, S.K. and Condon, R.E. (1986) Gastrointestinal motor correlates of vomiting in the dog: quantification and characterisation as an independent phenomenon. *Gastroenterology*, **90**, 41–47.

Lang, I.M. and Sarna, S.K. (1989). 'Motor and myoelectric activity associated with vomiting, regurgitation and nausea in *Handbook of Physiology*, The Gastrointestinal System Vol 1, Part 2 (ed. J.D. Wood). American Physiological Society, Bethesda, Maryland, pp. 1179–98.'

Lee, K.Y., Park, H.J. and Chey, W.Y. (1985) Studies on a mechanism of retching and vomiting in dogs. *Dig. Dis. Sci.*, **30**, 22–28.

Magendie (1824) Quoted in Alvarez, W.C. (1948) *Introduction to Gastroenterology*. Heinemann, London.

Miller, A.D. (1990) Respiratory muscle control during vomiting. *Can. J. Phys. Pharm.*, **68**, 237–41.

Miner, W. and Sanger, G.J. (1986) Inhibition of cisplatin-induced vomiting by 5 hydroxtryptamine M-receptor antagonism. *Br. J. Pharm.*, **88**, 497–99.

Miolan, J.P., Lajard, A.M., Rega, P. and Roman, C. (1984) 'Vagal control of the gastrointestinal tract during vomiting', in *Gastrointestinal Motility* (ed C. Roman) pp. 167–77, MTP, Lancaster.

Otterson, M., Sarna, S.K. and Moulder, J.E. (1988) Effects of fractionated doses of ionizing radiation on small intestinal motor activity. *Gastroenterology*, **95**, 1249–57.

Pilot, M.-A., Thompson, H.H. and Zara, G.-P. (1986) Intestinal motility produced following administration of clonidine in the conscious dog. *J. Phys.* 105P.

Quastel, M.R. (1968) Effect of whole body irradiation on spontaneous motility of rat isolated duodenum and its contractile response to acetylcholine and 5-HT. *Br. J. Rad.*, **41**, 142–46.

Racke, K. and Schwörer, H. (1991) Regulation of serotonin release from the intestinal mucosa. *Pharmacol. Res.* **23**, 13–25.

Roos, I.A., Fairlie, D.P. and Whitehouse, M.W. (1981) A peculiar toxicity manifested by platinum(II)amines in rats: gastric distension after peritoneal administration. *Chem. Biol. Int.*, **35**, 111–17.

Sanger, G.J, Wardle, K.A., Shapcott, S. and Yee, K.F. (1991) 'Constipation evoked by $5HT_3$ receptor antagonists', in *Serotonin: Molecular Biology, Receptors and Functional Effects.* (eds J.R. Fozard and Saxenap.) pp. 381–88. Birkhauser Verlag, Basel.

Sarna, S.K. (1985) Cyclic motor activity; migrating motor complex. *Gastroenterology*, **89**, 894–913.

Sarna, S.K. (1987) Giant migrating contractions and their myoelectric correlates in the small intestine. *Am. J. Physiol.*, **16**, G697–G705.

Sarna, S.K. (1989) Motor correlates of functional gastrointestinal symptoms. *Viewpoints on Digestive Diseases*, **2**, 122–26.

Schaeppi, U., Heiman, I.A., Fleischman, R.W., Rozencrantz, H., *et al.* (1973) *Cis*-dicholorodiammineplatinum (II) (NSC-119 875) preclinical toxicological evaluation of intravenous injection in dogs, monkeys and mice. *Toxicol. Appl. Pharmacol.*, **25**, 230–41.

Schemann, M. and Erhlein, H.J. (1986) Post prandial patterns of canine jejunal motility and transit of luminal content. *Gastroenterology*, **90**, 991–1000.

Schuurkes, J.A.J. and Van Nueten, J.M. (1990) 'Pharmacological modulation of gastro-duodenal coordination', in *Gastro-pyloro-duodenal Coordination*, (eds Van Nueten, J.M., Schuurkes, J.A.J. and Akkermans, A.) pp. 155–66, Wrighton Biomedical Publishing, Petersfield.

Smith, C.C. and Brizzee, R.R. (1961) Cineradiographic analysis of vomiting in the cat. *Gastroenterology*, **40**, 655–64.

Stern, R.M., Koch, K.L., Stewart, W.R. and Lindblad, I.M. (1987) Spectral analysis of tachygastria recorded during motion sickness. *Gastroenterology*, **92**, 92–97.

Stewart, J.J., Burks, T.F. and Weisbrodt, N.W. (1977) Intestinal myoelectric activity after activation of central emetic mechanism. *Am. J. Phys.*, **2**, E121–E137.

Stewart, J.J. (1983) Effects of emetic and cathartic agents on the gastrointestinal tract and the treatment of toxic ingestion. *J. Toxicol. Clin. Toxicol.*, **20**, 199–253.

Summers, R.W., Flatt, A.J., Prihoda, M.J. and Mitros, F.A. (1987) Effect of irradiation on morphology and motility of canine small intestine. *Dig. Dis. Sci.*, **32**, 1402–10.

Swann, M.B.R. (1924) A study of the immediate effects of X-rays on the functions of certain tissues and organs. *Br. J. Radiol.*, **29**, 210–19.

Wingate, D.L. (1981) Backwards and forwards with the migrating complex. *Dig. Dis. Sci.*, **26**, 641–66.

Wolf, S. (1965) *The Stomach*. p. 321, Oxford University Press, New York.

Wulschke, S., Ehrlein, H.-J. and Tsiamitas, C. (1986) The control of gastric emptying mechanisms cannot be overridden by motor stimulants. *Am. J. Phys.*, **251**, G744–G751.

Zara, G.-P., Qin, X.-Y., Pilot, M.-A. and Thompson, H. and Maskell, J. (1991) Response of the human gastrointestinal tract to erythromycin. *J. Gastrointestinal Motil.*, **3**, 26–31.

6

Neurotransmitters and receptors in the emetic pathway

R.A. LESLIE and D.J.M. REYNOLDS

6.1 INTRODUCTION

The study of the neuropharmacology of the mechanisms of nausea and emesis has gone through a period of rapid advancement since the realization in the mid-1980s that a class of pharmacological compounds, the relatively specific 5-HT_3 receptor antagonists (Fozard, 1989), have a profound effect on some forms of emesis (Miner and Sanger, 1986). Compounds that were known to antagonize one of the two original sub-classes of 5-HT receptor ('5-HTM'; Gaddum and Piccarelli, 1957) were found to alleviate the vomiting caused by administration of either ionizing radiation or cytotoxic drugs used to treat cancer patients (Miner and Sanger, 1986; Andrews and Hawthorn, 1987).

Before the discovery that 5-HT_3 receptor blockers could be so effective in alleviating some cases of nausea and vomiting, little was known about the role of 5-HT in this autonomic defence process. Early studies had shown that cells and varicose fibres showing characteristics of 5-HT neurons could be found in the caudal brainstem, including in and around the area postrema (AP) of some experimental animals such as rats (Fuxe and Owman, 1965). The AP, a small circumventricular organ located at the caudal margin of the fourth ventricle of the brain, has long been suspected as playing a role as a chemoreceptive trigger zone (CTZ) for the vomiting response (Borison, 1974). It is interesting to note that 5-HT-immunoreactive nerve fibres, but no cell bodies, have been described in higher mammals, including humans.

It is still far from clear that the 5-HT found in the caudal medulla oblongata plays a central role in the aetiology of nausea and emesis, although current circumstantial evidence suggests that it does. It is reasonably certain, however, that 5-HT_3 receptors which are located most probably on the sensory (distal) terminals of afferent fibres of the vagus nerve, play a crucial role in this process.

This chapter will review the evidence for the occurrence of the various neurotransmitters and neuromodulators and their receptors in regions of the nervous system implicated in the mediation of nausea and vomiting. It will examine in particular the recent studies that have focussed on the role of 5-HT in these processes.

6.2 CNS STRUCTURES INVOLVED IN NAUSEA AND EMESIS

The main central nervous system structures considered to play major roles in the mediation

Emesis in Anti-cancer Therapy
Mechanisms and treatment
Published in 1993 by Chapman & Hall, London
ISBN 0 412 37250 9

rhombocephalon = pons + cerebellum + medulla oblongata

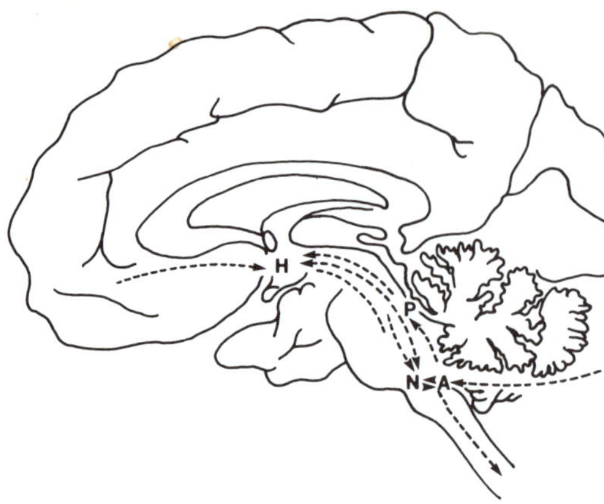

Figure 6.1 Diagram of a mid-sagittal brain section illustrating some important pathways involved in emesis. Although a human brain is depicted, it should be recognized that most of our current information about these pathways has been derived from animal studies. The area postrema (A) is located dorsally in the caudal medulla oblongata; it forms part of the lateral floor of the fourth ventricle. This nucleus is connected with multiple brainstem centres but its main outputs are to the subjacent nucleus of the *tractus solitarius* (N) and to the parabrachial nuclei (P) in the pontine region. These two centres, themselves interconnected, can affect motor centres involved in emesis: the nucleus of the *tractus solitarius*, for example, has connections with the nearby dorsal vagal motor nucleus as well as with the ventral grey matter of the spinal cord. The parabrachial nuclei are directly connected with the hypothalamus (H), especially its periventricular nucleus. The hypothalamus, in turn, receives cerebral cortical input and affects motor function via its autonomic connections.

of nausea and vomiting are clustered in the caudal brainstem and the central grey matter of the spinal cord (Fig. 6.1). They include (1) the chemoreceptive trigger zone for vomiting (the AP), (2) the major visceral sensory nucleus of the vagus nerve (the nucleus of the *tractus solitarius* or NTS), (3) the dorsal motor nucleus of the vagus nerve which sends parasympathetic efferents to the abdominal viscera, (4) a 'vomiting centre' which has been considered to act as an integrating motor centre or a central pattern generator for the emetic response and to lie in the dorsomedial medulla oblongata, and (5) and ventral horn of the spinal cord which contains lower motor neurons responsible for activating the somatic muscles which help to expel gastric contents.

6.2.1 THE VAGUS NERVE

The AP, NTS and dorsal motor nucleus of the vagus nerve (DMVN) together form the so-called 'dorsal vagal complex' (DVC) in the dorsal region of the rhombencephalon. The AP and NTS receive visceral afferents conveyed via the vagus nerve; together they may be thought of as the major sensory nuclear region of the vagus. As well as being involved in the mediation of nausea and vomiting, the DVC modulates other autonomic functions such as gastro-intestinal motility and secretion and respiratory and cardiovascular reflexes. The dorsal motor nucleus of the vagus, which contains many of the parasympathetic neurons of the vagus, innervates mainly gastro-intestinal and respiratory visceral structures.

The other vagal motor nucleus is the *nucleus ambiguus* which primarily innervates laryngeal and cardiac structures (Hopkins, 1987). Although autonomic motor fibres which innervate abdominal visceral structures are involved in the vomiting response, the major motor components responsible for expulsion of gastric contents during emesis are part of the somatic rather than the autonomic nervous system, and are located in the ventral grey matter of the spinal cord.

One of the main triggers of nausea and vomiting involves the ingestion of toxic substances; the expulsion of gastric contents resulting from such ingestion is a straightforward way for the body to rid itself of these toxins (Davis *et al.*, 1986). It has long been known that the vagus nerve provides a substantial proportion of the innervation of the abdominal viscera concerned with these processes. Although the vagus is recognized as a major parasympathetic motor nerve, most of its fibres are in fact sensory and terminate in the brainstem. Physiological studies have indicated that these fibres of the vagus provide the most important neural route for gastro-intestinal information to reach the brainstem and mediate, amongst other gastro-intestinal reflexes, the emetic response (Andrews, 1986; Barnes, 1984).

Recent advances in neuronal tract-tracing techniques have allowed the elucidation of the anatomical connections of the vagus nerve between the periphery and the central nervous system. The afferent fibres of the vagus terminate in the caudal portion of the NTS and in the AP (Leslie and Gwyn, 1984). A heavy concentration of these afferents is located in the most dorsomedial region of the NTS (Gwyn and Leslie, 1979) which is termed the *subnucleus gelatinosus* (Taber, 1961). The largest proportion of vagal afferents to this region of the NTS is derived from the stomach wall (Gwyn *et al.*, 1979; 1985; Kalia and Mesulam, 1980; Leslie *et al.*, 1982). Gastric afferents have also been described as projecting directly to the AP (Kalia and Meslulam, 1980).

6.2.2 THE AREA POSTREMA

The small brainstem nuclear structure, the AP (Fig. 6.2), must be intact in order for most stimuli to be effective in inducing emesis. Ablation of the AP, for example, will afford protection from vomiting due to parenteral application of certain drugs. One example is apomorphine, a synthetic opiate analogue that is pharmacologically more closely related to the catecholamine dopamine than to the opiates. Apomorphine given systemically is normally a very potent emetic, but is completely ineffective in this regard in animals that have undergone AP lesions (Borison, 1959; Lindstrom and Brizzee, 1962; Wang and Borison, 1952). Such brain lesions do not abolish the capability to vomit in response to all stimuli, however, as gastric irritants such as copper sulphate will still evoke emesis (Borison, 1959).

AP ablation can also protect against radiation-induced vomiting (Brizzee *et al.*, 1959; Chinn and Wang, 1954; Harding *et al.*, 1985) or motion sickness in some species (Brizzee *et al.*, 1980; Wang and Chinn, 1954). It may be, for example, that in the case of radiation-induced emesis, neuronal receptors within the AP (which would include receptors on neuronal elements of extra-AP origin such as vagus nerve afferent fibre terminals) detect humoral factors released by affected peripheral tissues and the resultant output from AP initiates the emetic response (Carpenter, 1989). Suggested possible candidates for such a humoral substance are prostaglandins, dopamine (Carpenter *et al.*, 1986), or a neuroactive peptide such as PYY (Harding *et al.*, 1985; see also below).

The structure and location of the AP makes it ideally suited to detecting either blood-borne or cerebrospinal fluid (CSF)-borne humoral information. It is one of a number of 'circumventricular organs', positioned around the ventricular system of the brain, that usually have a very poor blood–brain diffusion barrier to polar molecules (i.e. they 'lack a blood–brain barrier'). The main reason for this is the lack of endothelial occluding junctions in the microvasculature of these structures; the presence of such junctions is a normal feature of most brain parenchymal blood vessels. Furthermore, there are no effective intercellular occluding junctions between ependymal cells that cover the AP that might protect it from humoral effects of the CSF (Gotow and Hashimoto, 1979; Leslie, 1986). Hence, experiments with electron-opaque tracing substances indicate that the parenchyma of the AP is readily accessible to elements circulating in the blood or CSF (Gotow and Hashimoto, 1979; Torack and Finke, 1971). By virtue of its close proximity to the NTS, which receives direct

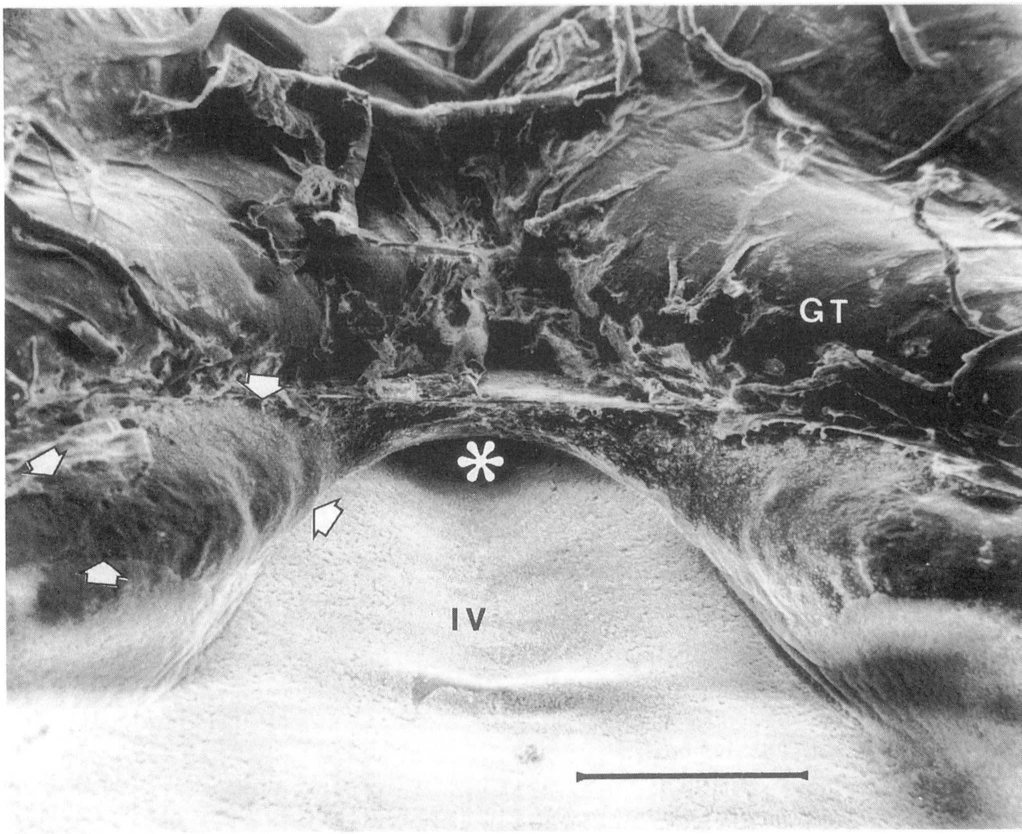

Figure 6.2 Scanning electron micrograph of the floor of the cat caudal rhombencephalon. The obex can be seen covering the entrance to the central canal (*) of the spinal cord. The *tela choroidea* has been removed from this specimen. Arrows indicate the boundaries of the area postrema (AP) which forms a bilateral structure in the floor of the fourth ventricle (IV). For further details, see Leslie *et al.*, 1978, the study from which this material was taken. Bar = 1 mm.

gastric afferent information, and the probability that such information is able to synapse directly upon its own cells, the AP is also well positioned to receive neural input that may result in nausea and/or vomiting.

The major efferent connection of the AP is to the parabrachial nuclei of the pontine region of the brain (Loewy and Burton, 1978; Shapiro and Miselis, 1985). The functional significance of this pathway is poorly understood at present but it may, amongst other things, help explain the way in which nausea reaches the cerebral cortex and conscious levels.

6.2.3 THE NUCLEUS OF THE *TRACTUS SOLITARIUS*

Although the AP receives direct sensory input from the vagus nerve, the NTS has long been recognized as the major site in the brain which receives vagal afferent information. Unlike the AP, the NTS has a normal well-developed blood–brain diffusion barrier, its blood vessels are lined by endothelial cells linked to each other by *zonulae occludentes* (tight junctions). Furthermore, no dilated perivascular spaces occur around the blood vessels in this nucleus, as they do in the AP. Notwithstanding these differences, however, a subdivision of the NTS, the *subnucleus gelatinosus* (SNG), and the AP appear to be remarkably similar structures. Their neurons have virtually identical ultrastructural characteristics (Leslie, 1986; Leslie *et al.*, 1982), and they also have many of the same connections, incorporated chemicals, and receptors. One can speculate that the AP is simply an extension of this part of the NTS into the fourth ventricular lumen that has over the course of time lost its blood–brain barrier. For all of the reasons mentioned above these two brainstem nuclei should be considered together in any examination of their physiological roles.

Anatomical, physiological and pharmacological studies on the NTS have shown that it mediates many autonomic functions. Anatomical tracing studies, aimed at localizing within the NTS neuronal components associated with discrete physiological functions, have revealed a topographical distribution of such components (Kalia and Mesulam, 1980). Thus, the localization of gastric vagal afferent terminals in the *subnucleus gelatinosus* of the NTS (Leslie *et al.*, 1982), suggests that this subdivision of the NTS may play an important role in mediating nausea and emesis.

6.2.4 THE VOMITING CENTRE

The concept of a vomiting centre existing as a discrete brainstem locus and responsible for initiating the stereotypical vomiting response, dates from work by Hatcher (1924). Wang and Borison carried this idea further by showing that two separate brainstem regions were responsible for (1) the detection of emetic substances and (2) the initiation of the motor events culminating in emesis (Wang and Borison, 1952; Borison and Wang, 1949; 1951). The chemoreceptive trigger zone is considered to lie in the AP. The vomiting centre, however, was thought to be located in the medullary reticular formation, somewhat ventral to the dorsal vagal complex (Borison and Wang, 1949). More recent studies, aimed at locating the vomiting centre with more precision, however, have been unable to elicit consistent emetic episodes from electrical stimulation of the region in question (Miller and Wilson, 1983). Thus the suggestion has been made that a somewhat diffuse collection of neurons in the region of the NTS acts as a 'central pattern generator' to co-ordinate the sequential firing of emetic motor units in an orderly and effective manner (Davis *et al.*, 1986; Carpenter, 1989). A similar group of neurons, thought to behave in this fashion to co-ordinate the stereotypical cascade of events involved in deglutition, is also localized in the region of the NTS (Kessler and Jean, 1985; 1986).

6.2.5 OTHER ANATOMICAL SITES ASSOCIATED WITH NAUSEA AND VOMITING

Apart from the sites mentioned above, there are undoubtedly other regions of the body that are important in the initiation and co-ordination of nausea and emesis. For example, in some species the splanchnic nerves appear to be implicated in the initiation of the emetic response (Wang and Borison, 1951). The precise nature of the sensory stimuli responsible for mediating emetic events, and the detailed anatomical course of fibres concerned, remain to be elucidated although the major route seems to involve the vagus nerve itself (Andrews, 1986).

Other possible sites should not be overlooked. The liver, for example, could well play a role as a 'chemoreceptor trigger zone' for the vomiting response. It quickly samples all the blood draining from the gastro-intestinal tract and could send afferent neuronal information to the brainstem via the vagal or other pathways. Humoral information, often thought to gain access to the brain via the AP, may use this visceral route instead, at least in some circumstances.

Finally, there are other circumventricular organs which, like the AP, have a poor blood–brain diffusion barrier and one or more of these could provide a 'window' directly into brain parenchymal tissue for humoral information. An obvious example would be the median eminence at the base of the hypothalamus which itself is largely involved in most autonomic responses and as yet has not been investigated thoroughly with regard to its possible role in the mediation of nausea and vomiting.

As can be seen from the above discussion, much information concerning the central nervous system pathways responsible for mediating the phenomena of nausea and vomiting is still lacking. Much more work needs to be done to discover the detailed connections and neurochemistry of these circuits. Clearly, the important question of where the 'vomiting centre' is located in the brainstem, or even whether such a discrete collection of neurons exists, should be addressed in future studies. If the neurons responsible for acting as a pattern generator for the emetic response can be characterized more exactly, and their output found to be amenable to pharmacological manipulation in a controlled way, it may yet be possible to design an effective and universal anti-emetic drug.

6.3 CLINICAL STRATEGIES FOR ANTI-EMETIC THERAPY

The lack of a unified approach to the management of cytotoxic drug-induced nausea and vomiting is reflected by the wide varieties of anti-emetic regimes which have been evaluated both experimentally and in clinical trials. Historically, studies of anti-emetics for use in cancer patients have centred on drugs which have known antagonist activity at dopamine D_2, muscarinic cholinergic and histamine H_1 receptors. No single agent has been found to be particularly effective and combinations of drugs have been used in an attempt to achieve better symptomatic control. Peroutka and Snyder (1982) tried to provide a rational approach for designing combinations of drugs by highlighting the relative potencies of different anti-emetics as antagonists at D_2, H_1, and muscarinic receptor sites. The range of clinical strategies employed up until 1984 has been well reviewed elsewhere (Barnes, 1984). In recent years one of the most common anti-emetic regimes used by oncology units has been 5-HT_3 receptor blockade (either in the form of high dose metoclopramide or, most recently, the more selective antagonists ondansetron or granisetron – see below). These regimes are used in combination with dexamethasone and a benzodiazepine, the latter aimed at reducing problems of anticipatory nausea and vomiting. Such strategies provide up to 70% protection against sickness due to cisplatin administration, one of the most emetogenic and widely used cytotoxic agents (Harris and Cantwell, 1986). The observation that no single agent or combination regimen affords complete protection may be because cytotoxic drugs exert their emetic effects at more than one site in the emetic cascade and a 'final common pathway' has so far eluded pharmacological characterization.

Table 6.1 shows the great variety of neurotransmitters and neuro- and vasoactive substances so far identified within the DVC. Many of these are undoubtedly involved with autonomic function such as cardiorespiratory control and gastro-intestinal reflexes relatively unrelated to emesis. Electrophysiological studies by Carpenter (1989) and others, however, suggest that many of these substances are, indeed, implicated in the emetic response. In the following section the neurochemistry of vomiting with a particular focus on 5-HT and its involvement in both the peripheral and central mediation of emesis is reviewed.

Table 6.1 Neurochemicals found in medium-to-high concentrations in the area postrema and the *nucleus tractus solitarius*

Area postrema	*Nucleus tractus solitarius*
alpha-neo-endorphin	acetylcholine
beta-neo-endorphin	ACTH
dopamine	adenosine
dynorphin A	adrenaline
dynorphin B	alpha-MSH
GABA	alpha-neo-endorphin
glutamate	angiotensin II
glycine	aspartate
leu-enkephalin	atrial natriuretic peptide
LH-RH	beta-neo-endorphin
met-enkephalin	bombesin
neurotensin	CCK
noradrenaline	CRF
serotonin	dopamine
VIP	dynorphin A
	dynorphin B
	FMRFamide
	GABA
	galanin
	gamma-MSH
	glutamate
	glycine
	histamine
	insulin
	leu-enkephalin
	melatonin
	met-enkephalin
	neurotensin
	noradrenaline
	NPY
	oxytocin
	PYY
	serotonin (5-HT)
	somatostatin
	substance P
	taurine
	TRH
	vasopressin
	VIP

6.4 THE NEUROCHEMISTRY OF CYTOTOXIC DRUG-INDUCED VOMITING

6.4.1 INTRODUCTION

Considerable amounts of information have become available in recent years concerning the types of neuroactive substances and their receptors that are located in brain regions implicated in the mediation of nausea and vomiting (Leslie, 1985). Barnes (1984) describes various techniques that have been used to identify receptor types in the AP. These include drug trial and behavioural monitoring studies, iontophoretic application of various compounds followed by behavioural or electrophysiological studies, and binding studies using radiolabelled ligands. Especially interesting is the observation of Carpenter and his colleagues (1983) that a very wide variety of pharmacological agents have excitatory or inhibitory effects on electrical activity of AP neurons. In many cases, a single neuron has been shown to be affected by iontophoretic application of many different drugs. Examples of such effective substances tested are: angiotensin II, apomorphine, dopamine, gastrin, glutamate, histamine, insulin, leu-enkephalin, neurotensin, noradrenaline, several prostaglandins, serotonin, substance P, TRH, vasopressin, and VIP (Carpenter *et al.*, 1983). Thus, many pharmacological substances may mediate the activity of AP neurons, and there is, as a result, little optimism that a universal anti-emetic drug that would act at the level of the chemoreceptor trigger zone will be found.

Since the subject of neurochemistry of the dorsal vagal complex was last reviewed in detail (Leslie, 1985; Palkovits, 1985), much more information has come to light on two aspects of the study in particular. These are the involvement of serotonin in this brain region and of the role of various neuropeptides, especially the opiates.

6.3.2 SEROTONIN (5-HT) AND THE VOMITING RESPONSE

Recent studies have given us a much better insight into the mechanism of action of 5-HT_3 receptor antagonist drugs in alleviating emesis and, to a certain extent, nausea following administration of either cytotoxic drugs or ionizing radiation. Previously, attention had been focussed on other neurotransmitters such as dopamine and acetylcholine and their various receptors. In particular, it was thought that dopaminergic mechanisms were responsible in large part for mediation of cytotoxic drug-induced emesis because large-dose metoclopramide is an effective treatment for cancer patients receiving such therapy (Harrington *et al.*, 1983). The effect of this compound on the dopaminergic system, however, often produces unwanted effects on the extrapyramidal motor system (Rawlins *et al.*, 1986). It is, of course, well known that apomorphine, a D_2 receptor agonist, can evoke emesis – presumably by acting upon dopamine D_2 receptors in the AP – and that this could be blocked either by ablation of the AP or by administration of domperidone. This is an effective D_2 receptor antagonist which does not easily cross the blood–brain barrier. Domperidone is, however, not a particularly effective drug for treating cytotoxic drug-induced vomiting. The observation that metoclopramide is more effective in treating this condition may now be explained by its action on the 5-HT_3 receptor over and above its activity at the dopamine D_2 receptor.

Sanger (1984) showed that metoclopramide in high concentrations has pharmacological actions unrelated to its dopamine D_2 antagonism; one of these was its ability to antagonize 5-HT_3 receptor activity (Fozard, 1984). Sanger (1987) tested the substituted benzamide BRL 24924 (renzapride) on cisplatin-induced vomiting in the ferret model. He suggested that its anti-emetic effect in that model was due to its action as a 5-HT_3 receptor antagonist. Furthermore, Miner and Sanger (1986) showed that the specific 5-HT_3 receptor antagonist MDL 72222 completely blocked cisplatin-evoked emesis in the ferret. When the potential for 5-HT_3 receptor antagonist compounds to be highly effective treatments for cytotoxic drug-induced vomiting was realized, a great deal of effort in the pharmaceutical industry was devoted to developing new, more specific 5-HT_3 receptor antagonist drugs. Some successful examples of these, now available for clinical use, are ondansetron (Zofran^R) and granisetron (Kytril^R).

It had previously been noted that 5-HT can be demonstrated to occur in fibres and varicosities in the dorsal vagal complex (Leslie, 1985) although 5-HT-containing cell bodies have only been shown to occur in lower mammals such as rats (Fuxe and Owman, 1965). There are relatively few 5-HT receptors in this part of the brain, with one notable exception. It has recently been shown by several groups that there are high numbers of 5-HT_3 receptor ligand binding sites in the NTS in particular (Pratt *et al.*, 1990) as well as in other regions of the DVC of several species, including man (Fig. 6.3) (Waeber *et al.*, 1989; Reynolds *et al.*, 1989; Leslie *et al.*, 1990; Reynolds *et al.*, 1991). There is now strong evidence to suggest that these 5-HT_3 receptor sites are located on the membranes of vagal afferent fibres terminating here and which derive largely from the wall of the proximal gut (Pratt and Bowery, 1989; Leslie *et al.*, 1990). It is, of course, possible that 5-HT_3 receptors may also be located postsynaptically on neuronal elements within the DVC but there is no direct evidence to support this.

There are several intriguing questions that remain concerning the physiological function of these binding sites in the caudal brainstem. For example, what is the source of the 5-HT that, presumably, is the endogenous ligand for these receptors? Serotonergic cell bodies in the nearby raphe nuclei probably send efferents to the NTS and adjacent regions. It is possible

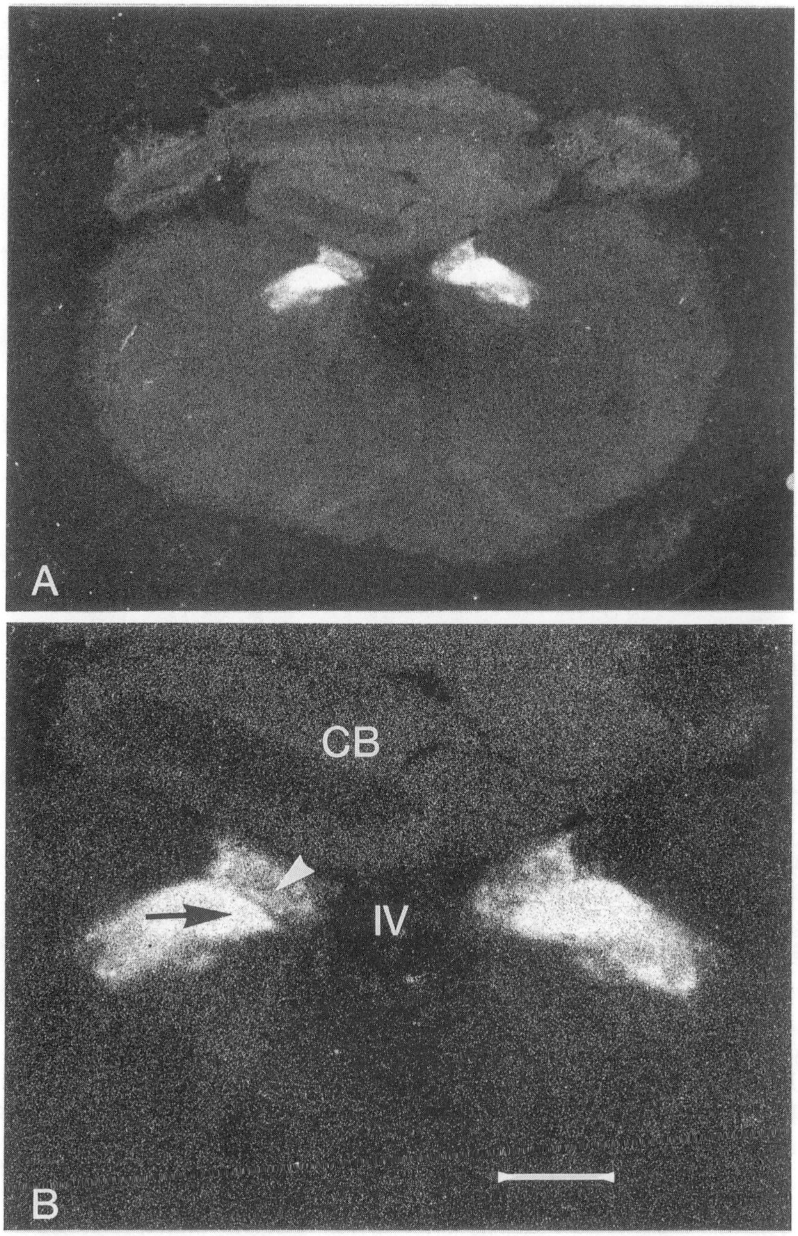

Figure 6.3 Autoradiograms generated over transverse sections of feline caudal medulla oblongata illustrating the binding of [^{3}H]-GR 65630 (New England Nuclear) to specific brain nuclei. Frozen sections were incubated in 1.0 nM ligand for 45 min and autoradiograms prepared on Amersham Hyperfilm to indicate total binding of the radioligand. Adjacent sections were incubated in the same solution with an excess of unlabelled zacopride to allow determination of specific binding (Reynolds *et al.*, 1991). A: low power micrograph showing the disposition of the heavily labelled regions within the section. B: at higher power, the relative densities of binding within the DVC can be seen, with the heaviest concentration (1.35 pmol/mg protein) being found in the subnucleus gelatinosus of the NTS (arrow) and much lighter labelling (0.29 pmol/mg protein) in the AP (arrowhead). CB = cerebellum; IV = fourth ventricle; bar = 1 mm.

that intrinsic serotonergic cell bodies in the AP, at least in lower mammals, could provide a source of 5-HT to be released locally in the DVC (Fuxe and Owman, 1965). Alternatively, these 5-HT_3 receptor binding sites may be acted upon by circulating humoral 5-HT (perhaps released from enterochromaffin cells in the stomach wall) that gains entry to the DVC through the AP (Fig. 6.4). This is, however, rather unlikely because of the rapid clearance of 5-HT from the systemic circulation (Leslie and Reynolds, 1991). A sub-population of neurons in the nodose ganglion, projecting to the DVC, is probably serotonergic (Gaudin-Chauzal *et al.*, 1982). It is possible, therefore, that the vagus nerve itself is the source of 5-HT that could act on these receptors. Finally, it could be that these binding sites are of no great physiologically importance. The very large amounts of this receptor protein in the DVC, however, would seem to argue against this latter suggestion and in a teleological sense it would seem to be a great waste of biological energy to manufacture and transport such a large amount of substance centrally. Indeed, the concentration of 5-HT_3 receptor ligand binding protein in the SNG of the NTS is the highest in the whole brain.

It thus remains to be determined with any certainty whether the 5-HT_3 receptor ligand binding sites in the caudal brainstem have anything to do with the vomiting response at all. Some evidence is available that suggests that they might; it has been shown that central administration of cisplatin causes emesis in cats (Smith *et al.*, 1988). This may be inhibited by intracerebroventricular injection of zacopride, a 5-HT_3 receptor antagonist (Smith *et al.*, 1988). The vomiting due to intraperitoneal injection of cisplatin in ferrets can also be inhibited by 5-HT_3 receptor antagonists administered directly to the brainstem in the vicinity of the DVC (Higgins *et al.*, 1989). It is possible, therefore, that both cisplatin and 5-HT_3 receptor antagonists may have a central site of action in addition to their peripheral

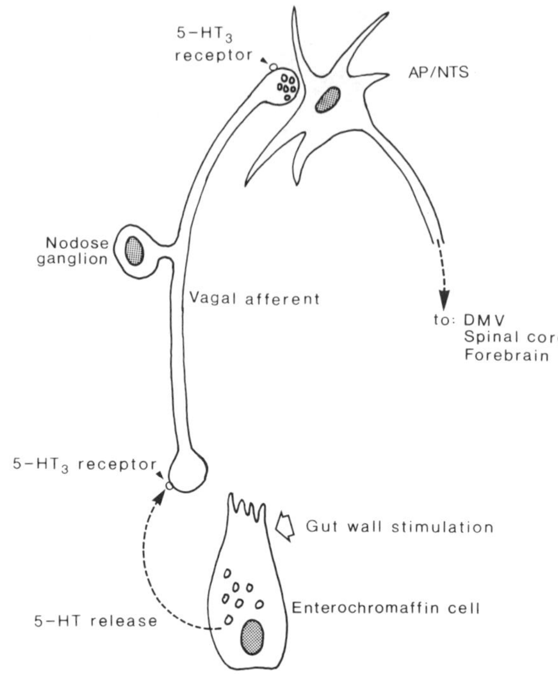

Figure 6.4 Diagram showing a schema which attempts to explain the action of 5-HT_3 receptor antagonist drugs acting at peripheral 5-HT_3 receptors to alleviate cytotoxic drug-induced vomiting. Enterochromaffin cells positioned in the mucosa of the gut wall are known to be filled with 5-HT-containing granules. It is hypothesized that cytotoxic drugs could cause release of this 5-HT into the gut tissue and act upon 5-HT_3 receptors positioned on the distal sensory terminals of vagal afferent neurons whose cell bodies are located in the nodose ganglion. Activation of these afferents is known to cause vomiting through a cascade of events mediated at the level of the DVC (particularly the subnucleus gelatinosus of the NTS). The function of the high concentration of 5-HT_3 receptors presumed to be on the proximal terminals of these vagal afferent fibres is at present unknown.

effects. The studies of Paul Andrews and his colleagues (Andrews and Hawthorn, 1987; Andrews *et al.*, 1988), on the other hand, have shown that 5-HT_3 receptors in the periphery (most probably on the distal terminal membranes of vagal afferent fibres in the gut wall) are crucially important in the mediation of cytotoxic- and radiation-induced emesis. This situation is still being actively investigated.

The most recent studies by Andrews *et al.* (1990) have suggested that an alternative site or pathway arises in the experimental animal as a result of plastic changes due to combined vagotomy and sympathectomy. Thus, 5-HT_3 receptor antagonists, which blocked all emesis under their test conditions in intact animals, were not totally effective in animals that had previously undergone visceral afferent nerve lesion. Another approach to these studies is to examine neuronal activity in the brainstem following emetogenic stimuli. Reynolds *et al.* (1991) have shown that the product of the immediate–early gene c-*fos* is expressed in specific cells in the NTS and AP following administration of cisplatin to experimental ferrets. The evidence suggests that these cells are neurons. In these animal experiments, pretreatment with granisetron abolishes the *fos*-like immunoreactivity in the NTS *but not in the AP*. Thus, the evidence suggests that cisplatin acts by involving vagal afferent pathways, but it may also act directly on the AP. It is not clear from these experiments that cellular activity in the AP, as a result of cisplatin administration, has anything to do with the vomiting response. It seems clear, however, that 5-HT_3 antagonist drugs do not act at the level of the AP in this regard.

If the hypothesis previously shown in Figure 2.4 is correct, how could blockade of *proximal* (i.e. at the DVC end of the vagal afferents) effect a control of emesis? One suggestion is that activation of these receptors could cause *release* of transmitter sequestered in these terminals which results in the initiation emesis and their subsequent antagonism then blocks that process.

Unfortunately, we still have very little idea of which transmitters might be contained in the vagal afferent neurons of the nodose ganglion or how the afferent information is processed at the level of the DVC once it arrives there from the periphery.

Yet another factor that may concern the role of 5-HT in the control of nausea and vomiting has recently come to light where a further separate 5-HT receptor has been discovered both in the peripheral and central nervous systems. This has been termed the 5-HT_4 receptor (Dumuis *et al.*, 1988); its functional aspects have been studied most extensively in the periphery with respect to its role in control of gastro-intestinal and cardiovascular systems.

Interestingly, some of the earliest 5-HT_3-active compounds studied, e.g. the substituted benzamide renzapride (BRL 24924), have now been shown to act as specific agonists at the 5-HT_4 receptor (Dumuis *et al.*, 1988). It may be that such action of these compounds may play a more important role in control of gastro-intestinal motility than does their 5-HT_3 antagonist effect. Nevertheless, reduced gastro-intestinal motility has often been shown to be associated with nausea although whether there is a cause and effect relationship is uncertain. 5-HT_4 receptor activity has been detected in several CNS structures such as the mesencephalic tectum and hypothalamus (Dumuis *et al.*, 1988); thus far, however, such receptors have not been reported as occurring in the human CNS. It is thus possible that 5-HT_4 receptors may have important roles to play in the control of nausea and emesis and it will be interesting to see if this idea is borne out when more pharmacological tools become available to study this 'new' receptor. Autoradiographic studies have demonstrated the presence of other 5-HT receptor binding sites in the DVC; for example, 5-HT_{1A}, 5-HT_{1C}, and 5-HT_2 (Pazos *et al.*, 1987a; 1987b). Lucot and Crampton (1987) showed in cats that the 5-HT_{1A} receptor ligand buspirone blocks nausea and vomiting due to cisplatin administration. However, buspirone has dopaminergic blocking properties as well (McMillen and Mattiace, 1983), and its metabolite 1PP is an adrenergic

α_2 receptor antagonist (Caccia *et al.*, 1986). In summation, then, the role of 5-HT_{1A} receptors in nausea and vomiting is far from clear.

6.3.3 CHOLINERGIC MECHANISMS

Historically, acetylcholine has been associated with the parasympathetic nervous system and its presence in the DVC might reasonably be anticipated. The evidence for acetylcholine being involved in emetic control, however, is, perhaps surprisingly, not at all clear cut. Indirect evidence for the presence of acetylcholine in the DVC comes from early studies which demonstrated the presence of the enzyme acetylcholinesterase, particularly within the subnucleus gelatinosus and the commissural subnucleus of the NTS (Gwyn and Wolstencroft, 1968; Palkovits and Jacobowitz, 1974). More recently, techniques using immunocytochemistry to identify the synthetic enzyme choline acetyltransferase (ChAT), have been used in an attempt to provide more reliable localization of cholinergic neurons. Vagal afferent denervation (following nodose ganglion excision) results in decreased ChAT levels in the NTS suggesting that some of the vagal sensory fibres are cholinergic (Helke *et al.*, 1983). In contrast, Armstrong and colleagues (1983) failed to identify any ChAT immunoreactivity in the NTS or the AP but were able to see activity in the DMV. The role of acetylcholine receptors (particularly muscarinic receptors) in the DVC that may be involved in nausea and vomiting has been more thoroughly studied.

6.3.3.1 Muscarinic cholinergic receptors

There is now a substantial literature devoted to the use of muscarinic cholinergic receptor antagonists, such as scopolamine, in the prophylactic treatment of space and motion sickness. Muscarinic receptor blockers in various species have been reported as effective in alleviating nausea and vomiting occurring post-operatively (Cookson, 1986), with apomorphine administration (Isaacs, 1956), cytotoxic drugs (Sawicka and Sallan, 1977), X-irradiation (Roylance *et al.*, 1989) and emesis due to peripheral administration of acetylcholine (Borison and Wang, 1953) or the central administration of muscarinic receptor stimulants (Beleslin *et al.*, 1989).

The undoubted efficacy of scopolamine as a prophylactic treatment for motion sickness has to some extent overshadowed the role which muscarinic receptors may play in other forms of emesis, particular that associated with the clinical use of cytotoxic drugs. It would appear from some studies that muscarinic receptor antagonism may afford some protection against vomiting due to cancer chemotherapy (Sawicka and Sallan, 1977) but other studies have shown no benefit (Longo *et al.*, 1985). In ferrets, the nonspecific muscarinic receptor antagonist atropine modified the emetic response to X-irradiation, the protein synthesis inhibitor emetine, and the cytotoxic agent cyclophosphamide (Roylance *et al.*, 1989). In 1989 Beleslin *et al.* demonstrated that muscarinic M_1 receptors are implicated in the control of emesis using 4-(m-chlorophenylcarbamoxyloxy)-2 butyryltrimethylammonium chloride, administered intracerebroventricularly in cats. Furthermore, autoradiographic binding studies utilizing the nonspecific muscarinic ligand [^{3}H]-QNB have demonstrated a high concentration of muscarinic receptor recognition sites in the brainstem (Pedigo and Brizzee, 1985; Leslie *et al.*, 1989), particularly in the subnucleus gelatinosus of the NTS, the principal site of termination of vagal sensory fibres emanating from the proximal gut (Leslie *et al.*, 1982). Following unilateral nodose ganglion excision, Leslie *et al.* (1989) observed a diminution of [^{3}H]-QNB binding site density ipsilateral to the lesion, suggesting that some of these receptor sites are located on vagal sensory fibre terminals.

This observation has recently been extended

and autoradiographic binding studies have been performed using [^{3}H]-QNB and the more M_1-specific ligand [^{3}H]-pirenzipine in the DVC of the ferret. Figure 6.5 shows [^{3}H]-QNB and [^{3}H]-pirenzipine binding in sham-operated animals and in animals that had received a unilateral nodose ganglion excision approximately two weeks before binding studies were performed. There is a clear reduction in the binding of both ligands suggesting that at least some of the terminal sensory vagal fibres bear M_1 receptor sites.

6.3.3.2 Nicotinic cholinergic receptors

There is some evidence, based mainly on the work of Beleslin and colleagues, to suggest that nicotinic cholinergic receptors may also be implicated in emetic behaviour, at least in the cat (Beleslin and Krstic, 1987). There are as yet no clear data from other species (and in particular no human data) to support this and there is no evidence to implicate nicotinic cholinergic receptor mechanisms in cytotoxic drug-induced nausea and vomiting.

6.3.4 CATECHOLAMINES

There is clear evidence of the existence of dopaminergic, adrenergic and noradrenergic neurons and fibres within the dorsal medulla oblongata (e.g. Kalia *et al.*, 1985). Although there may be some differences between species in the exact distribution within cytoarchitectonic subdivisions of the nuclei of the DVC, it is generally accepted that all three catecholamines are contained in neurons, fibres and terminals of this brain region. Receptor binding sites for dopamine D_2 ligands (Stefanini and Clement-Cormier, 1981; Schwartz *et al.*, 1986) and adrenergic α_2 ligands (Robertson and Leslie, 1985) have also been described in the DVC.

Noradrenaline and adrenaline when injected i.c.v. produce emesis (Feldberg and Sherwood, 1954) and this effect can be inhibited by AP ablation (Borison, 1959) or by α_2 adrenoreceptor antagonists (Beleslin and Strabac, 1987). The contribution of adrenergic or noradrenergic mechanisms to cytotoxic drug-induced nausea and vomiting is unknown.

In contrast, there is a considerable amount of literature relating to dopamine receptor antagonist drugs and the treatment of cancer therapy-associated emesis (Barnes, 1984). Despite their widespread use over many years, dopamine receptor antagonists provide only limited anti-emetic protection and this is particularly so for most emetic cytotoxic regimes including cisplatin (Chapter 9). High dose metoclopramide achieves a similar rate of protection against cisplatin-related vomiting as do the more specific 5-HT_3 receptor antagonists (Chevallier, 1990) which suggests, perhaps, that dopamine receptor blockers will have little to offer the nauseated and vomiting cancer patient over and above the 5-HT_3 receptor antagonists.

6.3.5 HISTAMINE

Low levels of histamine have been found within the DVC (Saavedra *et al.*, 1976) and histamine H_1 receptor binding sites have been localized in this brain region (Palacios *et al.*, 1981). Histamine itself is emetic when injected into the cerebral ventricles (Bhargava and Dixit, 1968), an effect which is abolished by ablation of the AP. H_1 receptor antagonists alone, however, do not completely abolish emesis due to i.c.v. histamine nor do H_2 blockers alone; when given in combination, however, they do and this suggests that H_2 as well as H_1 receptors in the AP are important in histamine-induced vomiting (Bhargava *et al.*, 1976). Histamine H_1 receptor antagonists have an established role in the treatment of motion sickness and, to some extent, in the sickness of pregnancy (Barnes, 1984). The inclusion of antihistamine drugs in combination anti-emetic therapies in cancer treatment has been advocated (Peroutka and Snyder, 1982) but as

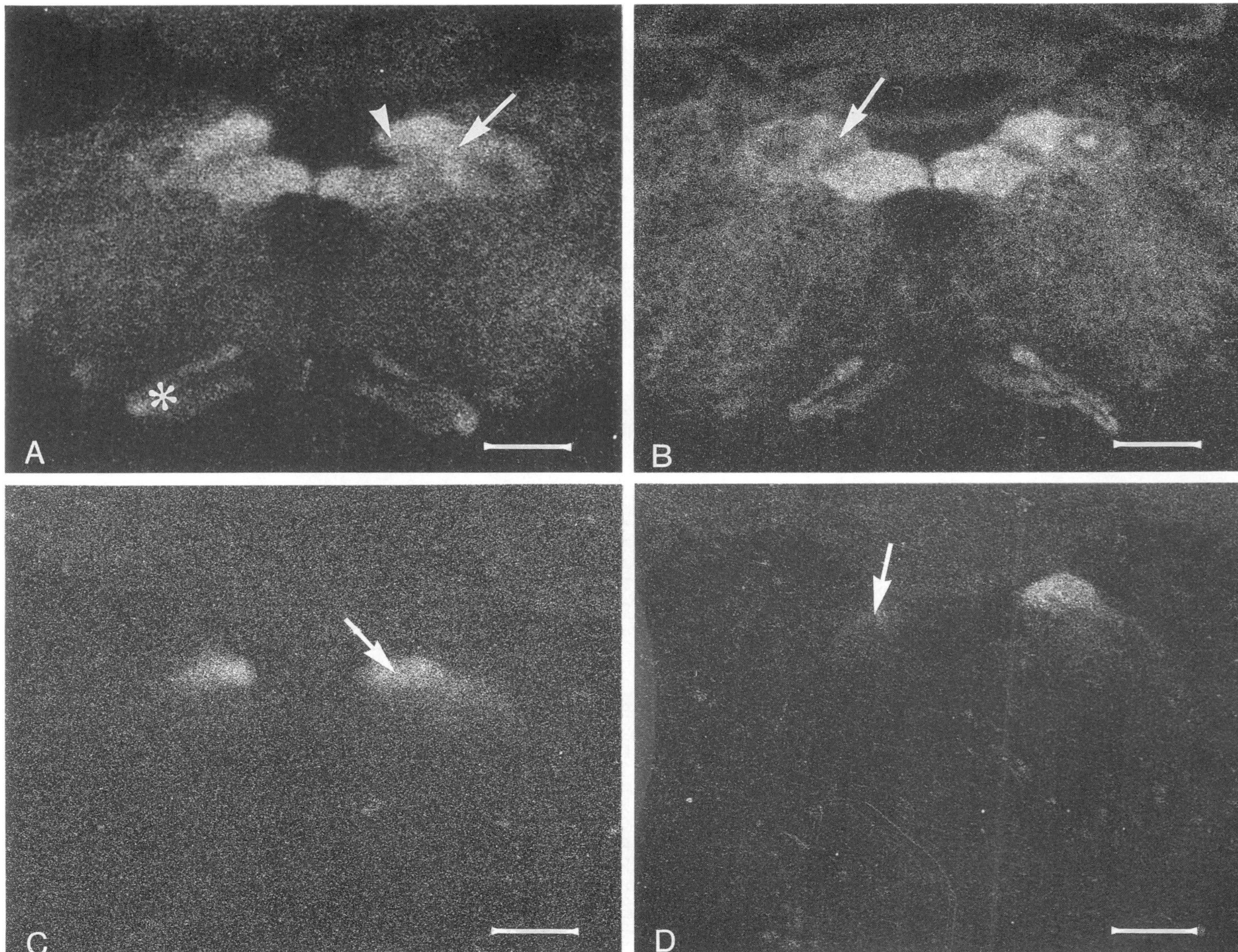
A
B
C
D

discussed by Sanger (Chapter 9), there is little clinical evidence to support their use. Any anti-emetic effects attributed to antihistamine drugs must be viewed in the light of their sedative actions and the knowledge that at least some of the commonly used antihistamines have significant potency at muscarinic receptors (Peroutka and Snyder, 1982).

6.3.6 OPIATES

It has been recognized for many years that opiate drugs can both provoke vomiting and prevent it (Leake, 1922). Costello and Borison (1977) suggested that the emetic action of morphine in the cat arose from activation of receptors within the chemoreceptor trigger zone for vomiting in the AP and the anti-emetic effects of morphine occurred within the 'vomiting centre'. This was supported by the observation (Bhargava *et al.*, 1981) that administration of met-enkephalin into the fourth ventricle caused emesis with a very short latency and that this did not occur in animals which had undergone prior CTZ ablation. Although the anatomical basis for a discrete vomiting centre is lacking (as discussed above), the concept of an anti-emetic action of opiates at a site further downstream of the CTZ in the 'emetic cascade' (Davis *et al.*, 1986) is supported by a number of observations.

Leake (1922) observed that morphine administered subcutaneously to dogs initially caused vomiting but then inhibited emesis due to emetine or apomorphine given 2–5 hours later. Costello and Borison (1977) observed that morphine, levorphanol, fentanyl and methadone given i.c.v. to cats inhibited emesis following i.c.v. apomorphine (a dopamine agonist). Furthermore, this anti-emetic action of the opiates could be prevented by pretreatment with the non-specific opiate antagonist naloxone suggesting that the anti-emetic effect is mediated through opiate receptors. Of the opiates used, when given alone, only morphine caused vomiting. However, when animals were pretreated with systemic naloxone, all the opiates tested were emetic. This emetic action could then be blocked by further naloxone administered i.c.v.

Figure 6.5 Autoradiograms of [^{3}H]-QNB and [^{3}H]-pirenzepine binding on transverse sections of ferret caudal brainstem. Bars = 1 mm. A: total binding of the non-specific muscarinic cholinergic radioligand [^{3}H]-QNB in the DVC of a control animal brain. Sections were incubated in 5 nM [^{3}H]-QNB (Amersham) for 60 min. Adjacent sections were incubated in the same solution containing unlabelled 10 μm atropine to determine nonspecific binding. Dense concentrations of binding are evident in the DVC including the AP (arrowhead) and NTS (arrow). Dense binding is also evident in the hypoglossal nucleus (double arrow). The binding seen in the inferior olivary nucleus (*) was not displaced by atropine. B: autoradiogram generated over a similar section from a ferret that had received a unilateral nodose ganglion lesion approximately two weeks prior to sacrifice for binding studies. The section was incubated in [^{3}H]-QNB in the same manner as that shown in A. A clear attenuation of binding is seen (arrow) in the DVC of the operated side. C: autoradiogram generated over a brainstem section taken from a control animal (the orientation and magnification are identical to those seen in A). This section had been incubated in 5 nM [^{3}H]-pirenzepine for 60 min. Dense binding can be seen in the DVC (arrow) but is clearly less extensive than that seen in sections incubated in [^{3}H]-QNB (compare with A). In particular, there is no binding visible in the hypoglossal nucleus and much less binding in lateral and ventral subdivisions of the NTS. D: autoradiogram similar to that shown in C, but generated over a section taken from a ferret that had received a unilateral vagus nerve lesion (nodose ganglion removal) approximately two weeks prior to the binding experiment. Binding ipsilateral to the lesion (arrow) has almost totally disappeared. Taken together, these studies indicate the strong possibility that M_1 muscarinic receptors are located presynaptically on proximal terminals of vagal afferent fibres in the AP and dorsomedial NTS of the DVC.

Other authors (Bhargava *et al.*, 1981) have shown that when naloxone is given alone and in high doses into the fourth ventricle, it causes vomiting which occurs even in animals which have had a previous CTZ ablation. How, then, can opiates exert both emetic and anti-emetic actions?

The realization that multiple opiate receptors exist (Lord *et al.*, 1977), and the development of more specific ligands for these receptors, provided the basis for reassessing this rather confused picture. Harris (1982) postulated that action at the *mu* opiate receptor might underly the anti-emetic effects of opiates and that the emetic effects are due to agonism at the delta receptor. With the advent of relatively selective *mu* and *delta* ligands, some evidence now exists to support this contention (Blancquaert *et al.*, 1986). These authors used morphine, fentanyl and methadone at doses aimed to achieve some degree of selective agonism at *mu* opiate receptors and found that they inhibited emesis due to apomorphine and copper sulphate in dogs. The *delta* opiate receptor agonist, [D-Ala^2, Met^5] enkephalinamide (DALA) had no anti-emetic activity but was emetic when given alone and the emetic response was diminished if animals were pretreated with naloxone.

The spectrum of anti-emetic activity of opiates is broad and includes vomiting due to opiates themselves as discussed above (Bhargava *et al.*, 1981; Costello and Borison, 1977; Lefebvre *et al.*, 1981), copper sulphate (Blancquaert *et al.*, 1986), apomorphine (Leake, 1922; Costello and Borison, 1977; Bhargava *et al.*, 1981; Lefebvre *et al.*, 1981; Blancquaert *et al.*, 1986), nicotine (Beleslin *et al.*, 1981), emetine (Leake, 1922) and cisplatin (Florczyk *et al.*, 1982).

The hypothesis that the emetic action of opiates is mediated via *delta* receptors in the CTZ and the anti-emetic action via *mu* receptors at a site within the emetic cascade sufficiently 'downstream' to affect such diverse emetic stimuli is far from clear and warrants further investigation.

6.3.7 OTHER NEUROMODULATORS

As already noted elsewhere (e.g. Barnes, 1984; Leslie, 1985) a majority of known neurotransmitters and neuromodulators has at one time or another been implicated in the control of function at the level of the DVC, and many of these have been suggested to be important in the modulation of nausea and/or vomiting.

Much recent work has focussed on the role of neuropeptides such as oxytocin, vasopressin (AVP), substance P, cholecystokinin (CCK), angiotensin II (AII) and neuropeptide Y (NPY) in the DVC. Clearly, the major role of these compounds is to mediate a variety of autonomic responses, and some may have little or nothing to do with gastro-intestinal control at all. For example, AII and AVP are implicated in the control of heart rate and blood pressure while substance P has been extensively investigated as a modulator of pain. On the other hand, some of these neuropeptides may be very important in the mediation of nausea and vomiting. For example, Hawthorn *et al.* (1988) have shown that vasopressin and oxytocin (both powerful stimuli that evoke vomiting in that experimental animal model) are released in response to abdominal vagal afferent stimulation or apomorphine administration in the ferret. CCK is also implicated in the control of satiety and as such may well play a role in modulation of nausea (Leslie, 1985). Many of the known neuromodulators and their respective receptors are found in considerable numbers in the DVC and reasonably direct pathways exist between elements of the DVC and the main autonomic control centres of the forebrain such as the hypothalamus (Sawchenko, 1983; Leslie *et al.*, 1992). Thus, some or all of these modulators may be involved in mediating some aspects of the 'quasi-autonomic' functions of nausea and emesis.

Table 2.1 (above) lists most of the neuroactive compounds that have been found by various techniques to be involved in the AP and NTS. Although not exhaustive, these lists indicate that most of the known neurotransmitters and neuromodulators are represented. As mentioned above, these brainstem structures are responsible for a wide range of physiological control processes, most having to do with aspects of the autonomic nervous system. The vomiting response, however, involves to a very large degree the activation of somatic musculature of the abdomen and thorax to effect expulsion of gut contents. The major function of the DVC and higher brain centres in this regard, therefore, appears to be to integrate the sensory information received from the periphery, via either vagal afferent nerve fibres or the bloodstream; this information is processed in the DVC and elsewhere and co-ordinated output to many other centres is made. These targets include (1) the spinal cord where phrenic nerve efferents along with motor fibres to the abdominal wall musculature are responsible for expulsion of stomach contents via the oesophagus, (2) cerebral cortex to notify conscious levels of events in the abdomen and elsewhere, and (3) higher autonomic nervous centres to co-ordinate cardiac, respiratory and gastric smooth muscle responses appropriate to cope with the complex process of vomiting.

6.5 CONCLUSIONS

Despite the large amount of research effort that has been devoted to the subject over the last decades, we are still little closer to an understanding of which specific neurotransmitters or neuromodulators (as represented in Table 2.1) are specifically linked with any of these processes. Indeed, it may well be that there is no one-to-one relationship between specific physiological functions and specific neuroactive substances; the failure to find a universally effective anti-emetic drug would support such a suggestion. As we have seen, even the most effective anti-emetic compounds yet found for cytotoxic drug-induced emesis, the 5-HT_3 receptor antagonists, seem to be ineffective in many other cases of emesis (motion sickness, for example) and are not even 100% effective in the chemotherapy clinic. The complexity of the processes would argue, in a teleological sense, against there being such simple relationships in any case. For instance, it is clearly necessary to inhibit respiratory reactions during the act of vomiting, and to limit gastro-intestinal mobility and co-ordinate peripheral blood flow to suit the circumstance. It is difficult to see how only one level of neurophysiological control (i.e. the level of transmitter and receptor distribution within the nervous system) could cope with such a task. Certainly many more levels of neurological control come into play to effect this co-ordinated integration of function: patterns of neuronal connectivity, differential receptor distributions, hormonal influence on neuronal firing, 'second' and 'third' messenger activity in the neurons involved – all probably play their part. Thus, intervention at any one of these levels (blocking all activity at 5-HT_3 receptors, for instance) may be a partially effective means of controlling inappropriate or unwanted activity such as chemotherapeutic-induced emesis, but the probability is that it will never provide the complete answer.

ACKNOWLEDGEMENTS

The authors wish to thank Dr Pedro Loewenstein who collaborated on the studies reported here on muscarinic receptor localization in the ferret dorsal vagal complex and generously allowed us to quote these results. We would also like to thank Ms Jenny Harvey who provided invaluable technical assistance and Dr H. McQuay for helpful discussions.

REFERENCES

Andrews, P.L.R. (1986) Vagal afferent innervation of the gastrointestinal tract. *Prog. Brain Res.*, **67**, 65–85.

Andrews, P.L.R. and Hawthorn, J. (1987) Evidence for an extra-abdominal site of action for the 5-HT_3 receptor antagonist BRL 24924 in the inhibition of radiation-evoked emesis in the ferret. *Neuropharmacol.* **26**, 1367–70.

Andrews, P.L.R., Rapeport, W.G. and Sanger, G.J. (1988) Neuropharmacology of emesis induced by anti-cancer therapy. *Trends Pharmacol. Sci.*, **9**, 334–41.

Andrews, P.L.R., Davis, C.J., Bingham, S., Davidson, H.I.M., Hawthorn, J. and Maskell, L. (1990) The abdominal visceral innervation and the emetic reflex: pathways, pharmacology, and plasticity. *Can. J. Physiol. Pharmacol.*, **68**, 325–45.

Armstrong, D.M., Saper, C.B., Levey, A.I., *et al.* (1983) Distribution of cholinergic neurons in rat brain: demonstrated by the immunocytochemical localization of choline acetyltransferase. *J. Comp. Neurol.*, **216**, 53–68.

Barnes, J.H. (1984) The physiology and pharmacology of emesis. *Molec. Aspects Med.*, **7**, 397–508.

Beleslin, D.B., Krstic, S.K., Stfanovic-Denic, K. *et al.* (1981) Inhibition by morphine and morphine-like drugs of nicotine-induced emesis in cats. *Brain Res. Bull.*, **6**, 451–53.

Beleslin, D.B. and Krstic, S.K. (1987) Further studies on nicotine-induced emesis: nicotinic mediation in area postrema. *Physiol. Behav.*, **39**, 681–86.

Beleslin, D.B. and Strbac, M. (1987) Noradrenalin-induced emesis: alpha-2 adrenoceptor mediation in the area postrema. *Neuropharmacol.*, **26**, 1157–65.

Beleslin, D.B., Strbac, M., Jovanovic-Micic, D. *et al.* (1989) Area postrema: cholinergic and noradrenergic regulation of emesis. A new concept. *Arch. Int. Physiol. Biochem.*, **97**, 107–15.

Bhargava, K.P. and Dixit, K.S. (1968) Role of the chemoreceptor trigger zone in histamine-induced emesis. *Br. J. Pharmacol.*, **34**, 508–13.

Bhargava, K.P., Dixit, K.S. and Palit, G. (1976) Nature of histamine receptors in the emetic chemoreceptor trigger zone. *Br. J. Pharmacol.*, **57**, 211–13.

Bhargava, K.P., Dixit, K.S. and Gupta, Y.K. (1981) Enkephalin receptors in the emetic chemoreceptor trigger zone of the dog. *Br. J. Pharmacol.*, **72**, 471–75.

Blancquaert, J.P., Lefebvre, R.A. and Willems, J.L. (1986) Emetic and antiemetic effects of opioids in the dog. *Eur. J. Pharmacol.*, **128**, 143–50.

Borison, H.L. (1959) Effect of ablation of medullary emetic chemoreceptor trigger zone on vomiting responses to cerebral intraventricular injection of adrenaline, apomorphine and pilocarpine in the cat, *J. Physiol. (Lond)*, **147**, 172–77.

Borison, H.L. (1974) Area postrema: chemoreceptive trigger zone for vomiting – is that all? *Life Sci.*, **14**, 1807–17.

Borison, H.L. and Wang, S.C. (1949) Functional localization of central co-ordinating mechanism for emesis in the cat. *J. Neurophysiol.*, **12**, 305–13.

Borison, H.L. and Wang, S.C. (1951) Quantitative effects of radon implanted in the medulla oblongata: a technique for producing discrete lesions. *J. Comp. Neurol.*, **94**, 33–56.

Borison, H.L. and Wang, S.C. (1953) Physiology and pharmacology of vomiting. *Pharmac. Rev.*, **5**, 193–230.

Brizzee, K.R., Calton, F.M. and Vitale, D.E. (1958) Effects of selective placement of lesions in lower brain stem structures on X-irradiation in the dog. *Anat. Rec.*, **130**, 533–41.

Brizzee, K.R., Ordy, J.M. and Mehler, W.R. (1980) Effect of ablation of area postrema on frequency and latency of motion sickness-induced emesis in the squirrel monkey. *Physiol. Behav.*, **24**, 849–53.

Brizzee, K.R. and Mehler, W.R. (1986) 'The central nervous connections involved in the vomiting reflex', in *Nausea and Vomiting*: Mechanisms and Treatment, (eds C.J., Davis, G.V. Lake-Bakaar and D.G. Grahame-Smith) pp. 31–55. Springer-Verlag, Berlin.

Caccia, S., Conti, I., Vigano, G. and Garattini, S. (1986) l-(2-Pyrimidinyl)-piperazine as active metabolite of buspirone in man and rat. *Pharmacology*, **33**, 46–51.

Carpenter, D.O. (1989) 'Central nervous system mechanisms in deglutition and emesis', in *Handbook of Physiology* Vol. 6: *Motility and Circulation* (ed. J.D. Wood), pp. 685–714. American Physiological Society, Bethesda, MD.

Carpenter, D.O., Briggs, D.B. and Strominger, N.

(1983) Responses of neurons of canine area postrema to neurotransmitters and peptides. *Cell. Molec. Neurobiol.*, **3**, 113–26.

Carpenter, D.O., Briggs, D.B., Knox, A.P. and Strominger, N.L. (1986) Radiation-induced emesis in the dog: effects of lesions and drugs. *Radiation Res.*, **108**, 307–17.

Chevallier, B. (1990) Efficacy and safety of granisetron compared with high-dose metoclopramide plus dexamethasone in patients receiving high-dose cisplatin in a single-blind study. *Eur. J. Cancer*, **26** (Suppl. 1), S33–S36.

Chinn, H.I. and Wang, S.C. (1954) Locus of the emetic action following irradiation. *Proc. Soc. Exp. Biol. Med.*, **85**, 472–74.

Cookson, R.F. (1986) 'Mechanisms and treatment of post-operative nausea and vomiting', in *Nausea and Vomiting: Mechanisms and Treatment*, (eds C.J. Davis, G.V. Lake-Bakaar, and D.G. Grahame-Smith), pp. 130–50. Springer-Verlag, Berlin.

Costello, D. and Borison, H. (1977) Naloxone antagonizes narcotic self blockade of emesis in the cat. *J. Pharmacol. Exp. Therap.* **203**, 222–30.

Davis, C.J., Harding, R.K., Leslie, R.A., and Andrews, P.L.R. (1986) 'The organisation of vomiting as a protective reflex', in *Nausea and Vomiting: Mechanisms and Treatment*, (eds C.J. Davis, G.V. Lake-Bakaar and D.G. Grahame-Smith), pp. 65–75. Springer-Verlag, Berlin.

Dumuis, A., Bouhelal, R., Sebben, M. and Bockaert, J. (1988) A 5-HT receptor in the central nervous system, positively coupled with adenylate cyclase, is antagonized by ICS 205–930. *Eur. J. Pharmacol.*, **146**, 187–88.

Feldberg, W. and Sherwood, S.L. (1984) Injections of drugs into the lateral ventricle of the cat. *J. Physiol. (Lond)*, **123**, 148–67.

Florczyk, A.P., Schurig, J.E. and Bradner, W.T. (1982) Cisplatin-induced emesis in the ferret: a new animal model. *Cancer Treat. Rep.*, **66**, 187–89.

Fozard, J.R. (1984) Neuronal 5-HT receptors in the periphery. *Neuropharmacology*, **23**, 1473–86.

Fozard, J.R. (1989) 'Agonists and antagonists at 5-HT_3 receptors', in *Cardiovascular Pharmacology of 5-hydroxytryptamine*, (ed P.R. Saxena, *et al.*) pp. 101–15. Kluwer, Dordrecht.

Fuxe, K. and Owman, C. (1965) Cellular localization of monoamines in the area postrema of certain mammals. *J. Comp. Neurol.*, **125**, 337–54.

Gaddum, J.H. and Picarelli, Z.P. (1957) Two kinds of tryptamine receptor. *Br. J. Pharmacol.*, **12**, 323–28.

Gaudin-Chazal, G., Seyfritz, N., Araneda, S. *et al.* (1982) Selective retrograde transport of [^{3}H]-serotonin in vagal afferents. *Brain Res. Bull.*, **8**, 503–9.

Gotow, T. and Hashimoto, P.H. (1979) Fine structure of the ependyma and intercellular junctions in the area postrema of the rat. *Cell Tiss. Res.*, **201**, 207–25.

Gwyn, D.G. and Wolstencroft, J.H. (1968) Cholinesterases in the area subpostrema. *J. Comp. Neurol.*, **133**, 289–308.

Gwyn, D.G. and Leslie, R.A. (1979) A projection of vagus nurve to the area subpostrema in the cat. *Brain Res.*, **161**, 335–41.

Gwyn, D.G., Leslie, R.A. and Hopkins, D.A. (1979) Gastric afferents to the nucleus of the solitary tract in the cat. *Neurosci. Lett.*, **14**, 13–17.

Gwyn, D.G., Leslie, R.A. and Hopkins, D.A. (1985) Observations on the afferent and efferent organization of the vagus nerve and the innervation of the stomach in the squirrel monkey. *J. Comp. Neurol.*, **239**, 163–75.

Harding, R.K. and McDonald, T.J. (1989) Identification of PYY as an emetic peptide in the dog. *Peptides*, **10**, 21–24.

Harrington, R.A., Hamilton, C.W., Brogden, R.N. *et al.* (1983) Metoclopramide. An updated review of its pharmacological properties and clinical use. *Drugs*, **25**, 451–94.

Harris, A.L. (1982) Cytotoxic therapy-induced vomiting is mediated via enkephalin pathways. *Lancet*, I, 714–16.

Harris, A.L. and Canwell, B.M.J. (1986) 'Mechanisms and treatment of cytotoxic-induced nausea and vomiting', in *Nausea and Vomiting: Mechanisms and Treatment* (eds C.J. Davis, G.V. Lake-Bakaar and D.G. Grahame-Smith), pp. 78–93. Springer-Verlag Berlin.

Hatcher, R.A. and Weiss, S. (1923) Studies on vomiting. *J. Pharmacol.*, **22**, 139–93.

Hawthorn, J., Andrews, P.L.R., Ang, V.T.Y. and Jenkins, J.S. (1988) Differential release of vasopressin and oxytocin in response to abdominal vagal afferent stimulation or apomorphine in the ferret. *Brain Res.*, **438**, 193–98.

Helke, C.J., Handelmann, G.E. and Jacobowitz, D.M.

(1983) Choline acetyltransferase activity in the nucleus tractus solitarius: regulation by the afferent vagus nerve. *Brain Res. Bull.*, **10**, 433–36.

Higgins, G.A., Kilpatrick, G.J., Bunce, K.T. *et al.* (1989) 5-HT_3 receptor antagonists injected into the area postrema inhibit cisplatin-induced emesis in the ferret. *Br. J. Pharmacol.*, **97**, 247–55.

Isaacs, B. (1956) The influence of hyoscine and atropine on apomorphine – induced vomiting in man. *Clinical Science*, **15**, 177–82.

Kalia, M. and Mesulam, M.M. (1980) Brain stem projections of sensory and motor components of the vagus complex in the cat. II Laryngeal, tracheo-brochial, pulmonary, cardiac and gastrointestinal branches. *J. Comp. Neurol.*, **193**, 467–508.

Kalia, M., Fuxe, K. and Goldstein, M. (1985) Rat medulla oblongata II. Dopaminergic, noradrenergic (A1 and A2) and adrenergic neurons, nerve fibres and presumptive terminal processes. *J. Comp. Neurol.*, **233**, 308–32.

Kessler, J.P. and Jean, A. (1985) Identification of the medullary swallowing regions in the rat. *Exp. Brain Res.*, **57**, 256–66.

Kessler, J.P. and Jean, A. (1986) Inhibitory influence of monoamines and brain stem monoaminergic regions on the medullary swallowing reflex. *Neurosci. Lett.*, **65**, 41–8.

Leake, C.D. (1922) The action of morphine on the vomiting centre in the dog. *J. Pharm. Exp. Therap.*, **20**, 359–64.

Lefebvre, R.A., Willems, J.L. and Bogaert, M.G. (1981) Gastric relaxation and vomiting by apomorphine, morphine and fentanyl in the conscious dog. *Eur. J. Pharmacol.*, **69**, 139–45.

Leslie, R.A. (1985) Neuroactive substances in the dorsal vagal complex of the medulla oblongata: nucleus of the tractus solitarius, area postrema, and dorsal motor nucleus of the vagus. *Neurochem. Internat.*, **7**, 191–211.

Leslie, R.A. (1986) Comparative aspects of the area postrema: fine-structural considerations help to determine its function. *Cell. Molec. Neurobiol.*, **6**, 95–120.

Leslie, R.A., Gwyn, D.G. and Hopkins, D.A. (1982a) The central distribution of the cervical vagus nerve and gastric afferent and efferent projections in the rat, *Brain Res. Bull.*, **8**, 37–42.

Leslie, R.A., Gwyn, D.G. and Hopkins, D.A. (1982b) The ultrastructure of the subnucleus gelatinosus of the nucleus of the tractus solitarius in the cat, *J. Comp. Neurol.*, **206**, 109–18.

Leslie, R.A. and Gwyn, D.G. (1984) Neuronal connections of the area posterma. *Fed. Proc.*, **43**, 2941–43.

Leslie, R.A., Shah, Y., Thejomayen, M., Murphy, K.M. and Robertson, H.A. (1989) The neuropharmacology of emesis: the role of receptors in neuromodulation of nausea and vomiting. *Can. J. Physiol. Pharmacol.*, **68**, 279–88.

Leslie, R.A., Reynolds, D.J.M., Andrews, P.L.R. *et al.* (1990) Evidence for presynaptic 5-HT_3 recognition sites on vagal afferent terminals in the brainstem of the ferret. *Neurosci.*, **38**, 667–73.

Leslie, R.A. and Reynolds, D.J.M. (1991) 'The area postrema and vomiting: how important is serotonin?' in *Current Aspects of the Neurosciences* Vol. 3, (ed N.N. Osborne), pp. 79–101, MacMillan, London.

Leslie, R.A., Reynolds, D.J.M. and Lawes, I.N.C. (1992) 'Central connections of the nuclei of the vagus nerve', P81–98. In Neuroanatomy and physiology of abdominal vagal afferents (eds. S. Ritter, R.C. Ritter and C.D. Barnes) CRC Press, Boca Raton, U.S.A.

Lindstrom, P.A. and Brizzee, K.R. (1962) Relief of intractable vomiting from surgical lesions in the area postrema. *J. Neurosurg.*, **19**, 228–36.

Loewy, A.D. and Burton, H. (1978) Nuclei of the solitary tract: efferent projections to the lower brain stem and spinal cord of the cat. *J. Comp. Neurol.*, **181**, 421–50.

Longo, D.L., Wesley, M., Howser, D. *et al.* (1985) Results of a randomized double-blind crossover trial of scopolamine versus placebo administered by transdermal patch for the control of cisplatin-induced emesis. *Cancer Treat. Rep.*, **66**, 1975–76.

Lord, J.A.H., Waterfield, A.A., Hughes, J. and Kosterlitz, H.W. (1977) Endogenous opioid peptides: multiple agonists and receptors. *Nature*, **276**, 495–99.

Lucot, J.B. and Crampton, G.H. (1987) Buspirone blocks cisplatin-induced emesis in cats. *J. Clin. Pharmacol.*, **27**, 817–18.

McMillen, B.A. and Mattiace, L.A. (1983) Comparative neuropharmacology of buspirone and MJ-13805, a potential anti-anxiety drug. *J. Neural. Trans.*, **57**, 25–265.

Miller, A.D. and Wilson, V.J. (1983) 'Vomiting

center' reanalyzed: an electrical stimulation study. *Brain Res.*, **270**, 154–58.

Miner, W.D. and Sanger, G.J. (1986) Inhibition of cisplatin-induced vomiting by selective 5-hydroxytryptamine M receptor antagonism. *Br. J. Pharmacol.*, **88**, 497–99.

Palacios, J.M., Wamsley, J.K. and Kuhar, M.J. (1981) The distribution of histamine H_1 receptors in the rat brain: an autoradiographic study. *Neurosci.*, **6**, 15–37.

Palkovits, M. (1985) Distribution of neuroactive substances in the dorsal vagal complex of the medulla oblongata. *Neurochem. Internat.*, **7**, 213–19.

Palkovits, M. and Jacobowitz, D.M. (1974) Topographic atlas of catecholamine and acetylcholinesterase-containing neurons in the rat brain. II. Hindbrain (mesencephalon, rhombencephalon). *J. Comp. Neurol.*, **157**, 29–41.

Pazos, A., Probst, A. and Palacios, J.M. (1987a) Serotonin receptors in the human brain. III. Autoradiographic mapping of serotonin-1 receptors. *Neurosci.*, **21**, 97–122.

Pazos, A., Probst, A. and Palacios, J.M. (1987b) Serotonin receptors in the human brain. IV. Autoradiographic mapping of serotonin-2 receptors. *Neurosci.*, **21**, 123–29.

Pedigo, N.W. and Brizzee, K.R. (1985) Muscarinic cholinergic receptors in area postrema and brainstem areas regulating emesis. *Brain Res. Bull.*, **14**, 169–77.

Peroutka, S.J. and Snyder, S.H. (1982) Antiemetics: neurotransmitter receptor binding predicts therapeutic actions. *Lancet* **II**, 658–59.

Pratt, G.D. and Bowery, N.G. (1989) The 5-HT_3 receptor ligand [^{3}H]-BRL 43694 binds to presynaptic sites in the nucleus tractus solitarius of the rat. *Neuropharmacol.*, **28**, 1367–76.

Pratt, G.D., Bowery, N.G., Kilpatrick, G.J. *et al.* (1990) Consensus meeting agrees distribution of 5-HT_3 receptors in mammalian hindbrain. *Trends Pharm. Sci.*, **11**, 135–37.

Rawlins, M.D., Taylor, W.B. and Bateman, D.N. (1986) 'Rational approaches to therapy for nausea and vomiting: two common solutions', in *Nausea and Vomiting: Mechanisms and Treatment* (eds C.J. Davis, G.V. Lake-Bakaar and D.G. Grahame-Smith), pp. 167–71, Springer-Verlag, Berlin.

Reynolds, D.J.M., Leslie, R.A., Grahame-Smith, D.G. and Harvey, J.M. (1989) Localization of 5-HT_3 receptor binding sites in human dorsal vagal complex. *Eur. J. Pharmacol.*, **173**, 127–30.

Reynolds, D.J.M., Leslie, R.A., Grahame-Smith, D.G. and Harvey, J.M. (1991) Autoradiographic localization of 5-HT_3 receptor ligand binding in the cat brainstem. *Neurochem. Internat.*, **18**, 69–73.

Reynolds, D.J.M., Barber, N.A., Grahame-Smith, D.G. and Leslie, R.A. (1991) Cisplatin-evoked induction of c-*fos* protein in the brainstem of the ferret: the effect of cervical vagotomy and the anti-emetic 5-HT_3 receptor antagonist granisetron (BRL 43694). *Brain Res.* **565**, 231–6.

Robertson, H.A. and Leslie, R.A. (1985) Noradrenergic $alpha_2$ binding sites in vagal dorsal motor nucleus and nucleus tractus solitarius: autoradiographic localization. *Can. J. Physiol. Pharmacol.*, **63**, 1190–94.

Roylance, R.R., Andrews, P.L.R., Hawthorn, J. *et al.* (1989) The antiemetic effects of atropine sulphate in the ferret. *Br. J. Pharmacol.*, **96**, 330P.

Saavedra, J.M., Brownstein, M.J., Kizer, J.S. and Palkovits, M. (1976) Biogenic amines and related enzymes in the circumventricular organs of the rat. *Brain Res.*, **107**, 412–17.

Sanger, G.J. (1984) 'Mechanisms by which metoclopramide can increase gastrointestinal activity', in (eds A. Bennett and G. Velo) *Mechanisms of Gastrointestinal Motility and Secretion*, pp. 303–24, Plenum Press, New York.

Sanger, G.J. (1987) Increased gut cholinergic activity and antagonism of 5-hydroxytryptamine M-receptors by BRL 24924: potential clinical importance of BRL 24924. *Br. J. Pharmacol.*, **91**, 77–87.

Sawchenko, P.E. (1983) Central connections of the sensory and motor nuclei of the vagus nerve. *J. Autonom. Nerv. Syst.*, **9**, 13–26.

Sawicka, J. and Sallan, S. (1977) Transdermal therapeutics system, scopolamine (TS): prevention of vomiting associated with cancer chemotherapy. *Soc. Clin. Oncol.* **18**, 302.

Shapiro, R.C. and Miselis, R.R. (1985) The central neural connections of the area postrema of the rat. *J. Comp. Neurol.*, **234**, 344–64.

Schwartz, J.C., Agid, Y., Bouthenet, M.L. *et al.* (1986) 'Neurochemical investigations into the human area postrema', in *Nausea and Vomiting: Mechanisms and Treatment*, (eds C.J. Davis, G.V.

Lake-Bakaar, and D.G. Grahame-Smith), pp. 18–30. Springer-Verlag, Berlin.

Smith, W.L., Callahan, E.M. and Alphin, R.S. (1988) The emetic activity of centrally administered cisplatin in cats and its antagonism by Zacopride. *J. Pharm. Pharmacol.*, **40**, 142–43.

Stefanini, E. and Clement-Cormier, Y. (1981) Detection of dopamine receptors in the area postrema. *Eur. J. Pharmacol.*, **74**, 257–60.

Taber, E. (1961) The cytoarchitecture of the brain stem of the cat. I Brain stem nuclei of cat. *J. Comp. Neurol.*, **116**, 27–69.

Torack, R.M. and Finke, E.H. (1971) Evidence for a sequestration of function within the area postrema based on scanning electron microscopy and the penetration of horseradish peroxidase. *Z. Zellforsch.*, **118**, 85–96.

Waeber, C., Hoyer, D. and Palacios, J.M. (1989) 5 hydroxytryptamine$_3$ receptors in the human brain: autoradiographic visualization using [^{3}H]ICS205 930. *Neuroscience*, **31**, 393–400.

Wang, S.C. and Borison, H.L. (1952) A new concept of organization of the central emetic mechanism: recent studies on the sites of action of apomorphine, copper sulphate and cardiac glycosides, *Gastroenterology*, **22**, 1–12.

Wang, S.C. and Chinn, H.I. (1954) Experimental motion sickness in dogs, Functional importance of chemoreceptive emetic trigger zone. *Am. J. Physiol.*, **178**, 111–16.

Wang, S.C. and Chinn, H.I. (1956) Experimental motion sickness in dogs. Importance of labyrinth and vestibular cerebellum, *Am. J. Physiol.*, **185**, 617–23.

7

The mechanism of emesis induced by anti-cancer therapies

P.L.R. ANDREWS and C.J. DAVIS

7.1 INTRODUCTION

The physiology of vomiting has been studied to varying degrees for several hundred years with the initial research focusing for the most part on the mechanics of the expulsion of gastric contents. This type of study is illustrated by the experiments of Magendie reported in his 'Memoire sur le Vomissement' (1813) in which the stomach of a dog was replaced by a pig's bladder and it was demonstrated that the contents of the bladder could be expelled when the animal was given an emetic. The identification of the mechanisms by which emetic agents trigger the emetic reflex began at the turn of the twentieth century with the studies of Magnus, Cannon, Hesse and Hatcher and Weiss (reviewed by Hatcher in 1924). Although these studies identified many of the fundamental aspects of the reflex (e.g. the co-ordinating action of the brainstem, defining gut irritation as a stimulus, and the sensitivity of the fourth ventricle to emetic stimuli) it was not until the studies by Borison, Brizzee and Wang in the late 1940s that the modern view of the emetic reflex, controlled by a 'vomiting centre', receiving inputs from various emetic detectors such as the gut, vestibular labyrinths and the chemoreceptor trigger zone, began to emerge. It is against this background of increased understanding of the physiology and pharmacology of the emetic reflex that the development of anti-cancer therapies should be considered. Although emesis was known to occur with therapeutic doses of X-radiation and following treatment with a number of the prototypical cytotoxic drugs such as nitrogen mustard, it was the introduction of the highly emetic but highly effective anti-tumour agent cisplatin which rekindled interest in the problem of chemotherapy-induced emesis. The importance of the problem was particularly apparent with cisplatin because at high doses it induces severe emesis in virtually all patients with some refusing further courses of potentially curative treatment because of this; this is a considerable problem as many of the patients receiving cisplatin are young men with testicular tumours. Our current understanding of the mechanism of emesis induced by both radio- and chemotherapy is based on the conceptual framework provided initially by the studies of Wang and Borison (1952) but extended by more recent studies of the emetic pathways (Andrews *et al.*, 1990b) and most recently by the critical insights into the pharmacology of these pathways that have been provided by the 5-HT_3 receptor antagonist drugs (Chapter 9).

Emesis in Anti-cancer Therapy
Mechanisms and treatment
Published in 1993 by Chapman & Hall, London
ISBN 0 412 37250 9

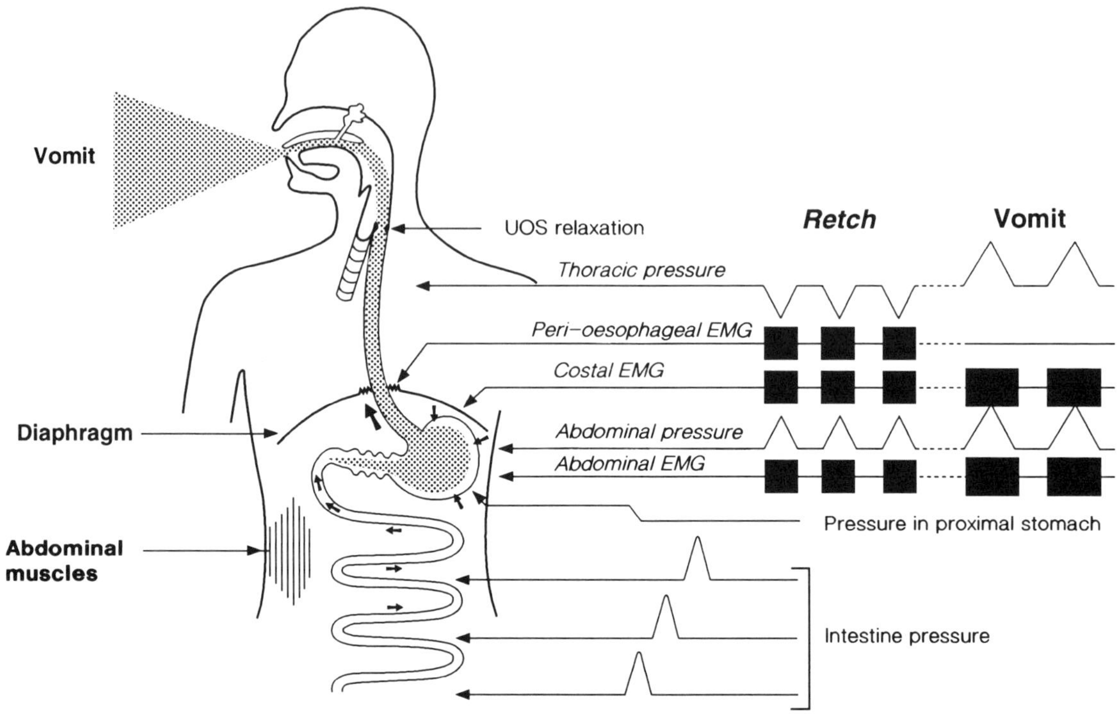

Figure 7.1 A summary of the major visceral and somatic motor events in retching and vomiting. (Adapted from Andrews and Hawthorn 1988, and Grundy *et al.*, 1991.)

Against such a background this chapter reviews the current hypotheses of the mechanisms by which cytotoxic drugs and ionizing radiation induce emesis and highlights a number of areas which still require experimental investigation.

7.2 GENERAL MECHANISMS OF EMESIS

For convenience, the three major components comprising the vomiting reflex, motor outputs, integrative mechanisms and emetic stimulus detectors will be discussed separately.

7.2.1 MOTOR COMPONENTS

The often spectacular expulsion of vomitus from the mouth is the most obvious motor component of the vomiting reflect but in fact it is only the last in a chain of events under the control of both the autonomic and somatic divisions of the nervous system. Almost irrespective of the cause of the emesis the pattern of motor activity described below is the same and hence the vomiting reflex may in some respects be considered as a 'stereotyped motor programme'. The motor components of the reflex can be conveniently divided into two separate but usually consecutive phases: a pre-ejection or prodromal phase and an ejection or vomiting phase; these will be discussed separately and are summarized in Figure 7.1.

7.2.1.1 Pre-ejection phase

This phase is usually accompanied by the sensation of nausea, the physiological basis of which, as has been said, is still poorly understood (see below and Chapter 4). Common signs associated with nausea are cold sweating, cutaneous vasoconstriction, pupil dilatation and tachycardia – all mediated by sympathetic nerve activation – and salivation mediated by parasympathetic nerves. These changes are probably a general indicator of autonomic arousal associated with the stressful nature of nausea. Of more significance are the changes that occur in the gut in the period immediately prior to the onset of retching and vomiting. The initial event appears to be a profound relaxation of the proximal stomach mediated by vagal efferent nerves supplying intramural non-adrenergic, non-cholinergic neurons (NANC). The transmitter used by these neurons is probably vasoactive intestinal polypeptide, although dopamine, purines and, most recently, nitric oxide have all been implicated (Andrews, 1986a; Lefebvre *et al.*, 1992). Gastric acid secretion also appears to be inhibited at this time. After the onset of the gastric relaxation a single contraction originates in the mid-small intestine and propagates in a retrograde fashion towards the stomach. Because of its large magnitude it is termed the retrograde giant contraction (RGC). The RGC is also under vagal control but the transmitter involved is acetylcholine.

While these two gastro-intestinal motor events do not lead to the direct expulsion of the gastric contents they do have important functions which are best appreciated when the vomiting reflex is viewed from its function as a protective reflex against the accidental ingestion of contaminated food (Davis *et al.*, 1986). The gastric relaxation probably serves to confine any ingested toxin to the stomach from where it can be readily ejected and in addition relaxation may place the stomach in the most mechanically advantageous position for compression by the diaphragm and abdominal muscles (see below). The RGC returns contaminated intestinal contents to the stomach ready for ejection. In addition, it has been suggested that the alkaline intestinal secretions may help to neutralize the acid gastric contents (Lang, 1990) so reducing damage to the teeth and oesophagus. While these motor changes have a clear function, they are not essential as they do not occur in animals with an abdominal vagotomy in which vomiting still occurs in response to central emetic stimuli (e.g. apomorphine).

Although nausea may continue in 'waves' for many hours and be accompanied by sweating, tachycardia and cutaneous vasoconstriction, the gastro-intestinal changes described above rarely occur without retching and vomiting ensuing. However, retching and vomiting will not begin until the RGC has reached the stomach, illustrating the complexity of the central co-ordinating mechanism (Lang, 1990).

7.2.1.2 Ejection phase

This phase consists of retching and vomiting both of which are under the control of the somatic division of the nervous system. The motor patterns are illustrated in Figure 7.1 (above) and may briefly be summarized as follows. During retching there is contraction of all parts of the diaphragm, synchronous with contraction of the *rectus abdominis* and the external intercostal muscles. The internal intercostal muscles contract out of phase. The net effect of this activity is to produce large rhythmic decreases in intra-thoracic pressure with concomitant increases in intra-abdominal pressure. Although there is intense muscle activity during retching, there is no ejection of gastric contents and it is even debatable whether gastric contents enter the oesophagus at this stage.

Retching is usually followed very shortly by vomiting. The major differences in the underlying motor patterns are that during vomiting there is a relaxation of the peri-oesophageal diaphragm facilitating the passage of gastric contents into the oesophagus; the contraction of the *rectus abdominis* muscles is more powerful and prolonged and the internal intercostal muscles are inactive (Miller, 1990). Thus the expulsive force (several hundred mm Hg) for vomiting is generated by the abdominal muscles and diaphragm which compress the stomach. The characteristic posture adopted by all animals during retching and vomiting is presumably to optimize this compression and to minimize strain on muscle groups and structures not involved in vomiting.

Although the function of vomiting is self-evident that of retching is far from clear. The observation that retching usually precedes vomiting indicates that in some way it is important for the final act of vomiting but this contrasts with the fact that vomiting can occur without any prior retching (e.g. in response to a sudden rise in intra-cranial pressure). In a study of a variety of emetic stimuli in the ferret, including X-radiation and cytotoxic drugs, the temporal pattern of distribution of retching alone and retching accompanied by vomiting was similar (Fig. 7.2) and comparing stimuli there was no marked variation in the number of retches preceding a vomit (Fig. 7.3). Some evidence has emerged suggesting that low intra-gastric volumes facilitate retching and large volumes reduce retching and facilitate vomiting (Andrews *et al.*, 1990b).

Various suggestions have been made about the function of retching including an involvement in overcoming the multi-component lower oesophageal sphincter anti-reflux barrier, sampling the nature of the gastric contents to see if it is sufficiently fluid for ejection, and 'winding up' the central emetic circuitry for conversion to the motor programme of vomiting (reviewed in Andrews *et al.*, 1990b).

It is essential that clinical studies include both retching and vomiting in the assessment of emesis because animal studies of cytotoxic drug- and radiation-induced emesis have shown that while retching in combination with vomiting accounts for about 53% of episodes, retching in isolation accounts for 40% of episodes and vomiting alone for only 7% (Andrews *et al.*, 1990a). Failure to record these separate events accurately can thus lead to distortion of the data, and possibly the drawing of incorrect conclusions as to the nature of the mechanisms involved.

7.2.1.3 Post-ejection phase

Following vomiting it is not uncommon for nausea to be alleviated and the subject to report feeling a little better. This does not occur following retching. Interestingly, vomiting may resolve a migraine attack (Blau, 1990). The mechanism is unknown but release of endorphins would be a logical possibility. Teleologically such a resultant sensation could be rationalized in the following way: nausea is highly aversive and is essential for animals to avoid future ingestion of the toxin but if the animal has already ingested the agent then it could be argued that vomiting should be encouraged and should in this case certainly not be aversive.

7.2.2 CENTRAL INTEGRATIVE MECHANISMS

The commonly used expression 'vomiting centre' originates from classical physiological experiments in which a 'centre' was the term used to describe a relatively discrete brain region from which a particular response could be elicited, usually by electrical stimulation. The existence of such a 'centre' co-ordinating all the aspects of emesis was proposed by Giannuzzi in 1865 (Wang and Borison, 1950). While it is no longer current in physiology to use the term 'centre', in the case of the emetic reflex, it provides a useful shorthand to describe the higher expression of the interactions between the brainstem regions involved in the integration of the inputs from the various emetic detectors and the co-ordination of the motor outputs (Davis *et al.*, 1986).

Two conceptual models have been proposed to describe the central neuronal circuitry

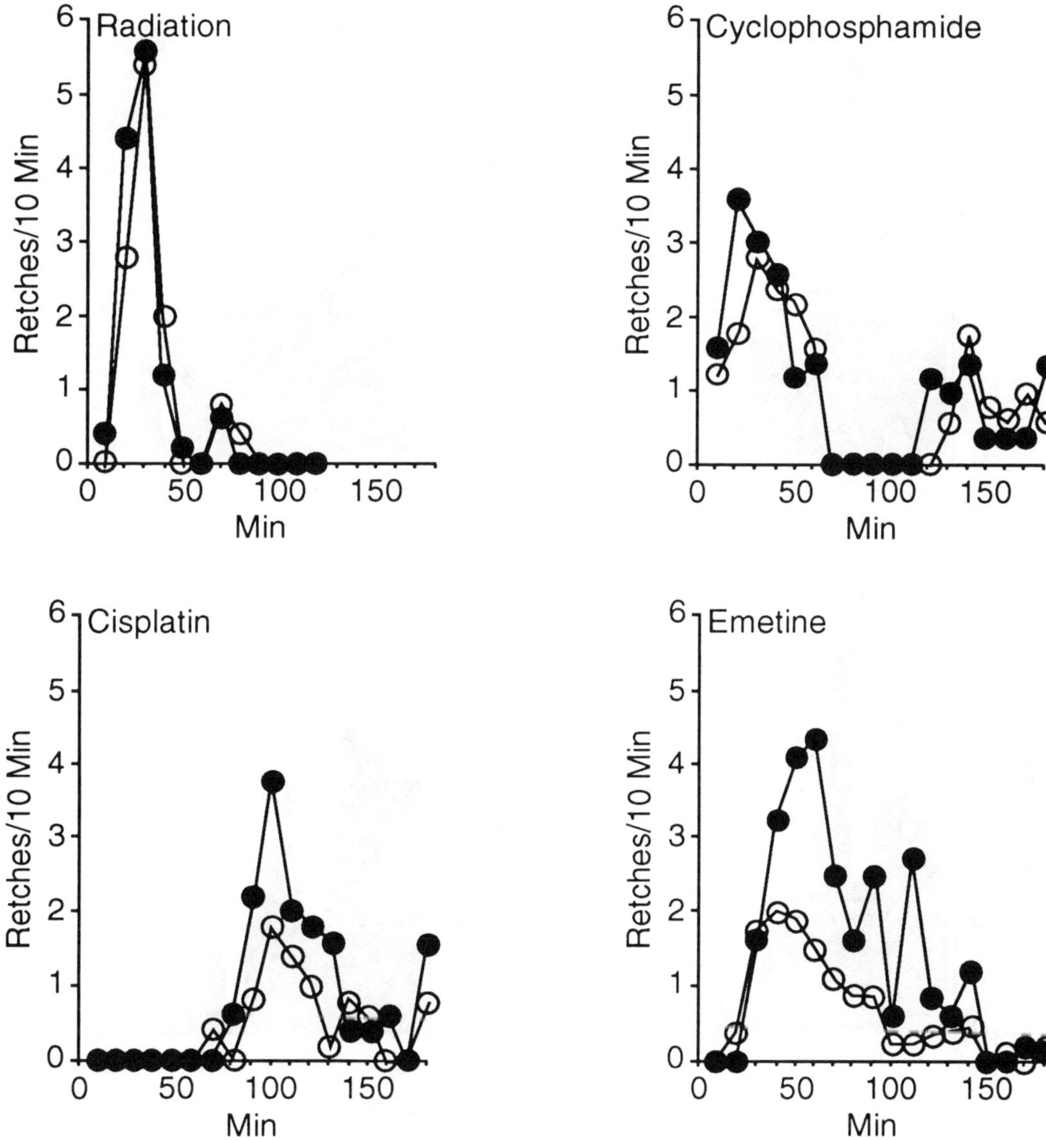

Figure 7.2 Temporal distribution of the incidence of retches alone (open circles) and retches followed by vomits (filled circles) in the ferret following a variety of experimental emetic stimuli. X-axis 10 min. time bins and the Y-axis is the incidence of retching/10 min. (Redrawn from Andrews *et al.*, 1990.)

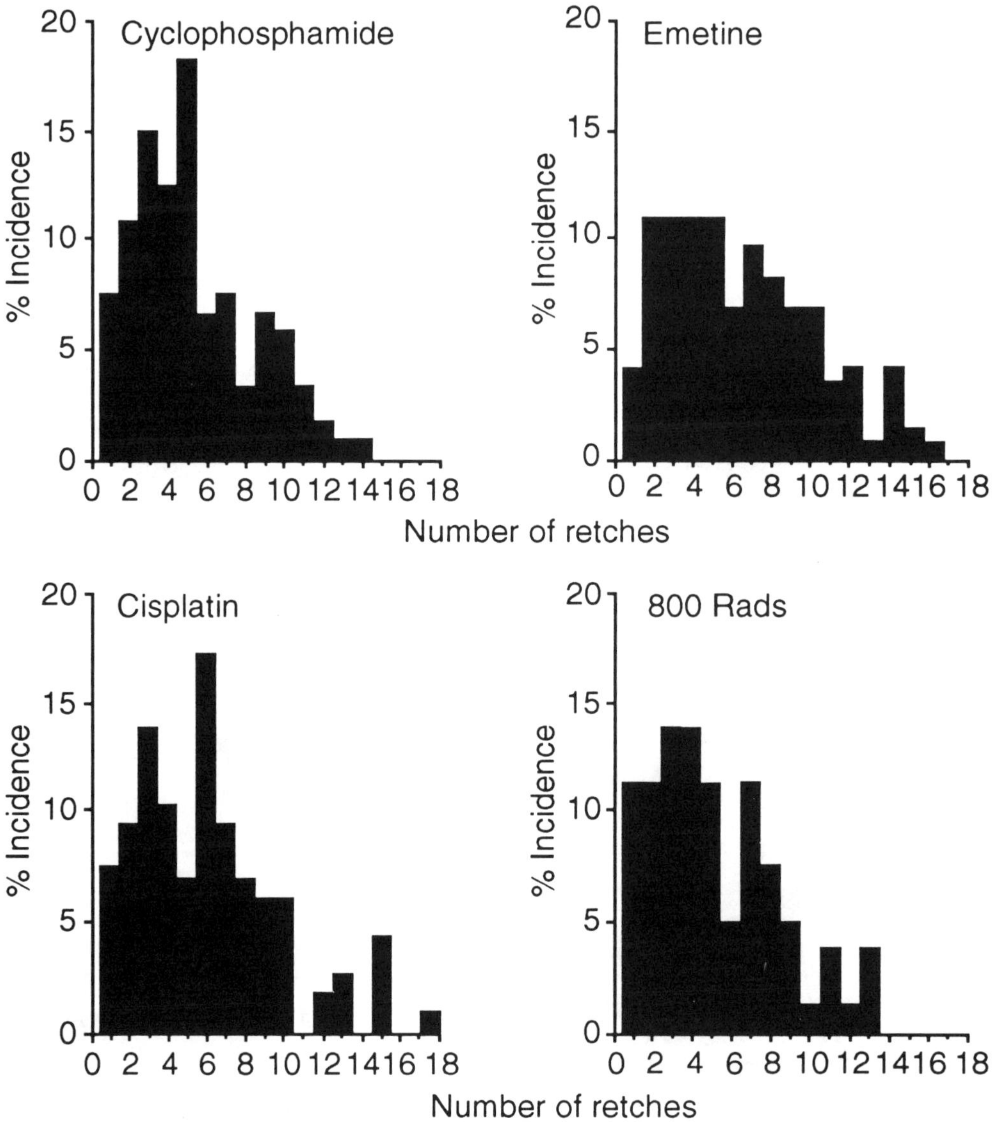

Figure 7.3 The distribution of number of retches preceding each vomit for cyclophosphamide (no. of animals, $n = 6$; total no. of vomits in whole group or total no. of data points in group, $d = 121$), emetine ($n = 6, d = 147$), cisplatin ($n = 6, d = 117$), and 800 rads ($n = 6, d = 80$) as emetic stimuli. The X-axis indicates the no. of retches preceding each vomit during the entire observation period. The Y-axis gives the frequency/incidence as a percentage. (Redrawn from Andrews *et al.*, 1990.)

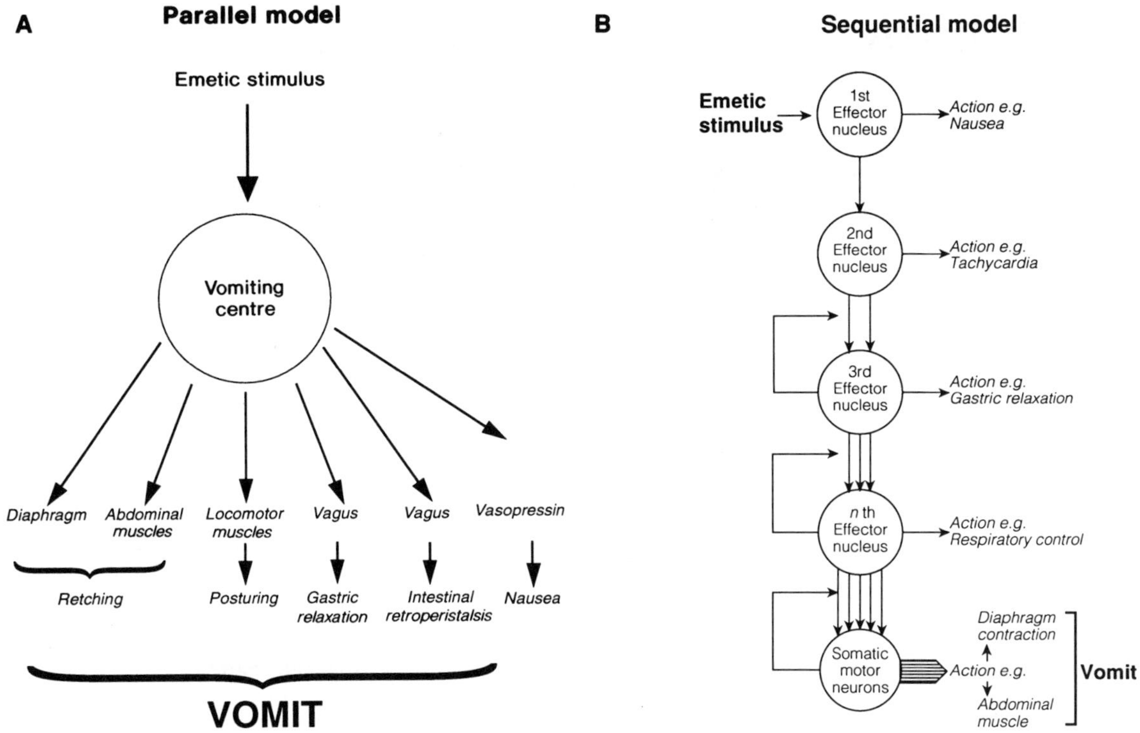

Figure 7.4 Two conceptual models (A and B) for the organization of the 'vomiting centre'. (Adapted from Davis *et al.*, 1986.)

responsible for organization of the motor outputs for vomiting (Fig. 7.4 A and B): a 'parallel' activation model (A) in which there is a single group of neurons, the 'vomiting centre', which co-ordinates the outputs, and a 'sequential' (B) model in which there is a cascade of activation of motor nuclei (probably with feedback) reflecting the gradual build-up of the prodromal phase and finally culminating in expulsion (Davis *et al.*, 1986). The latter model is attractive as it accounts for the experimental observation that it is possible to activate some of the epiphenomena of emesis (e.g. licking) without triggering expulsion (Miller and Wilson, 1983).

The co-ordination of the motor components of the vomiting reflex occurs in the brainstem. The vagal efferent neurons supplying the stomach and heart originate in the dorsal motor vagal nucleus and the *nucleus ambiguus* and the pre-sympathetic neurons which maintain sympathetic tone to the heart and blood vessels are located in the ventro-lateral brainstem. The dorsal and ventral respiratory groups involved in the regulation of the phrenic nerve output to the diaphragm, abdominal and accessory respiratory muscles are also located here (reviewed in Miller, 1990) (Fig. 7.5). It should be noted that all the nuclei involved in the motor pathways for emesis also have 'non-emetic' functions so emesis results from a uniquely co-ordinated *pattern and intensity* of activation of these nuclei when triggered by an appropriate stimulus. There is continuing debate about whether there may be a specific group of nuclei in the brainstem which orchestrates these outputs. It seems likely that there may indeed be such a region

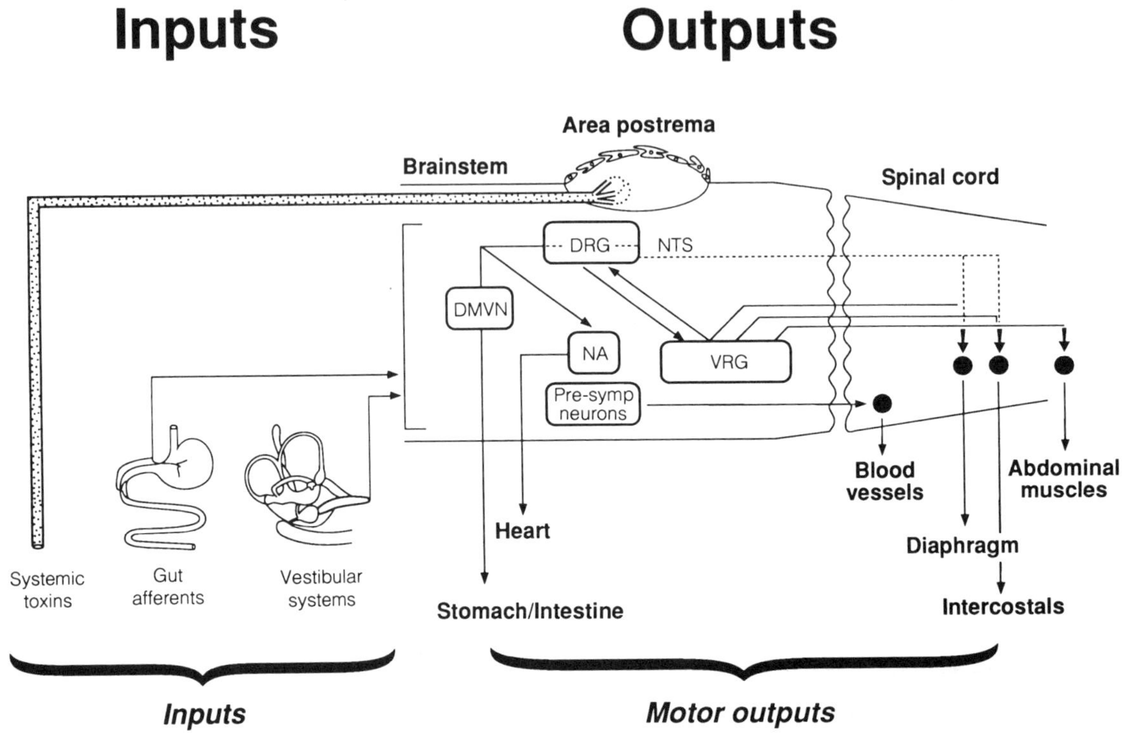

Figure 7.5 A diagram of the major visceral and somatic motor nuclei involved in emesis.

NA = nucleus ambiguus
VRG = ventral respiratory group
DRG = dorsal respiratory group
NTS = nucleus tractus solitarius
DMVN = dorsal motor vagal nucleus
Pre-sym = pre-sympathetic neurons

(Redrawn from Andrews and Bhandari, 1991.)

and two possibilities present themselves. Firstly, the *nucleus tractus solitarius* is the major integrative nucleus for incoming visceral information; it has outputs to the major motor nuclei involved in emesis (Leslie, 1986; Leslie *et al.*, 1990) and its ventral region forms the dorsal respiratory group of neurons (see above). The second possibility is the parvicellular reticular formation which has many of the neuroanatomical connections con-sistent with a co-ordinating function (Mehler, 1983). This proposal is also consistent with the region identified in the dorsolateral border of the lateral reticular formation by Wang and Borison (1950; 1951) and proposed as the 'vomiting centre'.

Whatever the neuroanatomical basis of the 'vomiting centre' the motor outputs require very careful co-ordination over a very short period of time to achieve the desired effect. For example, the activation of the somatic motor outputs to the diaphragm must be held in check until the retrograde intestinal contraction has reached the stomach; the peri-oesophageal diaphragm remains contracted until the transition from retching to vomiting, and any drive to inspire at the point of vomiting must be strongly inhibited.

In addition, prior to the onset of emesis the animal becomes aroused even from sleep and if this does not occur then there is a danger of death from aspiration of vomitus. The brainstem reticular formation is also involved in the regulation of arousal levels.

7.2.3 EMETIC DETECTORS

Whatever the nature of the emetic stimulus it must somehow be recognized as such by the body and activate a pathway with access to the central integrating systems described above. In this section four different inputs to the system are briefly outlined and the evidence for their involvement in emesis induced by anti-cancer therapies is reviewed below.

7.2.3.1 Abdominal visceral afferents

As the major function of the vomiting reflex is to protect against the accidental ingestion of toxins in food it is therefore not surprising that the gut should have detection systems capable of activating the reflex. Indeed the gut afferents may be viewed as the second line of defence against poisoning via food if it has circumvented detection by vision, taste and smell, all of which represent the first line (Davis *et al.*, 1986). The vagus is the major nerve involved in the detection of emetic stimuli and in its abdominal course contains about 80–90% afferent fibres (some of the roles of the vagal efferent fibres in emesis are discussed in section 7.4 and Chapter 6). Electrical stimulation of the abdominal vagal afferents is capable of inducing emesis within 20 seconds thus illustrating the potential of the pathway for rapid ejection of gastric contents (Andrews *et al.*, 1990b). Two types of vagal afferent fibre are involved in the emetic response:

1. Mechanoreceptors located in the muscular wall of the gut are activated by both contraction and distension of the gut (reviewed in Grundy and Scratcherd, 1989). Distension of the gastric antrum (e.g. by overeating) or proximal small intestine (e.g. by obstruction) may induce nausea and vomiting by stimulation of these afferents. As these afferents also respond to contraction of the gut muscle they can also signal the abnormal gastro-intestinal motility patterns that occur in the prodromal phase of emesis and hence could make a contribution to the genesis of abnormal visceral sensations associated with this phase (Chapter 5).

2. Chemoreceptors are located in the mucosa of the upper gut and monitor a number of features of the intra-luminal environment. They respond to mucosal stroking, acid, alkali, hypertonic solutions, temperature and 'irritants' (e.g. copper sulphate) (references in Grundy *et al.*, 1991). As lesion studies have shown that the emesis induced by intra-gastric hypertonic sodium chloride and copper sulphate is reduced or abolished by vagotomy, it is likely that it is these mucosal afferents that are responsible (Wang and Borison, 1951; Andrews *et al.*, 1990b). Emesis induced by intra-luminal bacterial toxins such as Staphylococcal enterotoxin can also be abolished by vagotomy (Sugiyama *et al.*, 1961) and it is likely that such agents can also activate the mucosal vagal afferents, although this has not been studied formally.

The anatomical substrate for the polymodal mucosal chemoreceptor is not known by the current hypothesis suggests an arrangement rather like that in the taste buds or carotid body with a 'detector cell' responding to a range of stimuli and releasing a neurotransmitter to discharge an afferent terminating in close proximity. In the intestine the enterochromaffin cell has been proposed as the 'detector cell', although this awaits experimental confirmation (see below).

Although cutting the abdominal visceral nerves is technically easier than AP ablation there are a number of factors which must be taken into account when interpreting the effects of such lesions and these are outlined below.

(a) The vagus and splanchnic nerves are mixed nerves containing both afferent and efferent fibres. In the case of the abdominal vagus >80% of the fibres are afferent (references in Andrews, 1986b). Thus surgical section will lesion both types of nerve and some account must be taken of this. While section of the vagal efferents will prevent most of the gastro-intestinal motor correlates of emesis, these are not essential for the ejection phase (Chapter 5). In addition, there is no evidence that vagal efferent stimulation can induce emesis since only afferent activation is capable of triggering the reflex.

(b) Care must be taken to ensure that the lesioned nerve does not regrow. This is not likely to occur when animals are tested at short intervals after surgery but it may be a problem if several months elapse, as has been found to occur in man following truncal vagotomy for duodenal ulcer. In view of this it is important that some attempt is made to confirm the extent of the lesion following emetic testing.

(c) Because animals are left for some time after the lesion before testing (usually at least a week) it is possible that there may be some reorganization (i.e. evidence of plasticity) in the emetic pathway. There may, for ex-ample be denervation sensitivity of the AP because of removal of the vagal afferent inputs; alternatively, the lesion may induce the expression of an emetic mechanism either not present in the intact animal or having a minor role (Andrews *et al.*, 1990b).

7.2.3.2 Area postrema

The studies of Wang and Borison (1950; 1951; 1952) brought about a major change in understanding the way in which emetic agents were detected and subsequently triggered the vomiting reflex. It has long been known that emesis can be induced by application of chemicals to the dorsal surface of the brainstem and it was assumed that this was through direct stimulation of the 'vomiting centre' which was understood to be located in this region. However, Wang and Borison (*ibid*) demonstrated that a number of stimuli were in fact detected by cells of the area postrema, termed the 'chemoreceptor trigger zone' for emesis, which in turn activated the 'vomiting centre'. While there is no doubt that the AP when appropriately activated can induce emesis, its description as the 'chemoreceptor trigger zone' has led to the assumption that *all* chemicals in the circulation must induce emesis by this route. As will become apparent from the discussions of the mechanisms by which X-radiation and cytotoxic drugs induce emesis (section 7.3) this is arguable and may indeed be erroneous.

The AP in man is a 'U'-shaped structure a few millimeters long located in the caudal part of the fourth ventricle in the region of the obex (Leslie, 1986 and Chapter 6). Significantly, the AP is present in animals with (e.g. ferret) and without (e.g. rat) an emetic reflex, which suggests that it has functions other than emesis (reviewed in Borison, 1989). The AP is one of the circumventricular organs of the brain (other examples are the subfornical organ and nucleus of the *stria terminalis*) and as such it is outside the blood–brain barrier because the capillaries lack endothelial occluding junctions, and outside the cerebrospinal fluid–brain barrier because the ventricular ependymal cells lack occluding junctions (Leslie, 1986). It is therefore relatively permeable to polar molecules in the blood or cerebrospinal fluid, a feature which makes it ideally suited for a general chemoreceptor function.

The AP has been implicated in emesis mainly by lesion studies but interpretation of these is complicated by a number of technical difficulties:

1. The AP is small, highly vascularized and relatively inaccessible as it is partly obscured by the cerebellum. The technical difficulties of the lesion make comparison of lesions between different research groups difficult and this may contribute to some of the confusion in the literature.

2. It is intimately related to the underlying *nucleus tractus solitarius*. This region is the main site for termination of visceral vagal afferents and is a co-ordinating area for integration of visceral information (Chapter 6). Also, it is involved in regulation of respiration as the ventral portion comprises the dorsal respiratory group of neurons. In lesioning the AP it is relatively easy to damage the underlying *nucleus tractus solitarius* making interpretation of the effects difficult. Histology will only identify structural damage but the area of functional damage may be more extensive. Some consideration should be given to assessment of functional collateral damage to the nucleus tractus solitarius.

3. Vagal afferents from the abdomen terminate in the area subpostrema also known as the *subnucleus gelatinosus* of the *nucleus tractus solitarius*. As its name implies, this structure is immediately subjacent to the AP and intimately related to it. In addition, some abdominal vagal afferents may terminate in the AP itself or be capable of activating it. The evidence for such effects comes from histological, neurophysiological and 2-deoxyglucose autoradiographic studies (reviewed in Davis 1988; Andrews *et al.*, 1990b).

The precise way in which the AP is activated by emetic agents is unknown but, as with the polymodal mucosal vagal afferent chemoreceptors, one possibility is via a chemodetector cell sensitive to a broad spectrum of agents which releases a transmitter to discharge nerves located in close proximity. It is by this mechanism that cytotoxic drugs may induce emesis. In addition, recordings from neurons in the AP have shown that they respond to a variety of endogenous agents many of which can induce emesis when given systemically (e.g. dopamine). Thus, if they were released into the blood or the cerebrospinal fluid by anti-cancer therapy and were not metabolized *en route* to the AP they could thereby induce emesis.

7.2.3.3 Vestibular system

The vestibular labyrinthine system is essential for the induction of emesis by motion stimuli but has never been implicated directly in emesis induced by radiation or cytotoxic drugs. However, there are two ways in which the vestibular system could be involved:

1. The evolutionary significance of an emetic response to motion is puzzling but Treisman (1977) proposed that when a toxin is ingested the animal may become unsteady on its feet and hence the labyrinths may be stimulated by such swaying motion. Studies of the effect of cyclophosphamide in cats reported neurotoxic effects within 10 minutes characterized by head bobbing, broad-based stance and falling (Fetting *et al.*, 1982). Obviously such a mechanism cannot apply to patients, although sudden movements of the head should be avoided

after treatment to minimize any labyrinthine input to the 'vomiting centre', particularly in patients who have for some time been relatively immobile in a recumbent posture such as might occur during total body radiation. The labyrinthine input should also be borne in mind when moving patients lying down on trolleys after radiation therapy, as this additional emetic input may induce emesis. Experimental studies in man suggest that the position of the head (and hence the degree of labyrinthine stimulation) can influence the emetic response to apomorphine which acts via the AP (Isaacs, 1957), and hence there is no reason why other emetic stimuli should not be affected in a similar way.

2. There is some evidence that the vestibular system may be more directly involved in the emetic response to certain drugs in particular. Studies in the dog reveal that removal of the vestibular system reduced the emetic response to lobeline, L-dopa and nicotine but not to pilocarpine or apomorphine (Money and Cheung, 1983). The most likely explanation is that these drugs are able to discharge vestibular afferents and to facilitate the primary effects that they have on the emetic mechanism.

   The possible involvement of this mechanism in the response to anti-cancer therapy has not been formally investigated and as other mechanisms (AP, vagal afferents) can account for the observed responses, such as involvement appears unlikely. However, a number of the cytotoxic drugs are ototoxic (e.g. cisplatin) indicating that they have access to the labyrinths so it would be unwise to exclude some involvement, particularly in the delayed types of emesis.

7.2.3.4 Higher influences

Studies in decerebrated animals have revealed that the integrative circuitry for the motor components of the emetic reflex reside in the brainstem and that such animals are capable of responding to emetic stimuli acting via the AP, vagus or even vestibular labyrinths. The role of 'higher' cerebral influences is at present unclear but there is little doubt that inputs from such areas can induce nausea and vomiting. Electrical stimulation of the amygdala in the macaque monkey, for example, evokes emesis (Smith and McHugh, 1967) and similar studies in man have demonstrated cerebral induction of nausea and vomiting (Thomas, 1968).

These higher inputs appear to have a mainly facilitatory role in modulating the sensitivity of the brainstem emetic mechanism (see below) rather than acting as primary detectors of the emetic stimuli. However, they clearly provide a substrate for anticipatory nausea and vomiting in chemotherapy patients and this could be argued to be an exaggerated form of the normal aversive responses seen in animals and man following exposure to contaminated food (Chapter 1). An understanding of the neuropharmacology of the pathways involved in these anticipatory responses is urgently required in order to provide a basis for the design of more rational drug therapy.

7.2.3.5 Miscellaneous inputs

Nausea and vomiting can be activated from several other regions of the body and they will be mentioned briefly here as there is a possibility of an involvement in radiation- and chemotherapy-induced emesis, although it is likely to be a minor one.

1. *Taste*
   Unpleasant tastes can induce nausea and retching, although whether this is a primary response or secondary to association with illness experienced as a result of prior exposure (a learned aversion) is unclear. A minority of patients report a bitter taste associated with chemotherapy and may

ascribe the induction of emesis to this (Fetting *et al.*, 1985). This response is interesting for several reasons: first, it is of short latency (30 min.) supporting the contention that cytotoxic drugs can have rapid effects in biological systems. Secondly, it raises the question of how these drugs specifically activate the 'bitter sensitive' taste-buds located in the posterior region of the tongue and the pharynx. A study of the effect of cytotoxic drugs on gustatory afferents may give insights into the neuroactive properties of these compounds. Thirdly, a bitter taste is usually associated with potential toxins in the food and hence the taste associated with chemotherapeutic agents is the 'correct' one.

The induction of a bitter taste is also of interest as it may be this that in part drives the lip-licking, and occasionally the salivation, seen in experimental animals given cytotoxic drugs (Bermudez *et al.*, 1988).

2. *Pharyngeal afferents*
   Nausea, and gagging in particular, can be readily evoked by mechanical stimulation of pharyngeal afferents projecting to the brainstem in the glossopharyngeal nerve. While there is no evidence for a direct involvement of such afferents in chemotherapy-induced emesis there may be a heightened awareness of this region associated with nausea.

3. *Auricular vagal afferents*
   After gastronomic overindulgence it was common practice for the Romans to retire to the 'Vomitorium' and stimulate their tympanum with a feather to induce prompt emesis. This procedure stimulates the auricular branch of the vagus nerve, also known as 'Arnold's nerve' or 'the Alderman's nerve'. The vomiting so induced may be due to a direct activation of brainstem pathways or secondary to a vaso-vagal attack also induced by stimulation of this nerve and resulting in a fall in blood pressure.

4. *Cardiac vagal afferents*
   Ventricular cardiac afferents are capable of inducing nausea and vomiting in man and experimental animals and their activation probably accounts for these symptoms (particularly nausea) prior to or in association with myocardial infarction (Abrahamsson and Thoren, 1973).

7.3 CYTOTOXIC DRUG- AND RADIATION-INDUCED EMESIS IN THE ANIMAL MODEL

As discussed in Chapter 1, there are a number of important clinical reasons why it is essential to understand the mechanisms by which cytotoxic drugs and ionizing radiation induce emesis. While some questions can be answered by careful quantitative clinical trials, the majority require the use of animal models. The major reasons for the use of animals in this context are: (1) to investigate the pathways by which the various stimuli induce emesis so that sites for anti-emetic therapy can be identified and, once a model is established, (2) to screen for novel anti-emetic agents and provide a basis for dose calculation in human Phase I trials.

The study of emesis is complicated by the fact that not all animals have a vomiting reflex. In particular, the common small laboratory rodents such as the rat and guinea-pig lack the reflex, as do lagomorphs (e.g. rabbits; Hatcher, 1924). The vomiting reflex is present in fish (e.g. the trout; Tiersch and Griffith, 1988), amphibia (e.g. the frog; Naitoh *et al.*, 1989), possibly some reptiles (e.g. the caiman; Schapiro, 1978), birds (e.g. pigeon; Chaney and Kare, 1966) and, among the mammals, insectivores (e.g. the house musk shrew; Ueno *et al.*, 1987), carnivores (e.g. the ferret and dog; Florczyk *et al.*, 1982; Wang and Borison, 1952) and primates (e.g. man, the macacque monkey; Brizzee 1956).

Studies of vomiting induced by cytotoxic drugs and radiation have in the main been confined to mammals, although pigeons respond to cisplatin (Preziosi *et al.*, 1989) and ducks to the trichothecine mycotoxin diacetoxyscirpinol (Ueno, 1983). Amongst the mammals the majority of studies have used carnivores, initially the cat and dog, but more recently the ferret, first used in this way by Florczyk *et al.* (1982). It is probably true to say that the vast majority of studies of emesis and anti-emetic drugs are now carried out in the ferret which has largely replaced the use of large numbers of cats and dogs. Studies over the past 10 years have shown that the ferret responds to a wide range of emetic stimuli (Davis, 1988) (Table 7.1) and hence is useful for studying a number of clinical problems involving emesis.

It is important to emphasize that these animal studies provide a **model** for components of the human situation and in no way attempt to mimic the entire clinical experience of receiving anti-cancer therapy. In the area of radiation- and cytotoxic-induced emesis, the animal studies have some limitations: two of these in particular should be highlighted and their implications discussed before reviewing the possible pathways and mechanisms involved.

7.3.1 SENSITIVITY TO THE STIMULUS

One striking feature about animal studies of cytotoxic drug-induced emesis is the difference in dose sensitivity between man and some animals. For instance, cisplatin in man causes nausea at doses as low as 0.08 mg/kg i.v. with vomiting occurring in a very high proportion of patients in the 'high dose' range of 1.3–3.0 mg/kg (approximately equivalent to 50–120 mg/m^2) (Von Hoff *et al.*, 1979). Dogs and monkeys respond in the same dose range (Schaeppi *et al.*, 1973) but cats, ferrets and the insectivore *Suncus murinus* all require higher doses on a per kilogram basis (McCarthy and Borison, 1984; Florczyk *et al.*, 1982; Matsuki *et al.*, 1988). Where a range of species have been studied, a similar pattern emerges for other agents such as cyclophosphamide, mustine, and anguidine (diacetoxyscirpinol) (references in Davis, 1988) (Table 7.2). One difficulty in comparing drug dosages in man and laboratory animals is with the basis for dose calculation. Taking cyclophosphamide as an example, studies of its toxicity and metabolism show that these correlate with body surface area rather than body weight (Gershwin *et al.*, 1974). This observation has important implications for studies using the smaller species such as *Suncus* and the ferret which have a higher surface area to body volume ratio. Calculating the doses of cyclophospha-mide on a surface area basis, a 'moderate' dose in man is 20–50 mg/kg, corresponding to about 1–2 g/m^2. In the ferret, the lowest dose inducing emesis was 100 mg/kg, corresponding to 1.4 g/m^2. Thus the clinical and experimental doses may be more comparable when recalculated on the basis of body surface area and this factor should not be neglected when attempting comparison of the sensitivity of animals and man to the same agent. Interestingly, dogs being treated with cisplatin for a variety of malignancies (mostly osteosarcomas) have a very similar sensitivity to man when the dose is administered on a surface area basis, with emesis occurring in >50% of animals at doses >50 mg/m^2 (about 2 mg/kg i.v.) even in the presence of anti-emetic therapy (Ogilvie *et al.*, 1989). The probability of vomiting at a dose of 70 mg/m^2 was almost thirty times that at 10 mg/m^2.

A somewhat different picture emerges using radiation with the dose of X-radiation inducing emesis being lowest for the ferret, followed by man, dog and monkey (Chapter 8). The cat is relatively insensitive to radiation requiring about 4500 rads to induce emesis in

Table 7.1 Effective emetic agents in the ferret

Subcutaneous	Intravenous/intraperitoneal	Per oral	Other
Apomorphine	Adriamycin	Calcium glucuronide	X-radiation
Lisuride	Apomorphine	Choline chloride	Vagal afferent stimulation
Loperamide	Cisplatin	Copper sulphate	
Morphine	Cisplatin analogues	Emetine	
Morphine-6-glucuronide	Cyclophosphamide	Glucose	
	Cyclohexamide	Ipecacuanha	
	Diacetoxyscirpinol	Mannitol	
	Emetine	Potassium chloride	
	Enkephalin	Sodium chloride	
	Hyperammonaemia	Syrup BP	
	Mustine	Veratridine	
	para-chlorophenylalanine	Zacopride	
	Trimelamol	2-Methyl 5-HT	
	Urethane	Phenyl biguanide	
	Theophylline		
	Enprofylline		
	8-Phenyl theophylline		
	Isobutylmethylxanthine		
	2-Methyl 5-HT		
	Phenyl biguanide		

(For references see Andrews *et al.*, 1990 a,b, Bhandari and Andrews 1991, Bhandari *et al.*, 1992, Davis 1988, Thompson *et al.*, 1992.)

Table 7.2 Comparison of emetic sensitivity of man and some laboratory animals

	Emetic stimulus				
Species	Apomorphine (μg/kg)	Cisplatin (mg/kg)	Mustine (mg/kg)	X-radiation (cGY)	Copper sulphate (mg %)
Man	20–30	2.5	0.4	800 [ED_{80}]	400
Monkey	unresponsive	1.25	NT	800 [ED_{80}]	NT
Dog	2.5–15.0	3.0	0.5	600	40–160
Cat	>4000	7.5	5.0	4500	1000–2000
Ferret	50–100	6.0–10.0	1.2	125	20–150
Suncus	unresponsive	40	NT	429 [ED_{50}]	40 mg/kg

NT = not tested
The doses stated are those evoking emesis in all animals tested unless otherwise stated (see text Andrews *et al.*, 1990b and Davis, 1988 for references).

all animals in contrast to 125 rads for the ferret and 800 rads for man [ED_{80}]. Such differences apply not only to cytotoxic drugs and radiation but also to other common experimental emetic stimuli such as apomorphine and copper sulphate. The dopamine D_2 receptor agonist apomorphine is particularly interesting in this respect as it is commonly used to activate emesis via the AP but while man, dog, cat, ferret and birds all respond, the insectivore *Suncus murinus* and the monkey are unresponsive (Ueno *et al.*, 1987; Brizzee *et al.*, 1955). This provides a striking example of a case where a non-human primate may not always be the best model for man. Indeed, care must be taken in the selection of the species of primate as studies of motion sickness indicate that while the squirrel monkey is very sensitive the macaque monkey may be resistant (reviewed in Daunton, 1990). In the same way as we have seen that different species are differentially sensitive to the various cytotoxic stimuli, the same is true when different types of motion are considered: the dog is moderately susceptible to vertical motion whereas the squirrel monkey is only slightly susceptible. In contrast, the monkey is highly sensitive to rotation but the dog is only slightly sensitive (reviewed in Daunton, 1990).

7.3.2 THE PATTERN OF EMETIC RESPONSE

Unfortunately it is very difficult to obtain precise data from human studies that are directly comparable to the animal studies. This is because such measurements have rarely been made in any formal way; the rate of cytotoxic drug administration is usually modified in an attempt to minimize emesis (e.g. slow infusion for cisplatinum). In patients, some form of anti-emetic treatment is always given; the patient may be receiving multiple drug therapies and, in the case of cisplatin, will be specifically hydrated. In addition, the presence of a tumour may also modify the response. Bearing these limitations in mind three features of the emetic response may be considered: latency, pattern, and duration of response.

7.3.2.1 Latency

Considering the limited number of stimuli for which comparative data are available, the onset of emesis in the animal models fall essentially in the same range as that reported for man (Table 7.3). The only major discrepancy to date is with cyclophosphamide which

Table 7.3 Man and ferret compared with respect to vomiting latency to various emetic agents (see text, Andrews *et al.*, 1990b, Davis 1988 for refs).

	Vomiting latency (min) Man	Ferret
Adriamycin	120–720	84 ± 6
Apomorphine	9.5 ± 0.9*	4.8 ± 3.6
Cisplatin	60–360	69 ± 6 to 99 ± 4
Cyclohexamide	5–60	17 ± 5
Cyclophosphamide	120–720	22 ± 8
Copper sulphate (PO)	2–5	6.8 ± 2.5
Ipecacuanha (PO)	5–40, 16.9 ± 3.2	8.4 ± 0.2
Mustine	30–120	28 ± 7
X-radiation (ED_{50})	~30	~30

* Nausea Latency.

in man may have an even longer latency than cisplatin; whereas in animals the latency is considerably shorter. These differences may reflect the different doses of cyclophosphamide used in man (animal studies have shown that the latency is dose-related), or possibly the hepatic metabolism of cyclophosphamide to its emetic metabolite phosphoramide mustard.

7.3.2.2 Pattern

Animal studies in general, and in particular the more recent studies in the ferret, have facilitated detailed analysis of the pattern of emesis which can give important insights into the precise way in which these compounds induce emesis. In addition, it is only by having a detailed knowledge of this pattern that it is possible to analyse properly the effects of nerve lesions and anti-emetic drugs. For example, are the early and later phases of the response affected to the same extent by a drug or can an apparently homogeneous response be resolved into two or more components?

Studies in the ferret of a range of emetic agents carried out under similar conditions have enabled a direct comparison of the responses. Examples of the responses to cisplatin, cyclophosphamide, radiation and emetine are shown in Figure 7.6. This analysis indicates that the pattern differs between agents and that in general the duration of the emetic response in the ferret is shorter than that in man but is comparable to that seen in other laboratory species. One question which arises is why the duration of emesis should be briefer in animals using the same drugs but usually at higher doses than in man? Is this a reflection of pharmacokinetic and pharmacodynamic differences? Does it suggest that aspects of the emetic mechanism are not the same in animals and man or is it due to additional clinical factors?

7.3.2.3 Anticipatory and delayed emesis

These two types of emesis represent a major unresolved clinical problem, especially with respect to cisplatinum. Delayed emesis is of particular concern because it is not very effectively treated with the current anti-emetic regimes. One difficulty in identifying the mechanism responsible is that none of the animals in which cisplatin is an effective emetic agent exhibit a delayed response. Although the definition of delayed emesis in man as starting 24 hours after drug administration is somewhat arbitrary, there is no indication that animals continue to vomit after the initial acute phase, which lasts in most cases only a few hours (Fig. 7.6). There is no obvious explanation for this lack of response but it is worth noting that the doses of cisplatinum in the cat and ferret which induce emesis are lethal in 3–7 days and thus the animal may be in a weakened state and unable to vomit. In the ferret an emetic dose of cisplatinum of 8 mg/kg i.v. reduced the white blood cell count by 89% within 3–4 days of administration (Florczyk *et al.*, 1982). In the dog, however, the emetic dose (3 mg/kg) is survivable by the vast majority of animals but delayed emesis is still not reported to occur.

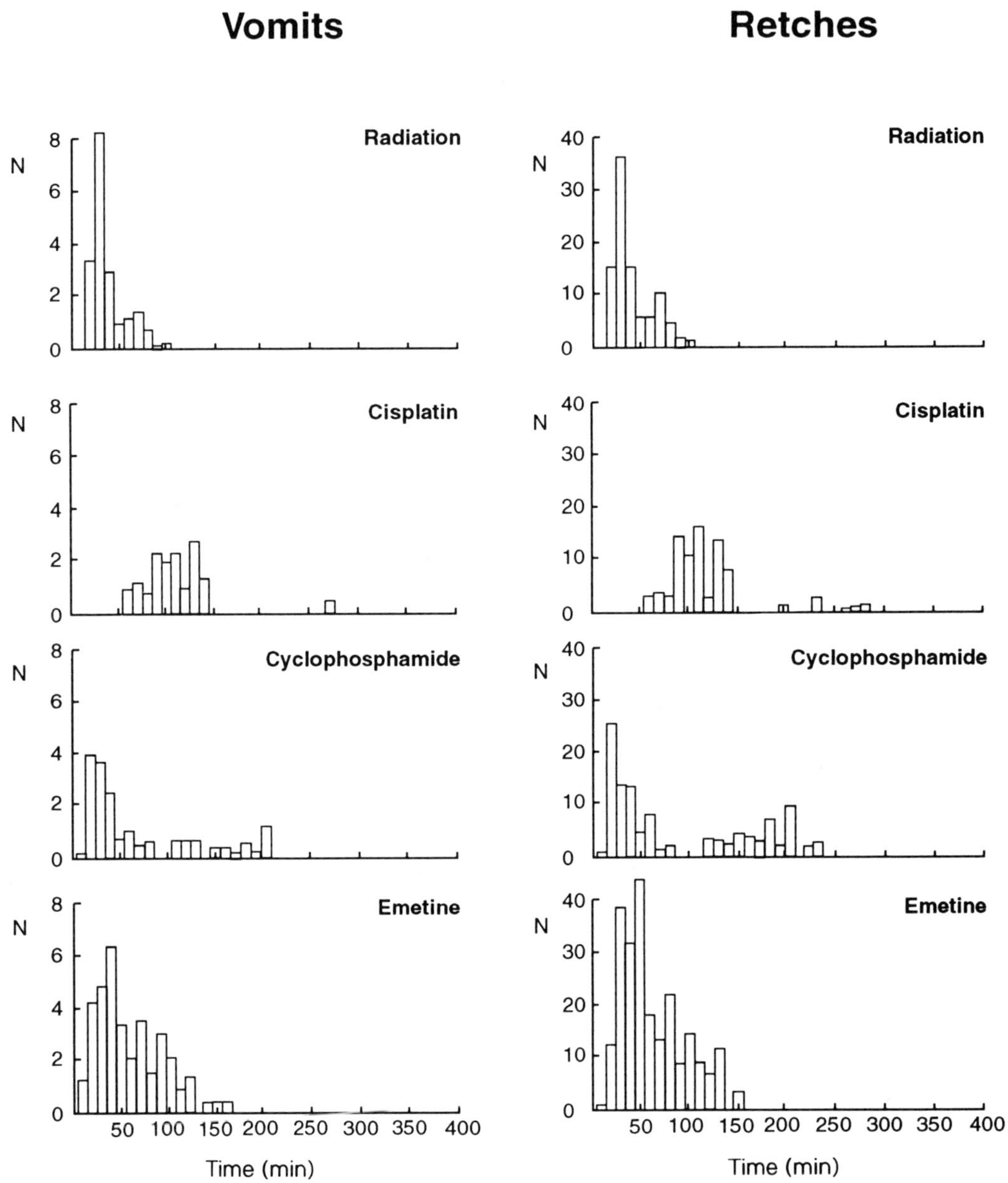

Figure 7.6 The pattern of retching and vomiting in the ferret in response to a variety of emetic stimuli. The values are the mean number of retches of vomits in 10 min. time bins. The values are from the authors' unpublished experiments with at least 6 animals/stimulus. The doses of the various stimuli are: radiation 200 rads whole body, 250 kV, 15 mA; cisplatin 10 mg/kg i.p.; cyclophosphamide 200 mg/kg i.p.; emetine 20 mg/kg i.p.

Anticipatory emesis is another problem where little is known of the underlying mechanism. The development of anticipatory nausea and vomiting following cytotoxic drug administration has not been investigated in animals but it is likely that such a model could be developed using classical conditioning paradigms. In studies of motion sickness there is some evidence for conditioning of the response (e.g. a decrease in latency) but only in highly susceptible individual animals (Daunton, 1990). It must be borne in mind that this anticipatory response, and in particular the nausea, is an attempt by the body to avoid exposure to a stimulus which on a previous occasion induced illness. The response relies on retaining a memory of the original experience and perhaps the only way of treating anticipatory emesis once established may be to delete this memory using drugs that interfere with the development of long-term potentiation (e.g. amino acid receptor antagonists such as MK-801).

7.3.4 IMPLICATIONS OF THE DIFFERENCES BETWEEN MAN AND ANIMALS

From the foregoing discussion it is clear that animal models of cytotoxic drug- and radiation-induced emesis have a number of limitations, particularly in terms of dose sensitivity and the pattern of response. The question that should be addressed is do these differences matter in terms of the usefulness of such models for understanding the mechanisms involved in man?

The dose of a drug required to induce a particular effect in any animal including man is going to depend upon a large number of factors many of which (e.g. genetic predisposition) may be out of the control of the investigator. In studying the mechanism by which cytotoxic drugs induce emesis, for example, the question of the dose required to induce the effect is irrelevant **provided that the dose activates the same pathways as in man and does not recruit additional mechanisms**. Identification of mechanisms in animals often relies on lesion studies and hence it may never be possible to test the predictability of the animal model in man, but, fortunately, the study of anti-emetic agents provides another means of testing the validity of a model. Recent studies with the 5-hydroxytryptamine$_3$ receptor subtype (5-HT$_3$) antagonists have demonstrated that, using the ferret as the model of cytotoxic- and radiation-induced emesis, it was possible to identify a novel class of anti-emetic agent (Bermudez *et al.*, 1988), predict its efficacy against a range of cytotoxic drugs in man, and, in the case of at least one agent (Granisetron; proprietory name Kytril), predict accurately the dose range for human use.

When an animal requires a different dose of an agent from that required by man to induce an effect this is often used to question the validity of the model. While this is an obvious criticism it neglects the insights that can be gained from understanding the reasons for the different sensitivities. For example, what features of the ferret make it so sensitive to radiation and the cat so insensitive? Studies of these phenomena may increase understanding of the factors determining the radiosensitivity of tissue itself.

The reason for the shorter duration of the emetic response in animals as compared to man is difficult to understand but may be a reflection of different metabolism of the agents. For example, with cyclophosphamide, estimates of the plasma half-life in man (2–10 hr) are much greater than in animals, where the value is 15–60 min. (Friedman *et al.*, 1979). Although, ideally, the pattern of emesis should mimic that in man this is probably an unrealistic expectation when all the confounding factors of the clinical situation are considered. In some respects the lack of exact mimicry does not matter as the short duration emesis seen in animals (a few hours) is representative of the acute (<24 hrs.) phase of emesis in man. However, the lack of a delayed emetic response, especially with cisplatinum, is a major disadvantage of the current models. A detailed comparative study of the pharmacokinetics, pharmacodynamics and pharmacological effects of cisplatin in man and, for example, the ferret may give insights into the mechanism involved. Possible reasons for the lack of delayed response in animals could be depletion of an essential neurotransmitter or irreversible damage to the emetic mechanism by cisplatinum but neither appears to be the case as animals treated with cisplatinum on consecutive days retain an emetic response (Gunning *et al.*, 1987). Early studies in the monkey showed that its sensitivity to cisplatinum was comparable to man but these studies were aimed at examining the general toxic effects of the drug and not its emetic characteristics. Therefore it is not known with certainty whether delayed emesis is a feature only of the primate response.

7.4 PATHWAYS INVOLVED IN ACUTE CYTOTOXIC EMESIS

This section attempts to identify which of the emetic pathways described above are involved in the acute emetic response to cytotoxic drugs and radiation.

Although many studies of the effects of AP ablation and visceral nerve lesions have been undertaken, the overall picture is still somewhat confused. This is mainly because a variety of species have been studied using an array different cytotoxic drugs. This situation further compounds inherent difficulties in the interpretation of the lesion studies outlined above. The effects of these lesions are summarized in Table 7.4. This indicates that it is not possible to make a definitive statement about the pathway activated by cytotoxic drugs in general even in the same species: compare, for example, the effects of AP ablation on the response to cisplatinum and cyclophosphamide in the cat. Furthermore, the pathway involved in one species cannot be extrapolated to another: compare, for example, the effects of AP ablation and visceral lesions on the response to irradiation in the cat and dog. In addition, in some species (e.g. ferret) it appears that the emetic response to a particular stimulus can be affected by a lesion at either site.

How then can these apparently discordant observations be reconciled? Two factors are probably involved.

7.4.1 THE RELATIONSHIP BETWEEN THE AREA POSTREMA AND VISCERAL AFFERENTS

One difficulty in resolving these discrepancies is that in few cases have both AP ablation and vagotomy been studied in the same species using the same emetic stimulus. In the ferret the emetic response to 200 rads total body radiation can be abolished by abdominal vagotomy or AP ablation; similarly, in the dog the response to cisplatinum is abolished by either lesion. These observations can be reconciled if the abdominal vagal afferents are proposed as the prime site at which the stimuli are detected and these afferents in turn activate the AP which then triggers the motor components of the emetic reflect. The projection of abdominal vagal afferents to the AP is supported by evidence from fiber-tracing studies (Leslie, 1986) and an increase in glucose utilization (i.e. metabolism) in the AP induced by vagal afferent stimulation (Davis, 1988; Andrews *et al.*, 1990b).

Such an organization of the pathway could account for the abolition of the response by both AP ablation or vagotomy. However, there are two other possibilities which should also be examined.

7.4.1.1

The vagal afferents may be the prime detectors and project to the medulla but terminate instead in the *nucleus tractus solitarius* in the

Table 7.4 Effect of area postrema ablation and abdominal visceral nerve lesions on the emetic response to different emetic stimuli

Lesion	Species	Apomorphine	Radiation	Cisplatin	Cyclophosphamide	Chloromethine
Area postrema ablation	Human	Abolished				
	Cat	Abolished	Present	Abolished	Present	Present
	Dog	Abolished	Abolished	Abolished	Present	Abolished
	Monkey	Abolished	↓/Abolished			
	Ferret	Abolished	↓/Abolished			
Abdominal visceral nerve lesion (vagotomy ± splanchnic section)	Human	Present				
	Cat	Present	↓/Abolished			↓/Abolished
	Dog	Present	Present/↓	Abolished		
	Monkey	Present	↓/Abolished			
	Ferret	Present	↓/Abolished	Abolished	Abolished	↓/Abolished
	Suncus		Abolished	Abolished		

(For references see Andrews and Hawthorn, 1988; Andrews *et al.*, 1990; Davis, 1988; Matsuki *et al.*, 1992. Sanger, Chapter 9, Reynolds and Leslie, Chapter 6.)

part immediately subjacent to the AP in a region termed the area sub-postrema (Leslie, 1986). This projection has in fact been demonstrated and it is difficult to envisage how some collateral damage to this area would not occur during thermocautery of the AP. Unfortunately, assessing the functional extent of such damage would be impossible without a detailed neurophysiological study of vagal reflexes as such a lesion would be the equivalent of a 'central' vagotomy.

Using induction of c-*fos* protein as an index of neuronal activity it has been shown in the ferret that cisplatinum increases the number of c-*fos* positive cells in both the *nucleus tractus solitarius* and the area postrema (Reynolds *et al.*, 1991). However, only the staining in the *nucleus tractus solitarius* was significantly reduced by vagotomy or administration of the 5-HT_3 receptor antagonist anti-emetic granisetron (section 7.3.4, above).

Other studies have shown that vagotomy abolishes the emetic response to cisplatinum in this species (Hawthorn *et al.*, 1988). The c-*fos* study is of particular interest as it shows an effect of cisplatinum on the AP which is probably unconnected with emesis. Could it be that it is this action on the AP that is involved in the anorexic effects of cytotoxic drugs? Overall, these studies indicate a relatively minor role for the AP in emesis, mainly as a relay for the primary signal. However, it is not clear why this particular type of emetic signal should be relayed as lesion studies have shown that the gastro-intestinal vagal afferents activated by copper sulphate can activate the emetic mechanism via their normal pathway through the *nucleus tractus solitarius* (Wang and Borison, 1952). It remains a possibility that there are subtypes of gastro-intestinal afferents whose central projection depends upon the type of information carried or their precise site of origin in the gut.

Studies in the ferret where abdominal vagotomy or AP ablation (validated by post-surgical abolition of the emetic response to the opiate loperamide) (Bhandari *et al.*, 1992) both abolish the response to 200 rads total body irradiation, electrical stimulation of the abdominal vagal afferents still induces retching in the AP-ablated animal (Bhandari and Andrews, unpublished observations). This result suggests that the sub-population of vagal afferents activated by radiation projects to the AP while another sub-population, also capable of inducing emesis, bypasses the AP.

7.4.1.2

Some of the recorded discrepancies could be explained if emesis was only induced when the stimulus directly or indirectly activated both sites or if the vagus somehow regulated the sensitivity of the AP or vice-versa. In any of these models lesion of either structure would certainly modify the emetic response.

The present types of experimental study make it difficult to distinguish between the above models proposed to account for the experimental observations in individual species where lesion of either the AP or vagus influences the response. Indeed, how can we account for apparent differences between the pathways used for the same stimulus in different species? Some possibilities are outlined below.

7.4.2 RATIONALIZATION OF APPARENT DIFFERENCES IN EMETIC PATHWAYS

Differences between the effects of lesions in different species are often simply dismissed as 'species differences' with little attempt to explain the basis of such differences or their possible physiological relevance. The most likely explanation is that different animals exploit the various pathways to different extents and even the same stimulus (e.g. chloromethine) may not activate the same pathway in different species. Initially it would appear that the main reason for attempting an understanding of the pathways is to

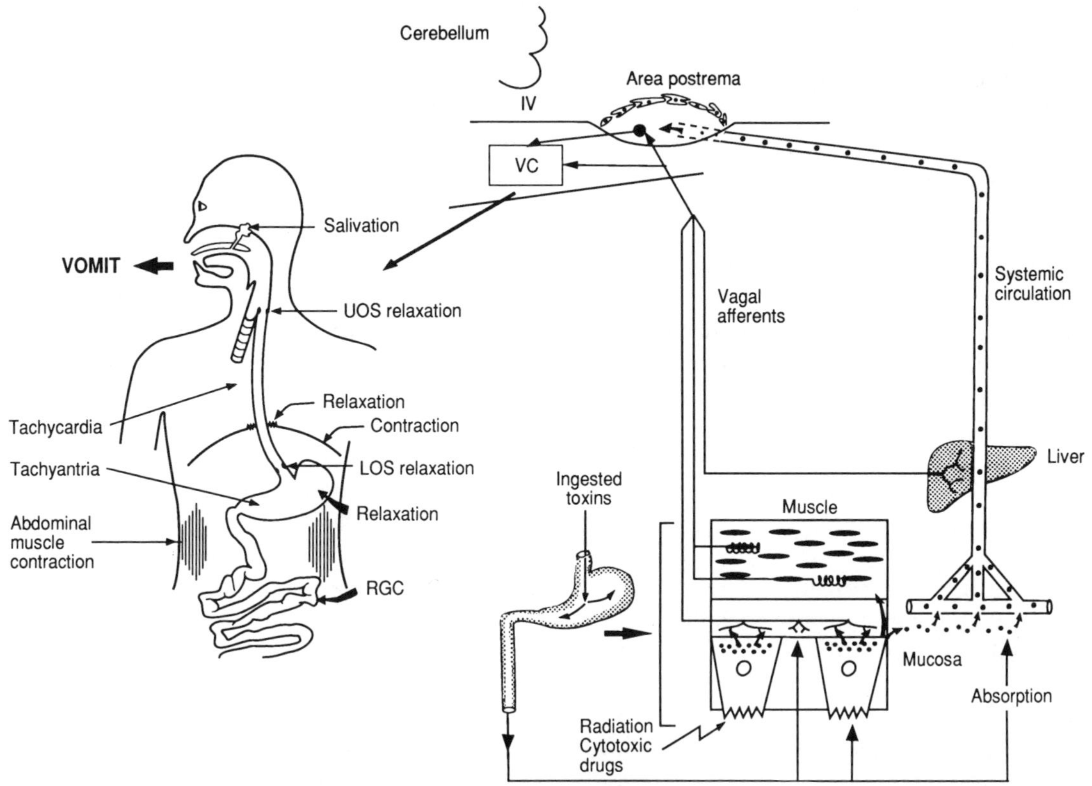

Figure 7.7 A summary of the main inputs to the 'vomiting centre' (VC) involved in the emetic response to systemic cytotoxic drugs and radiation. (Adapted from Andrews *et al.*, 1988.)

identify the best model for man. This is to some extent true but in the case of emesis induced by anti-cancer therapies there is a particular problem. Unlike many clinical situations, we do not have a human model against which to test the accuracy of the animal models: for such studies we would require humans with either a truncal vagotomy (an increasingly rare operation having its own emetic side effects) or an AP ablation. The latter has been performed successfully in man for intractable vomiting (Lindstrom and Brizzee, 1962) but only one series of operations has been reported. In addition to these surgical requirements, the patient should be receiving chemo- or radiotherapy, although not for a tumour as this may in itself be inducing emetic symptoms! It is therefore improbable that we will ever be able to validate the animal models in man. So are they of any use? The answer is, in the affirmative, of course, provided that the pathways activated in the animals can be clearly identified. For example, it may be that the ferret is the most suitable model for studying the ways in which radiation and cytotoxic drugs activate abdominal afferents whereas the dog, being perhaps more reliant on the area postrema, would be the best model for studying that aspect.

The pathways involved in the emetic response to radiation and cytotoxic drugs are summarized in Figure 7.7 to provide a basis for discussion of the cellular mechanisms of activation. This diagram should be regarded as a 'working hypothesis' that will need continual updating in the light of more experimental information as it becomes available, particularly from man.

7.5 CELLULAR MECHANISMS

How can a wide range of structurally dissimilar cytotoxic drugs and ionizing radiation activate the emetic pathways described above? An understanding of this may help to identify sites for novel approaches to anti-emetic therapy and also to provide insights into the physico-chemical features of the cytotoxic drugs responsible for emetic as opposed to the anti-tumour activity. It may even lead to the possibility of 'designing out' the unwanted effects.

The mechanisms considered will focus on the role of the vagus for the reasons outlined above but the role of the AP will also be reviewed and indeed many of the mechanisms discussed could equally apply to both sites. The two main possibilities – direct and indirect activation – will be considered separately.

7.5.1 DIRECT ACTIVATION OF EMETIC PATHWAYS

This is taken to mean that the ionizing radiation (considered here as a cellular poison; Chapter 8) and cytotoxic drugs act directly upon either the neurons in the AP or the vagal afferents to cause their activation and hence trigger the emetic pathway. This effect could be due either to a direct effect on the permeability of the neuronal membrane leading to depolarization and discharge or indirectly through an effect on intracellular systems such as protein kinase C, cyclic nucleotides or calcium which regulate membrane ionic permeability. While such mechanisms are appealing, a number of pieces of evidence argue against this occurring at either membrane or intracellular sites.

7.5.1.1

Cytotoxic drugs are a structurally diverse group of compounds and it appears unlikely that membrane receptors are present on the AP neurons or the vagal afferents that can respond to the native compounds or their metabolites. This situation has parallels in the olfactory and gustatory systems where several thousand substances can be distinguished and yet there appears to be little 'structure-sensation' relationship. Alternatively, as the anti-cancer compounds (and radiation) share the common feature that they are cytotoxic, it is possible that this feature alone may be associated with the common action of increasing neuronal membrane permeability. This appears, however, to be unlikely as recordings from single vagal afferents in the ferret have failed to find any evidence for direct effects of cisplatinum (Davidson and Andrews, 1990). However, cisplatinum may have effects on some neurons such as those in the enteric nervous system (Chapter 5) and its well-known neurotoxic effect suggests that such direct effects cannot yet be entirely excluded at least with respect to this particular agent. Indeed, perhaps direct neuronal effects cannot be excluded for all the cytotoxic drugs as some plant alkaloids (e.g. veratridine) and antibiotics (e.g. vallinomycin, a crown either with potent ionophore properties) can modify the ionic permeability of neuronal membranes.

Although the immediate effects of radiation on nervous tissue have been studied, they have not been studied in systems implicated in emesis or at doses relevant to clinical therapy. The overall impression is that with conventional types of radiation nervous tissue is relatively radio-insensitive. A recent study in man of stereotactic radiosurgery of the fourth ventricle showed a relationship between the dose to the AP and the incidence of nausea and vomiting during the first six post-operative hours (Alexander *et al.*, 1989). The median dose to the AP in the patients with symptoms was 618 rads (range 275–1257 rads) whereas in symptom-free patients the dose range was <5–184 rads. The authors concluded that the emesis was most likely due to vasogenic oedema of the brainstem induced by the radiation, a conclusion supported by a study of a single patient receiving 1088 cGy who was protected from nausea and vomiting by a combination of droperidol and dexamethasone.

7.5.1.2

If cytotoxic drugs or radiation had direct effects on the emetic detectors then one might expect the onset of emesis to be very rapid, particularly with radiation, and in the case of cytotoxic drugs to have some temporal relationship to the plasma levels of the drug. The relatively long latency observed in man has been used to argue in favour of indirect effects of these stimuli but the data from man are difficult to use for such comparisons because of confounding factors such as the imprecision of latency measurements, patient differences, and the range of doses and rates of administration used. For these reasons this discussion will confine itself to the use of data from the ferret.

Apomorphine (a dopamine D_2 receptor agonist) and morphine when given subcutaneously or intravenously to the ferret are generally agreed to induce emesis by a direct effect on dopamine receptors located in the AP (Schwartz *et al.*, 1986). The latency of emesis is short, usually less than 5 minutes. In man, similar short latencies have been reported. Electrical stimulation of abdominal vagal afferents in the ferret induces emesis in conscious or anaesthetized ferrets in less than one minute. Thus, if suitably activated, the emetic detectors can trigger emesis very rapidly.

The latency values for a range of cytotoxic drugs and radiation are longer in the ferret, although in most cases not as long as those in man. If emesis can be induced rapidly once the detectors are activated then what factors contribute to these 'long' latencies?

In the case of cyclophosphamide there is a requirement for conversion to its active metabolites, but in the ferret the latency is shorter than for cisplatin suggesting that this is not a major factor. Again in the ferret the route of administration has little effect on the latency: when cyclophosphamide or cisplatin are given by intravenous or intraperitoneal routes at the fully emetic dose, the latencies are similar (Hawthorn *et al.*, 1988).

It is possible that the cytotoxic drugs have a slow rate of access to the emetic detectors. This is a difficult issue to resolve as few studies have examined the relationship between plasma levels, tissue levels and emesis in animals let alone man. From studies in man of cyclophosphamide and cisplatin it appears that emesis begins long after drug plasma levels have peaked and in the case of cisplatin when blood levels have in fact fallen to <10% of initial levels (Carl *et al.*, 1989). Although these observations are suggestive that it is not merely the presence of a suitable level of the agent that induces emesis, caution must be exercised in making such a conclusion as it is the **tissue level** of agent that is likely to be the critical factor. Access to the central emetic detectors in the AP is unlikely to be a problem as this region is outside the blood–brain barrier.

When cisplatin is given intravenously to the cat the latency to emesis is 100.6 ± 32.1 minutes whereas when given into the cerebral ventricles, whence it can rapidly access the AP, the latency is 4.0 ± 5.2 minutes (Smith *et al.*, 1988). This large difference in latency suggests that either cisplatin given intravenously does not act via the AP to induce emesis or that the emesis induced by the central administration of cisplatin is due to a different effect of the drug from that when it is given intravenously. It should be noted that this does not exclude all possible effects of cisplatin on the AP. Indeed, studies by Reynolds *et al.* (1991) have shown an increase in c-*fos* gene expression in the AP following cisplatinum administration. Differences in emetic latency similar to those described above have been reported for central and peripheral injections of mustine (Papp *et al.*, 1966).

There is also evidence to suggest that cisplatin gains rapid access to the neuronal plexuses in the gut wall as stimulation of gastro-intestinal motility has been reported in the ferret with a latency of <5 minutes (Chapter 5). In addition, studies of 5-hydroxytryptamine release in the guinea-pig ileum have shown an increased release within 5 minutes of administration (Schwörer *et al.*, 1991). Further evidence for rapid access of cytotoxic drugs to the tissues comes from reports of patients receiving cyclophosphamide, 5-fluorouracil and methotrexate who report bitter taste sensations within 30 minutes of drug administration (Fetting *et al.*, 1985). A study of the mechanism by which the cytotoxic drugs induce activation of taste buds may possibly give some insights into the transduction mechanisms occurring in the emetic detectors as parallels have been drawn between the two systems.

From consideration of the above studies the overwhelming impression is that neither the intensely emetic cytotoxic drugs nor radiation have direct effects on the emetic detectors. The section below discusses the possible mechanisms of indirect activation of emetic pathways by these stimuli.

7.5.2 INDIRECT ACTIVATION OF EMETIC PATHWAYS

Harris (1982) was the first to propose an indirect mechanism of action of the cytotoxic drugs in activating the AP. It was suggested that cytotoxic drugs inhibit the activity or synthesis of a rapidly turning over enzyme (in the AP or closely related structure) which is responsible for the breakdown of a tonically released neurotransmitter. A build-up of the transmitter would then cause activation of neurons which in turn would trigger emesis. The evidence for this hypothesis was that the latency of emesis appears related to the differing sub-cellular effects of the cytotoxic drugs; the more emetic agents have a shorter latency because of a primary effect on RNA and protein synthesis (e.g. cisplatin) and the less emetic drugs have an effect on *de novo* DNA synthesis and mitosis (e.g. vinca alkaloids) with a correspondingly longer latency. While this hypothesis is attractive and could apply equally to gut mechanisms as well as the AP it has never been tested experimentally. If disturbance of such a fundamental cellular mechanism is responsible for the emesis then in view of the biochemical similarities of these cellular processes in mammals it would not be unreasonable to expect at least the rank order of latency or emetic activity to be similar across a range of species. Unfortunately this does not appear to be the case. Taking the ferret as an example (because it has been used to study a variety of agents under similar conditions), it can be seen that when doses of emetics are used that induce emesis in all animals tested, then cisplatin has one of the longer latencies and is a relatively weak emetic. In fact, cisplatin and adriamycin are notable because of their 'long' latency whereas all the other cytotoxic agents induce emesis in a relatively narrow latency band or 'window' of 17–40 minutes (Table 7.3, above). This comparison between the ferret and man may not be fair, however, as Harris's (1982) hypothesis is based on ranking the drugs according to their emetic potential at average clinical doses; the comparison being between the probability of a patient vomiting and the actual number of emetic episodes induced in an animal. The precise relationships between cellular effects of the drugs, emetic activity and latency can only be resolved when there

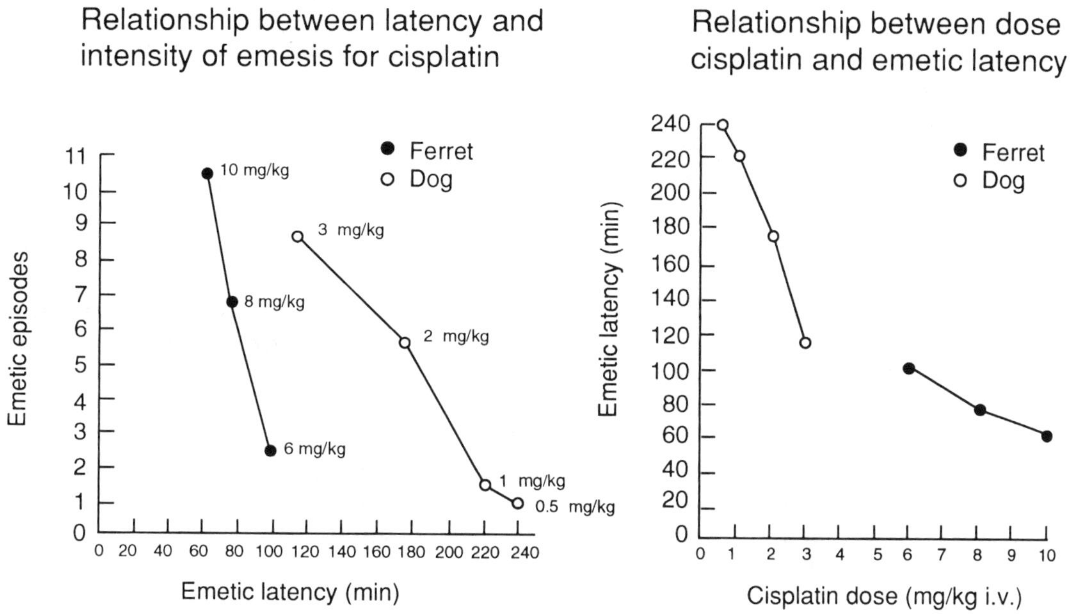

Figure 7.8 The relationships between the latency of the response to cisplatinum and the magnitude of the emetic response (left-hand panel). The dose-response relationship for cisplatinum in the dog (data from Bhandari *et al.*, 1988) and ferret (data from Schurig *et al.*, 1984).

is better quantification of human data so that more justified comparisons can be made.

In the development of cisplatin a range of structural analogues were produced with the aim of reducing the emetic effects and increasing the anti-tumour effects of the drug (Schurig *et al.*, 1984). Amongst the analogues that passed a murine anti-tumour assay some were more emetic than cisplatin (e.g. TNO-37) while others were less so (e.g. JM8) and, although no clear structure-emetic activity relationship was identified, the analogues with bi-dentate-leaving ligands were less emetic than cisplatin whilst those with mono-dentate-leaving ligands were comparable. Using the results presented in their study it is possible to examine the relationship between latency and emetic potential of the platinum analogues revealing a trend towards an inverse relationship between the latency to emesis and the number of emetic episodes, that is the more emetic agents tend to have a shorter latency. For cisplatin itself we see that as the dose of drug is increased the latency decreases and the number of emetic episodes rises, a relationship which holds true for the dog and ferret even though they differ markedly in their sensitivity to the drug (Fig. 7.8).

Two main conclusions about emetic mechanisms can be drawn from the above studies. Firstly, as pointed out by Harris and Cantwell (1986), the more emetic drugs tend to have a shorter latency and this appears to be the case even for the analogues of a single agent (e.g. cisplatin). In addition, it suggests that the latency of the emetic response is contributed to not only by its major biochemical effect (all the platinum analogues presumably have the same basic action due to effects on protein synthesis and DNA) but also by other characteristics (e.g. cell penetration) that may modify the time taken to activate the emetic mechanisms. Secondly, even with cisplatin itself, the latency can be reduced by increasing the dose of drug (Fig. 7.8, above) and this is also the case for radiation in man (Chapter 8) and in the ferret (range 50–400 rads) (Davis, 1988). Both these observations indicate that the latency is not only determined by how the emetic pathway is activated by these stimuli but also by the intensity of activation. Curiously, with emetic stimuli such as apomorphine, morphine and loperamide, which act directly on the AP by an agonist effect at receptors, there is little effect of drug dose on latency. This is also the case for intragastric emetic stimuli (e.g. copper sulphate) acting via vagal afferents. The latter observations provide further support for a substantial contribution to the latency by the time interval required for mobilization of cellular mechanisms.

If the key events inducing emesis are unlikely to occur either in the cells of the AP or vagal afferent axons themselves then how can the biochemical effects of the cytotoxic drugs described above cause activation of these pathways? For both pathways the proposed mechanism is that radiation and the cytotoxic drugs induce the release of a neuroactive agent which in the case of the vagal afferents acts locally and for the AP reaches it via the circulation.

7.5.2.1 Indirect activation of abdominal vagal afferents

Nerve lesion studies in animals (sections 7.3 and 7.4) have implicated the abdominal vagus in both radiation- and cytotoxic drug-induced emesis. The mechanism by which these stimuli activate the afferents was proposed by Andrews *et al.* (1988) and was based on the growing evidence for the involvement of 5-hydroxytryptamine (5-HT) and 5-HT_3 receptors in emesis. In this model it is proposed that the enterochromaffin cells (containing abundant 5-HT) in the mucosa of the upper gut are exquisitely sensitive to cytotoxic drugs and radiation and release their 5-HT when appropriately challenged. The 5-HT so released activates vagal afferents known to terminate in close proximity (reviewed in Grundy *et al.*, 1991) and hence induces emesis. This model is discussed more extensively in Chapter 9 together with a consideration of the site of anti-emetic action of the 5-HT_3 receptor antagonists.

The enterochromaffin cell–vagal afferent unit is thought to be the anatomical substrate for the gastro-intestinal mucosal chemoreceptors described above which is involved in monitoring the chemical nature of the intraluminal contents of the gut. It is these mucosal chemoreceptors that are involved in the emetic response to oral copper sulphate, hypertonic solutions and food toxins. Thus radiation and systemic cytotoxic drugs in fact induce emesis via activation of the system which functions to trigger emesis in response to potentially toxic agents in food. At this point it is perhaps worth recalling that in broad terms the body's response to food poisoning and anti-cancer therapy are in essence the same, that is nausea, vomiting, transient anorexia, and learned aversive responses. Indeed, even animals without a vomiting reflex such as the rat show similar responses to poisoned food and cytotoxic drugs. For example, rats will ingest clay when poisoned and the rationale is assumed to be an attempt to adsorb the toxin before absorption but such behaviour can also be induced by cytotoxic drugs (e.g. cyclophosphamide) with the consumption being related to the drug dose. Could a similar mechanism be the basis of the geophagy seen in some women in the first trimester of pregnancy?

7.5.2.2 Indirect activation of area postrema

In this model, instead of acting locally, the agent released by radiation or the cytotoxic drug enters the circulation to act at a distant

Table 7.5 A summary of the neurochemistry and neurophysiology of the area postrema. (For references, see Leslie *et al.*, 1985; 1986; Carpenter, 1990; Carpenter *et al.*, 1988.)

Present in AP	Activates AP neurons (% neurons activated)	Receptors binding sites and type	Induces emesis and route
Acetylcholine	√ (38)	√ Musc, Nic	√ i.c.v.
Adrenaline/ Nor-adrenaline	√ (32–40)	√ α_2	√ i.c.v
Angiotensin II	√ (47)	√	√ i.c.v., i.c.t.; i.v.
Cholecystokinin-8	√ (26)	?	√ i.v., X i.c.v.
Dopamine	√ (73)	√ D2	√ i.v.
Enkephalin	√ (53)	√ μ,δ	√ i.c.v., i.v., s.c.
GABA	?	?	?
Glutamate	√ (99)	?	√ i.v.
Histamine	√ (64)	√ H_1	√ i.c.v., X i.c.t.
LHRH	×	?	?
Neurotensin	√ (25)	?	√ i.c.t., i.c.v., i.v.
Substance P	√ (48)	?	√ i.v., X i.c.t.
Serotonin	√ (66)	√ $5\text{-}HT_3$	×
TRH	√ (66)	?	√ i.v.
VIP	√ (46)	?	√ i.v.

√ = function or effect demonstrated
X = function or effect shown to be absent
? = not studied
i.v. = intra-venous
i.c.v. = intra-cerebro-vertricular
i.c.t. = intra-cisternal

site assumed to be the AP, although other possibilities (e.g. hypothalamus) cannot be excluded.

Several sources of such an endogenous emetic factor have been proposed. In 1984 Harding *et al.* proposed that the gut mucosa was the most probable source of such an endogenous emetic 'hormone' and indeed several gut hormones are emetic when given intravenously or into the cerebral ventricles; these include neurotensin, cholecystokinin and vasoactive intestinal polypeptide (Table 7.5). At present the most promising candidate is peptide PYY. This peptide can induce emesis at a lower dose than other peptides, requires the presence of the AP for the response and AP neurons have been shown to be activated by the closely related compound neuropeptide NPY (reviewed in Kucharczyk and Harding, 1990). It is interesting to note that in addition to blocking the emesis induced by radiation and cytotoxic drugs, at least one of the $5\text{-}HT_3$ receptor antagonists, zacopride, can block NPY-induced emesis in the dog (Smith *et al.*, 1989). This work has yet to be repeated but it suggests that some of these agents may have broader effects. Further support for some interaction between NPY/PYY and $5\text{-}HT_3$ receptors comes from studies in man in which the $5\text{-}HT_3$ receptor antagonist ondansetron (proprietory name Zofran) reduced the post-prandial release of PYY (Talley *et al.*, 1989). The mechanism underlying these observations and their clinical significance remains to be elucidated.

It is unlikely that the 5-HT released from

the gut mucosa into the systemic circulation is involved in activation of the AP primarily because of the effect of the uptake mechanism in the platelets but also because of its metabolism during passage through the liver. Although some studies in man have reported an increase in plasma 5-HT concentration following cisplatin, the changes do not correlate with either the occurrence or pattern of emesis (Barnes *et al.*, 1990). In addition, large intravenous doses of 5-HT fail to induce emesis and although AP neurons are activated by iontophoretically applied 5-HT (Carpenter *et al.*, 1990), when given into the ventricles (Feldberg and Sherwood, 1954) or when analogues are injected into the AP (Higgins *et al.*, 1989) emesis is not induced. The role of 5-HT in emesis is discussed in more detail in Chapter 9.

Anti-tumour treatments may also induce the release of hormones with emetic activity from other sites. For example, both TRH and vasopressin (ADH) from the pituitary activate AP neurons and may be emetic (Carpenter *et al.*, 1984; 1988; 1990; Carpenter, 1990). In theory, these could gain access to the AP either via the blood or the cerebrospinal fluid. Vasopressin is a particularly promising candidate as plasma levels are vastly elevated in patients and animals receiving cytotoxic drugs (Cubeddu *et al.*, 1990) and experimental emetic stimuli including apomorphine and motion (Feldman *et al.*, 1988; Koch *et al.*, 1990).

The mechanism for vasopressin release may be indirect as a large release of vasopressin (but not oxytocin) can be induced by activation of abdominal vagal afferents in the ferret (Hawthorn *et al.*, 1988). Thus it is possible that the primary site of action of radiation and cytotoxic drugs is the gut which then releases a locally acting agent (e.g. 5-HT). This agent then fires vagal afferents which can directly activate the emetic reflex and which also induce the release of vasopressin from the posterior pituitary to enhance the emetic response. Although vasopressin has been shown to induce emesis, it has so far been implicated more in nausea and this is discussed in more detail below.

Other systemic factors implicated in emesis are prostaglandins (Carpenter *et al.*, 1983). Although there is some evidence for increases in circulating levels caused by radiation in nonvomiting animals, this is not supported by studies of irradiated monkeys (Dubois *et al.*, 1987) or patients receiving cisplatinum (Curry *et al.*, 1981). In the irradiated monkey there is a large increase in the plasma level of β-endorphin within two hours of exposure which returns to normal within two days (Dorval *et al.*, 1985).

A further endogenous factor, lipopolysaccharides (LPS) derived from the gut microflora, has been proposed as being involved in post-radiation induced nausea and vomiting as there is an increase in plasma levels following cervical radiotherapy (Maxwell *et al.*, 1986). The time course of the release is more suggestive of an involvement in the later components of emesis rather than in the more acute phase. The involvement of LPS in emesis has not been directly investigated in animals, although of interest are studies in the rat which demonstrated an increase in vasopressin by lipopolysaccharide from *E. coli* (Kasting *et al.*, 1985).

Although initially it may appear relatively straightforward to elucidate the role of putative endogenous emetic agents, the process is fraught with technical difficulties not the least of which is the temporal correlation of the plasma levels with the pattern of emesis. There is an expectation that the pattern of emesis will mirror the levels of an emetic agent in the plasma but, in fact, of more significance will be the levels of drug in the tissue compartment where the emetic detectors are located and which may not be in simple equilibrium with the plasma compartment. Some of the difficulties involved in such studies have been reviewed by Carl *et al.* (1989). From experiments in cross-circulated animals they concluded that 'neither in cats nor dogs was there significant evidence of a blood-borne humoral substance inducible upon cisplatin treatment'.

Although there appears to be little evidence to support a primary role for endogenous systemic agents in the induction of the acute phase of emesis (this does not exclude a sensitizing role), an involvement in the later phase should not be discounted, and such aspects are discussed in more detail below. Systemic factors may also be involved in the other effects of these therapies.

7.5.3 HUMORAL AGENTS AND PLASTICITY OF THE EMETIC PATHWAY

Studies of the effect of nerve lesioning in the ferret have suggested that under certain circumstances there may be involvement of an endogenous emetic agent that in the intact animal is either absent or has a minor role. In the intact ferret exposure to a 'high' dose of total body radiation (e.g. 800 rads) induces an emetic response that can be blocked by the 5-HT_3 receptor antagonist granisetron (proprietory name Kytril), a response which can also be blocked by acute abdominal vagotomy (Andrews and Bhandari, unpublished observations). From these studies it is concluded that the response is entirely dependent upon vagal and 5-HT_3 receptor activation. Three weeks after vagotomy, exposure to 800 rads results in a modified emetic response but it is not sensitive to blockade via 5-HT_3 receptor antagonism (Andrews *et al.*, 1990b). These observations, taken together, suggest that a novel mechanism is expressed following vagotomy and that it may take some time (a few weeks) to develop. The mechanism is not known but one of the most likely explanations is the release of an endogenous agent from the gut which then acts on the AP to induce emesis. The release can only be reliably accomplished by 'high' (i.e. more damaging) dose of radiation as the response to exposure to the lower dose of 200 rads is abolished in most animals following chronic vagotomy (Andrews *et al.*, 1990b).

These preliminary indications of 'plasticity' or reorganization in the emetic pathway may be of some clinical relevance. For example, in animal studies it is possible to achieve a complete block of emesis induced by X-radiation or a cytotoxic drug (e.g. cisplatin, cyclophosphamide) in all animals studied using a 5-HT_3 receptor antagonist. In patients given cisplatinum without prior chemotherapy, a complete response in 70% of patients is considered excellent for a 5-HT_3 receptor antagonist (Chapter 11). Although there are obvious differences between the clinical and experimental animal studies (section 7.3), could it be that the real difference in the response is due to the presence of additional non-5-HT_3 sensitive pathways in the patients who fail to respond on this type of therapy? The relative degree of expression of pathways may be a reflection of genetic differences (Japanese, for example, appear to be more radiosensitive than Westerners) or previous emetic experiences that are reflected more formally in predisposing factors such as a history of motion sickness or pregnancy sickness.

7.5.4 OTHER MECHANISMS

In using the term cytotoxic drug to describe the entire spectrum of anti-cancer chemotherapeutic agents there is a danger of assuming that in demonstrating a mechanism by which one agent induces emesis that such a mechanism applies to all. While the above discussions have focused on identification of common mechanisms it is worth drawing attention to two cytotoxic drugs which may illustrate other possibilities.

Animal studies with the potently emetic classical alkylating agent nitrogen mustard have revealed multiple sites of action including an apparent effect on the cerebral cortical pathways that influence the brainstem emetic co-ordinating areas (Borison *et al.*, 1958). The cholinergic receptor agonist pilocarpine is reported to induce emesis by an action at a forebrain site (Borison, 1959) and as nitrogen mustard is reported to induce the release of acetylcholine from neurons it is a distinct possibility that such as action contributes to the emetic effect of this agent.

Another example of a more direct pharmacological action comes possibly from procarbazine which probably exerts its anti-tumour effect by alkylation of DNA (Chapter 2). This agent was originally developed as a monoamine oxidase (MAO) inhibitor for use as an antidepressant. Severe nausea and vomiting are a problem with high bolus doses or infusions even though there is no myelotoxicity or anti-tumour effect, suggesting a dissociation between the true cytotoxic effects and the emesis. With oral doses, nausea and vomiting are initially moderately severe but subside with continued dosing. This pattern is typical of the side-effect profile of MAO inhibitors.

7.6 THE PATTERNS OF ACUTE AND DELAYED EMESIS: IS 5-HT THE SOLE MEDIATOR?

Thus far we have only considered the mechanisms responsible for initiating emesis but how is the response sustained over a period of hours or days and what determines the intensity and pattern of retching and vomiting throughout this time?

7.6.1 ACUTE PHASE

From detailed analysis of numerous records of the pattern of emesis in animals and a few similarly quantified studies in man the typical pattern is of a rapid build-up in retching and vomiting followed by a longer lasting 'tail' during which emesis gradually declines (Fig. 7.6, above). This would indicate that the intensity of the emetic stimulus is greatest soon after administration of the stimulus – as might generally be expected. Similar profiles are found for non-cytotoxic emetic stimuli such as apomorphine, morphine and loperamide acting at the level of the AP and those such as copper sulphate acting primarily via vagal afferents in the gut. In the case of the latter one might expect the response to decline as the vomiting thus triggered gradually removes the stimulus responsible for its initiation, but what is the explanation for the other stimuli?

There is little evidence that the overall pattern relates to either the plasma levels of the native drug or its metabolites, e.g. cyclophosphamide (Chapter 2) so how is the cytotoxic stimulus related to the intensity of emesis? If it is accepted that the final triggering of emesis is via the release of an intermediate agent (e.g. 5HT, PYY) rather than a primary direct action of the cytotoxic drug, then we can go some way towards answering these questions. Let us consider cisplatin as an example. A body of evidence has been presented suggesting that it is the gut enterochromaffin cell that transduces the effects of the cytotoxic drug into an emetic signal; thus we need to consider what happens to the enterochromaffin cell when exposed to the drug. So far this has only been studied in the guinea-pig but the results provide a conceptual framework for discussion of possible mechanisms (Schwörer *et al.*, 1991). On exposure to cisplatin there is a prompt release of 5-HT but even though the exposure is continuous, the release declines. Thus when the enterochromaffin cell is first exposed to cisplatin at a suitable concentration (the critical concentration is determined by the pharmacokinetics and pharmacodynamics) it will release 5-HT onto the vagal afferents which terminate in close proximity. The release will continue but if the *in vitro* studies can be extrapolated to the *in vivo* situation, this will not continue even if the cisplatin concentration is above the critical level. This could reflect a cellular toxicity of the cisplatin possibly interfering

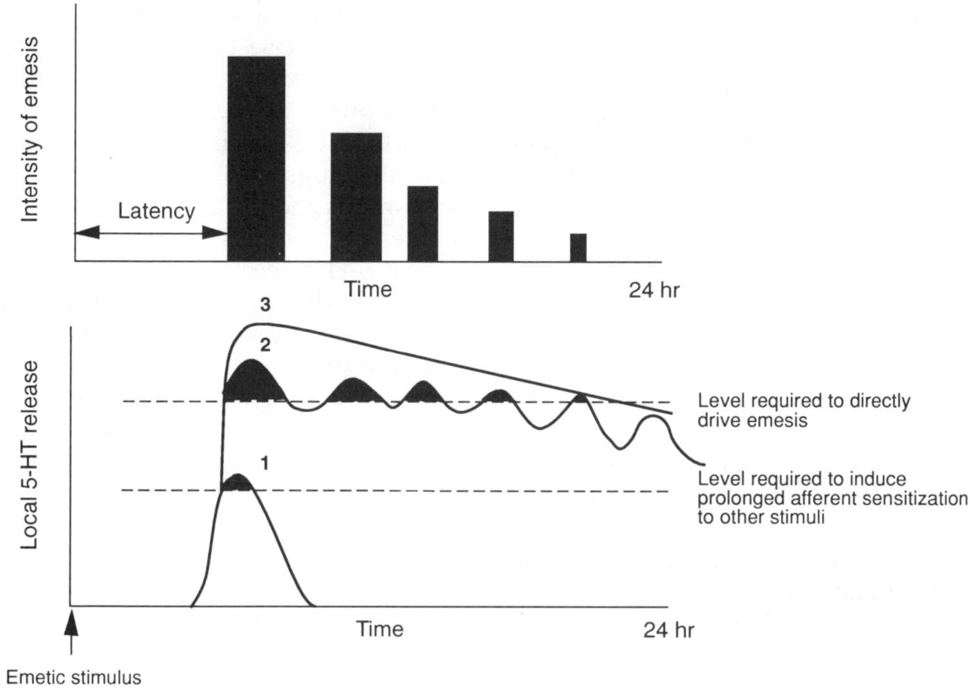

Figure 7.9 Three conceptual models of the possible release pattern of 5-hydroxytryptamine (5-HT) from the gut enterochromaffin cells following exposure to radiation or a cytotoxic drug. *Model 1*: The 5-HT is released in burst but only to a level that sensitizes the afferents to other stimuli which actually 'drive' the emesis. The rhythmicity of the bursts of emesis is either regulated centrally or by a bursting pattern of secretion of the other stimulus. *Model 2*: The 5-HT is released in such a quantity that it can directly drive emesis and induce sensitization. The pattern of emesis is essentially determined by the phasic secretory pattern of 5-HT. *Model 3*: Essentially as for model 2 except that the secretion of 5-HT is continuous and hence the pattern of emesis is determined by other factors.

with synthesis of 5-HT or the vesicular release mechanism, the latter requiring *de novo* protein synthesis. Is this perhaps the explanation for the increased levels of 5-HT in the gut mucosa 24 hours after cisplatin reported by Gunning *et al.* in 1987? It could also, of course, simply be due to an imbalance between the rate of synthesis and release due to intense activation of the release mechanism. From this discussion at least three models of the role of 5-HT can be proposed and the merits of each will be discussed in turn (Fig. 7.9). It should be borne in mind that each model should be able to account for the observation that an injection of a 5-HT_3 receptor antagonist can abort the established emetic response rapidly in animals (Bermudez *et al.*, 1988) and man (Cassidy *et al.*, 1988). In addition, while the discussion focuses on cisplatin there is only a reflection of the availability of data and the mechanisms could equally apply to many other emetic stimuli.

Firstly, there may be a single pulsed release of 5-HT with no continued release because of the limiting toxic cellular effects of the cisplatinum or because the cell is only exposed to the critical stimulus (e.g. radiation) or critical drug concentration (e.g. nitrogen mustard,

$t_{\frac{1}{2}}$ *in vitro* 9 min.) briefly. Could this single pulse of 5-HT trigger or sustain emesis? Well, it could trigger emesis; comparison of the time course of emesis, however, using large doses (5–10 mg/kg) of potent 5-HT_3 receptor agonists given orally or intraperitoneally in the ferret reveals that it is unlikely that such a release could account for the prolonged time course of emesis seen with anti-cancer therapies (Andrews *et al.*, unpublished observations). One role for such a brief release of 5-HT would be to sensitize the vagal afferents (or indeed other structures) to other stimuli. Although initially this may appear an unlikely effect, it is known that a single exposure to 5-HT can modify sensitivity in some systems for up to 48 hours (Sicuteri, 1968). In addition, neurophysiological studies of small diameter afferents in somatic muscle have shown that exposure to levels of 5-HT that do not in themselves cause neuronal activation can potentiate the nerve discharge induced by bradykinin (Mense, 1981). Secondly, the cisplatin may induce a continued release of 5-HT which then oscillates because of the time taken for the enterochromaffin cell to recharge its stores. Thus each time there is a release of 5-HT the afferents are discharged or are sensitized and emesis ensues.

Thirdly, the cisplatin may induce a truly continuous release of 5-HT which progressively declines with time after the stimulus. This 5-HT activates the afferents and triggers emesis but the pattern of emesis is phasic because of tachyphylaxis (desensitization) of the vagal 5-HT_3 receptors. Studies of another vagal reflex, the von Bezold-Jarisch reflex (Chapter 9) have shown that this reflex becomes desensitized if the 5-HT is administered at intervals of <12 minutes. The pattern of emesis may also be phasic because of the organization of the emetic circuitry as evidenced during experiments using continual electrical stimulation of vagal afferents (Andrews *et al.*, 1990).

A more detailed insight into the involvement of 5-HT can be gained from studies of the dose response curves of 5-HT_3 receptor antagonists against various emetic stimuli. As pointed out in the section on animal models, the intensity of emesis differs between cytotoxic drugs. If 5-HT is the link between the stimulus and the emetic response then the more emetic regimes should require a higher dose of 5-HT_3 receptor antagonist to reduce emesis. Studies with ondansetron (Zofran) in the ferret have shown that this does appear to be the case, with the highly emetic drug emetine requiring a higher dose of antagonist than radiation (Andrews and Bhandari, 1992). Further support for this linkage comes from studies using 5-HT_3 receptor antagonists of differing potencies tested against the same emetic stimulus. These studies show that the degree of reduction in emesis is related to the potency of the drugs as assessed using other assays of 5-HT_3 receptor antagonist activity.

The observation that an injection of a 5-HT_3 receptor antagonist can promptly stop emesis induced by X-radiation or cytotoxic drugs once established indicates that some form of continuous activation of 5-HT_3 receptors is required for emesis. Initially, this would appear to argue against the hypothesis that the 5-HT acts only as an initial sensitizing agent but this need not be the case if the 5-HT_3 receptors on the vagal afferent terminals have a very high affinity and a slow turnover rate. Some insight into the temporal involvement of 5-HT could be gained by careful studies of the dose of antagonist required to block emesis when given at different time points after administration of the emetic. It may also be possible to collect such data from some of the clinical intervention trials of 5-HT_3 receptor antagonists by monitoring the effectiveness of such administration with respect to time after cytotoxic administration. Such studies may also allow better definition of the transition point between 'acute' and 'delayed' phases of genesis. From the data obtained from prophylactic 5-HT_3 receptor antagonist administration

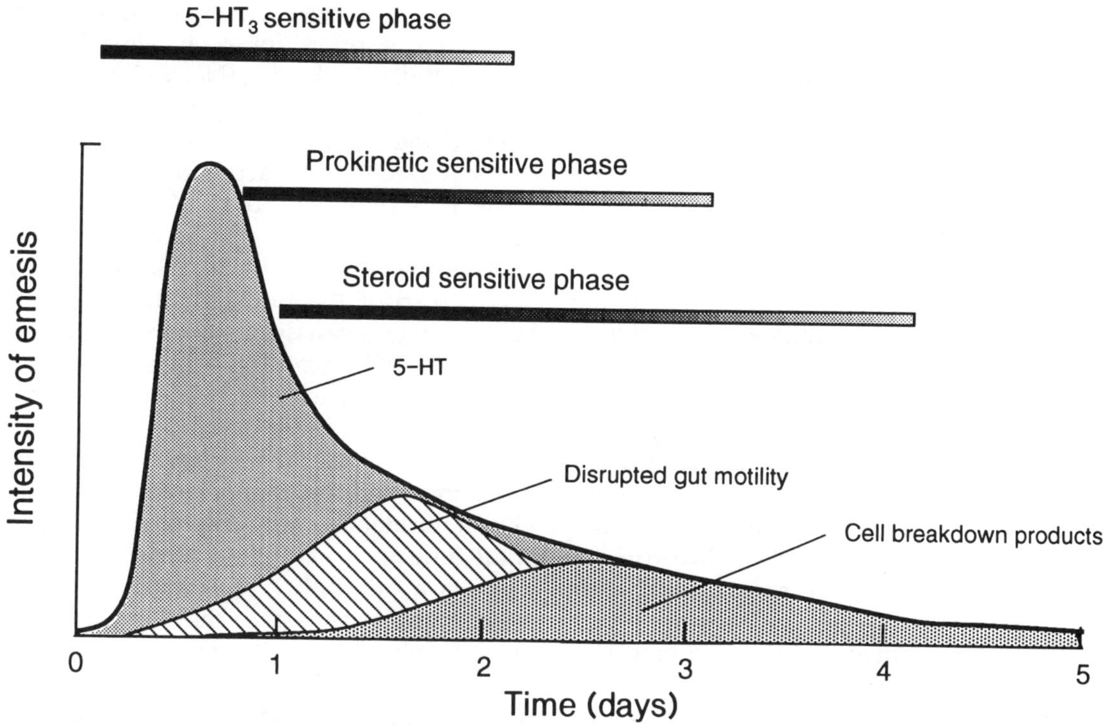

Figure 7.10 A conceptual model of the mechanisms that may be involved in the 'acute' and 'delayed' emetic effects of cisplatin. The model is intended to illustrate the multiplicity of mechanisms and how the predominant cause of emesis may be different for each phase accounting for the changing efficacy of various anti-emetic agents with time.

it would be expected that intervention would be less efficacious the nearer to the transition point that it was given.

7.6.2 DELAYED EMESIS

Understanding the mechanism of the delayed emesis – a particular problem with cisplatin and cyclophosphamide – has become a more pressing problem because of the high degree of success in the treatment of acute emesis. Conventionally, 'delayed emesis' is taken as starting about 24 hours after the administration of therapy but it should be remembered that this is a somewhat arbitrary distinction. The clinical trials to date using 5-HT$_3$ receptor antagonists have shown that these agents alone probably have only a minor effect on the delayed emesis (in contrast to their effects in the acute phase). This type of observation, although disappointing clinically, provides concrete evidence that the two phases involve different mechanisms (Fig. 7.10). It should be emphasized that this does not mean that there is no involvement of 5-HT$_3$ receptors (or indeed 5-HT) in the delayed phase but only to say that after the first 24 hours their role may diminish progressively.

The elucidation of the mechanism of delayed emesis will probably have to await human clinical trials as there is no currently available animal model for the study of this condition (as discussed above). One difficulty is that there are few descriptions of the 'natural' time course of delayed emesis. In one study with cisplatin, where patients recorded their own symptoms, 60 of the patients reported vomiting in the 48–72 hours following therapy (Kris *et al.*, 1985). One well-quantified study by Martin *et al.* (1990) monitored the course of emesis induced by carboplatin (300–400 mg/ m^2) in the absence of any anti-emetic therapy. It should be noted that although the time frame is different, the overall profile of the response showing a rapid rise to peak emesis and a prolonged decline is similar to that seen with cytotoxic drugs in animals (see Fig. 7.6, above). Although delayed emesis is less of a problem with this agent than cisplatin, the time course of the response is similar to high dose cyclophosphamide and FAC (5-FU, doxorubicin, cyclophosphamide combination) and thus provides a useful background against which to consider the problem of delayed emesis.

A number of mechanisms have been proposed many of which could be tested with carefully controlled clinical trials using well characterized pharmacological therapies. The mechanisms outlined below should not be viewed as alternatives; they could all be involved, contributing to different extents at different periods. The discussion will focus on cisplatinum and cyclophosphamide because, as has already been pointed out, delayed emesis is a particular problem with these agents.

7.6.2.1 Cerebral oedema, raised intra-cranial pressure and the blood–brain barrier

Nausea and vomiting can be induced by both cerebral oedema and raised intra-cranial pressure, particularly if they occur in the region of the brainstem. Is there then any evidence that the cytotoxic drugs with which delayed emesis is a problem have such effects? We are not aware of any formal studies in this area but two indirect pieces of evidence provide some support for such a mechanism. Firstly, studies in the dog (Neuwelt *et al.*, 1983) have shown that cisplatin given via the carotid artery (1 mg/kg, 28 mg/m^2) induced opening of the blood–brain barrier as indicated by Evans Blue staining of the brain parenchyma. There was associated neuropathology. This study shows that cisplatinum has the potential to disrupt the blood–brain barrier and hence may induce a degree of cerebral oedema. When given intravenously (2 mg/kg) there was no neurotoxicity or evidence of barrier disruption; however, if the blood–brain barrier was opened using mannitol then intravenous cisplatinum induced significant neurotoxicity. Thus if the blood–brain barrier is compromised at the time of cisplatinum administration then there is a possibility of central neurotoxic effects. Similar studies in the dog with cyclophosphamide (20 mg/kg i.v.) have revealed that it has only minor neurotoxic effects even with the blood–brain barrier disrupted (Neuwelt and Barnett, 1989). Although these observations would suggest that toxic effects of these agents on the central nervous system may not be of significance it should be borne in mind that what is being proposed is the induction of a mild, reversible cerebral oedema that may potentiate other emetic inputs.

One other piece of evidence supporting some involvement of blood–brain barrier disruption, oedema and raised intra-cranial pressure comes from the clinical experiences with corticosteroid analogues such as dexamethasone and methylprednisolone in delayed emesis. These agents have been used for over thirty years to treat cerebral oedema (reviewed in Yamada *et al.*, 1988) but their use as anti-emetics was based on the initial empirical observation that steroid pre-treatment reduced post-operative nausea and vomiting. The mechanism of the anti-emetic effect of the steroids is unknown but their anti-inflammatory effects mediated by modification of prostanoid turnover has attracted most attention (A review of mechanisms is given in Chapter 9). An additional possibility, particularly in delayed emesis, could be the well-known effects of the corticosteroids in reducing capillary permeability and hence oedema. In studies of the capillary permeability of brain tumours, steroids were shown to have little effect on permeability in normal tissue but reduced it in the immediate region of the tumour where permeability was increased. A similar observation has been made in studies of the delivery of methotrexate into the brain where dexamethasone reduced methotrexate delivery but only when the blood–brain barrier had been disrupted using mannitol (Neuwelt and Barnett, 1988). As pointed out above, the degree of disruption of the blood–brain barrier by conventional doses of cytotoxic drugs given intravenously is unclear and hence it is difficult to assess the contribution of such a capillary permeability effect to the overall anti-emetic action of steroids. One possibility that has not been investigated is whether the steroids have an effect on capillary permeability in parts of the brain where the capillaries are already relatively permeable, such as the AP. An effect here could limit the access of emetic stimuli, particularly large molecules such as lipopolysaccharides, and hence reduce any emetic effects. Such an effect on capillaries or even intercellular pathways could also occur in the gut.

7.6.2.2 Disordered gut function

Disturbances of gastro-intestinal tract function, particularly antral hypomotility and gastroparesis, are known to be capable of inducing protracted nausea and vomiting (Kerlin, 1989; Wengrower *et al.*, 1991). Therefore, if such changes in the gut were induced by cytotoxic drugs they could be implicated in the genesis of delayed emesis. In rats and mice treated with single doses of cisplatin there is a dose-related inhibition of gastric emptying reflected in an accumulation of food in the stomach (Bradner and Schurig, 1981). Following a single dose of cisplatin this gastroparesis may last several days, resolving spontaneously; a transient reduction in food intake occurs over a similar time course. The mechanism is not known but it can be reduced by prokinetic drugs, although not by selective 5-HT_3 receptor antagonists (Eeckhout, 1989). The effect of dexamethasone is not known. The rat does not vomit so the applicability of this model to delayed emesis in man is unclear. In addition, measurements of gastric emptying have not been made following administration of cisplatin which further complicates comparison.

Damage to the intestinal mucosa has been implicated in the genesis of disrupted gastro-intestinal motility produced by a number of agents such as Norwalk virus and coronavirus (Meeroff *et al.*, 1980; Burrows and Merritt, 1984). The functional and structural changes induced in the small intestine by the cytotoxic drugs cisplatin and the CMF combination may therefore induce a secondary change in motility (Cunningham *et al.*, 1985; Allan and Smyth, 1986). In the mouse the structural damage induced by cisplatin was not ameliorated by dexamethasone (Allan and Smyth, 1986).

If impaired gastric emptying or abnormal intestinal motility patterns are involved in the induction of delayed emesis then this can be tested relatively easily in man by judicious use of prokinetic agents such as cisapride and conventional dose metoclopramide. In using a gut motility stimulating drug it is critical that in the initial phase of delayed emesis (day 2/3) the stimulation is mild in order to avoid triggering emesis through excessive increases in motility under conditions where the emetic reflex may still be sensitized by the 5-HT released in the first 24 hours and the mucosa is damaged. As many patients who have been treated with 5-HT_3 receptor antagonists in the first 24 hours feel like eating, it may also be advisable to give some advice on diet over the following days. For example, small, frequent, low-residue meals will minimize the chances of developing gut stasis, a potent emetic stimulus in the sensitized state. In addition, fatty food and hypertonic drinks should be avoided as both slow gastric emptying and can induce emesis even in healthy subjects.

7.6.2.3 Products of cell breakdown

The gut mucosa normally provides an effective barrier against the entry of macromolecules into the bloodstream. Both radiation (Michalowski and Hornsey, 1986) and some cytotoxic drugs (e.g. cisplatin; Allan and Smyth, 1986) have toxic effects on the intestinal crypt cells and hence as these cells are sloughed there may be a breach in the integrity of the mucosa. This may allow access of endotoxin lipopolysaccharides (LPS) to the bloodstream. Intravenously administered *E. coli*-derived LPS endotoxins can induce emesis in animals and a dramatic rise in plasma LPS has been reported in radiotherapy patients receiving 1000 rads to the cervix. The rise in plasma LPS reached a peak over four days and was related to the morbidity index (Maxwell *et al.*, 1986). It is possible that although dexamethasone does not prevent the crypt cell damage induced by cisplatin, it may somehow reduce the permeability of the intestinal capillaries to some of the larger molecules that enter the interstitium via breaches in the mucosa.

The gut mucosa is a rich source of hormones many of which in higher doses can induce emesis and release of these as part of the cytotoxic effects of cisplatin and radiation should not be overlooked.

Protecting the gut against these damaging effects may offer a therapeutic approach to delayed emesis. In one study some of the intestinal damage induced by cisplatin was reduced by 2-mercaptoethane sulphonate (Allan *et al.*, 1986). A study of diethyldithiodicarbamate (DDTC) used as a 'rescue' treatment in cisplatin-induced toxicity, demonstrated a reduction in acute cisplatin emesis in the dog (Bhandari *et al.*, 1989). While DDTC has a number of actions (e.g. as an antioxidant, chelating agent for platinum) which may contribute to this effect, it is possible that it is also cytoprotective.

The above discussion illustrates that delayed emesis is probably multifactorial with the relative contribution (if any) of each of the above factors not yet determined. In the absence of a suitable animal model for this type of emesis, elucidation of the mechanism will probably depend upon clinical studies. Use of dexamethasone clearly offers one approach and better characterization of its effects in man will give important pointers to mechanisms and perhaps ways of improving its efficacy. Apart from studies of dexamethasone in delayed emesis, investigation of its interactions with 5-HT_3 receptor antagonists in the acute phase of emesis will also give important insights into its pharmacology. In addition to studies of dexamethasone, the involvement of disrupted gastro-intestinal motility is also relatively amenable to study in man using prokinetic drugs.

7.7 THE MECHANISMS OF NAUSEA

The mechanism of nausea is not known and hence this section is probably the most speculative part of our review. Nausea might be defined as an unpleasant, but not painful, sensation associated with a heightened awareness of the upper gut (throat, oesophagus, stomach) and the conviction that vomiting is imminent. The nauseated subject tends to focus on their own lack of well being and become disinterested in the external surroundings giving rise to problems if they are engaged in tasks requiring a high level of concentration such as flying an aeroplane. Stimuli which evoke vomiting usually evoke nausea prior to vomiting but it is possible in some cases (e.g. motion) to adjust the stimulus to produce only nausea whereas with some stimuli (e.g. suddenly raised intra-cranial pressure) vomiting may occur without nausea.

The factors determining the duration of nausea before the onset of vomiting are not known but even with the same stimulus (e.g. motion) there are considerable individual variations in the time taken to evoke vomiting and the reported intensity of the attendant nausea. The nausea may be ameliorated by vomiting but subsequently it is likely to increase in intensity again until the next vomiting episode, particularly if the stimulus continues. However, the nausea may also continue after stimulation has stopped, a phenomenon particularly easy to demonstrate with motion sickness (Reason and Brand, 1975).

Nausea is often accompanied by cold sweating, skeletal muscle vasodilatation, licking, salivation, cutaneous vasoconstriction, headache or tightness in the temples, decreased urine production, decreased glucose utilization, increased lactic dehydrogenase levels, hyperventilation, decrease in end tidal CO_2 percentage and increased blood pH (Reason and Brand, 1975). The proximal stomach is relaxed, gastric acid and pancreatic secretion are decreased, antral tachygastria and retrograde contractions or spasm may be present in the duodenum, and gastric emptying is decreased (Andrews and Hawthorn, 1988; Eversham *et al.*, 1978). Plasma vasopressin (anti-diuretic hormone, ADH) is elevated 20–50 times above basal level in response to some emetic stimuli such as motion (Eversham *et al.*, 1978), chemotherapy (Fisher *et al.*, 1982), apomorphine, and abdominal vagal afferent stimulation (Hawthorn *et al.*, 1988), but not to others such as ipecacuanha (Nussey *et al.*, 1988). Beta-endorphin but not met-enkephalin levels increase in the plasma about 30 minutes prior to the onset of nausea induced by chemotherapy (Pisher *et al.*, 1972), and growth hormone, prolactin and cortisol increase in response to motion stimuli but these changes are delayed in comparison to ADH secretion and hence they are considered to be a consequence of the stress induced by the stimulus (Eversham *et al.*, 1978).

Two major problems have hampered our understanding of the mechanism of nausea. It is possible, in man and animals, to monitor a number of physiological variables such as cutaneous blood flow, skin resistance, respiration rate, gastric electrical activity, blood pressure, heart rate, and the levels of a number of agents in the plasma in the period after emetic administration and before retching and vomiting start. While a number of these parameters change during the nauseous phase, and with a number of emetic agents, the major questions are: which actually contribute to the generation of the sensation of nausea, which are components of the body's preparation for vomiting (e.g. retroperistalsis, salivation), and which are reflections of the physiological response of the body to the stress of an unpleasant stimulus (e.g. β-endorphin, cortisol)?

Although we can make a number of deductions about which parameters fall into each category we cannot be certain of the answers without more careful studies in which a battery of variables (physiological and biochemical) are monitored **continuously** and related to reported symptoms. Second, while in experimental animals the number of retches or vomits can easily be quantified, the measurement and interpretation of behaviour in the pre-ejection phase is a difficult task. For example, in the ferret a number of behaviours have been identified which increase in intensity after an emetic agent is administered (Hawthorn and Andrews, unpublished observations; Davis, 1988). However, while these behaviours occur when we would expect nausea to be reported in man with the same treatments, we do not actually know whether the ferret actually perceives a sensation that we would recognize as nausea; this is similar to the way in which we can only observe how animals respond to noxious stimuli but have no concept of the sensation perceived by them. For the present it may be advisable to regard these pre-emetic behaviours as 'nausea-equivalents'.

Unfortunately, very few animal studies comment in detail, or indeed at all, on the behaviour of animals treated with emetic agents, particularly following such frequently used lesions as AP ablation. Thus even if we treated the pre-emetic behaviour as a 'nausea-equivalent', considerably more animal studies are required before any conclusions could be drawn. Nevertheless, animal studies have revealed a considerable amount of information about the gastro-intestinal motor changes which occur prior to vomiting and it is the possible role of these changes in the generation of nausea that the remainder of this section will address (see also chapter 4).

7.7.1 WHAT CONSTITUTES A NAUSEOGENIC STIMULUS AND HOW AND WHERE IS IT INTERPRETED?

Virtually any agent that evokes vomiting can also produce nausea. It has often been stated that nausea represents a low level activation of the emetic pathways and this idea has some merit if nausea is regarded as a warning signal (of, for example, pain); nausea is often evoked in isolation using low doses of emetic agents (e.g. apomorphine) in animals, including man. However, we should remember that retching and vomiting can be mediated via pathways involving only the brainstem, as decerebrated animals have the ability to vomit, whereas the generation of nausea presumably requires access of information to higher regions of the CNS. Thus it may be that not only is the stimulation at a low level but its central processing may be different from that which finally triggers the ejection of gut contents. A consideration of the properties of visceral afferents and the functions they subserve shows, however, that this is too simple a view.

As an example of this, mechanoreceptors under basal conditions signal the prevailing level of motor activity in the gut muscle and distension causes further activation which evokes a reflex to relax the muscle. Further distention may evoke a pleasurable sensation of fullness but, if continued, will evoke sensations of nausea, bloating or pain and finally vomiting may ensue. Thus while in one sense nausea may represent 'low level' activation of the vomiting pathway it represents a 'high level' of activation of other systems. A similar argument could be made for the vestibular system with low levels of stimulation giving information on head position and producing vestibulo-visual and vestibulo-colic reflexes whereas higher levels evoke nystagmus, nausea and vomiting. Although such 'intensity' theories are easy to understand, a more complex explanation may in fact be involved. Thus if the gut afferents form part of the pathway (see below) then it could be that it is not the signal carried by one group that is important but the pattern of signals reaching the CNS via a number of nerve fibres, as with taste coding (Ogawa *et al.*, 1968).

One feature that is common to nausea whatever the stimulus and which makes a marked contribution to this unpleasant sensory experience is the heightened awareness of the gut sometimes referred to as a 'visceral aura'. While this sensation may of course originate from the gut, an alternative possibility that may apply in some cases is that the sensation is actually 'referred to' the gut, rather as cardiac pain may be referred to the left arm. As most toxins in the natural world enter the body via the gut it would be appropriate to refer the sensation to that site even if the toxin has a central effect. How then could the 'processing' of this information be organized? Sensations from the gut must in the final analysis be the result of afferent signals from the abdomen (conveyed in the vagus or splanchnic nerves) being interpreted at a conscious level. The pathways involved are not precisely known but the *nucleus tractus solitarius* (NTS) in the brainstem certainly serves as a major integrating area for visceral afferent information and by virtue of its outputs (Chapter 6) could relay (directly or indirectly) such information to the 'higher' regions of the CNS.

Pathways have also been described by which information from vagal afferents and the AP could reach the visceral area of the sensory cortex in the granular portion of the insular region (Cechetto and Saper, 1990). Thus suitable afferent activation of the NTS and hence its output pathways could give rise to a pattern of activity which the cerebral cortex interprets as nausea. If, instead of being activated by visceral afferents, the pathway from the NTS to the cerebral cortex is activated in an **identical** manner by other inputs then the sensation produced (nausea) will be the same as if the abdominal afferents were activated (compare with convergence projection theory of referred pain). The AP has direct projections to the NTS and could be involved in nausea produced by emetic agents acting at this site. In considering this scheme we should also remember that the NTS sends outputs to the brainstem nuclei which are involved in regulating the autonomic nervous system and hence many of the physiological changes which accompany nausea. While this scheme has a number of flaws it does at least provide a framework for understanding how nausea generated either by gut or CNS stimulation both give rise to a similar spectrum of sensations and effects. In the sections below two of the better understood aspects of the physiology of nausea are discussed.

7.7.2 THE ROLE OF THE GUT IN NAUSEA

From the arguments presented in Chapter 5 it appears unlikely that the gastro-intestinal motor events seen prior to retching or vomiting are the main source of the sensation of nausea, although they may well reinforce the sensation, possibly contributing to the 'wave-like' nature of the nausea and the increase in intensity which is often described as vomiting becomes imminent. We have already stated that exogenous or endogenous (those from the gut) agents acting probably on the AP could evoke nausea referred to the gut by activation of the CNS pathways stimulated by visceral afferent activation. But we should also consider whether the CNS itself undergoes changes in response to incoming nauseogenic stimuli.

Two examples are relevant here. First, afferent activity from the gut is continually reaching the medulla in the many thousands of afferents which are active even in the interdigestive state, but in normal circumstances this activity does not enter consciousness. One aspect of nausea is a heightened awareness of the gut and this may occur not only as a result of an increase in gut afferent activity but also by 'allowing' more of the afferent barrage to enter consciousness. The function of this may be to enhance the association between the gut (the site at which the nauseant stimulus would usually act in nature), the sensation of nausea, and possibly the taste (if any) of the causative agent. In this respect it is particularly relevant that in man and rats nausea is the most potent stimulus for the production of acquired dislikes for the tastes of foods with other gut-related disorders (heartburn, bloating, pain, cramp, diarrhoea) being much less effective (Pelchat and Rozin, 1982). Secondly, it has been shown that the AP can influence cerebral cortical EEG activity (Bronzino *et al.*, 1972) and hence agents acting on the AP may influence the arousal level of the animal and thus its perception of visceral events.

7.7.3 THE POSSIBLE ROLE OF VASOPRESSIN

Considerable interest has focused on the endocrine changes associated with nausea.

Vasopressin has been the hormone most consistently associated with nausea. Massive increase (over 50-fold) in plasma vasopressin have been measured in response to a number of experimental stimuli (e.g. apomorphine; Feldman *et al.*, 1989; motion; Koch *et al.*, 1990) and clinical (e.g. chemotherapy; Edwards *et al.*, 1989) stimuli in both man and laboratory animals (e.g. monkey, Verbalis *et al.*, 1987; dog, Carl *et al.*, 1989). In general these studies indicate that in man vasopressin only rises in those subjects who experience nausea; in animal studies it begins in fact to rise before the onset of vomiting. It is of course impossible to identify whether vasopressin is the cause of nausea or a consequence of the generally stressful nature of the experience. Studies in which levels of 'stress' hormones such as cortisol have been monitored indicate that the release occurs later than that of vasopressin (Eversham *et al.*, 1978). In addition, vasopressin can activate AP neurons (Carpenter, 1990) and infusions can induce nausea and vomiting (Thomford and Sirinek, 1975), although in neither of these aspects is it unique. It should be emphasized that a universal causal link between vaso-pressin and nausea is far from proven as is illustrated by the following study with ipec-acuanha and apomorphine. Oral ipecacuanha is a potent nauseogenic and emetic stimulus and yet it failed to induce a rise in vasopressin in human subjects in which apomorphine induced a large increase (Nussey *et al.*, 1988). In addition, in patients with idiopathic diabetes insipidus, apomorphine failed to induce an increase in vasopressin, although nausea was induced.

Although there are gaps and some inconsistencies in our understanding of the role of vasopressin in nausea, it could possibly have other functions in the emetic reflex. For instance, the release of vasopressin has been suggested as an agent to promote water conservation in anticipation of the fluid and ionic losses caused by vomiting. While this hypothesis is not unreasonable, it is unclear why such a massive release of vasopressin of up to 30 times maximal anti-diuretic levels should be required to achieve this end.

Vasopressin has also been shown to facilitate memory consolidation and possibly the retrieval process by modulation of noradrenergic transmission in the limbic midbrain terminals of the dorsal noradrenergic bundle (De Weid, 1980). Since one of the functions of nausea is to induce an aversive response to the nauseating agent it is possible that the large quantities of vasopressin released during nausea may facilitate the formation of the aversive memory.

7.8 CONCLUSIONS

In recent years there have been considerable advances in our understanding of the relative contributions of the area postrema and the abdominal visceral afferents to the induction of emesis by anti-cancer therapies. The identification of the selective anti-emetic effects of the 5-HT_3 receptor antagonists has further facilitated knowledge of the mechanisms and provided a focus for research as well as greatly improving the quality of life for patients undergoing treatment for cancer. Inevitably there are still major gaps in our knowledge, particularly in the identification of the precise mechanisms by which anti-cancer therapies activate serotonergic systems, the mechanism of delayed emesis, and the neuropharmacology of the sensation of nausea. The solution to these problems requires a combination of fundamental studies with appropriate animal models and carefully designed clinical studies so that novel therapies can be designed based on a rational understanding of mechanisms.

ACKNOWLEDGEMENTS

The authors wish to thank SmithKline Beecham, Glaxo Group Research and the MOD (Procurement Executive) for financial support of their studies reported in this chapter. In addition, we acknowledge our co-workers, in particular Drs P. Bhandari, S. Bingham, I. Davidson and J. Hawthorn who participated in the studies and in discussions of the problems. Finally, we thank Mrs E. Town for patience in typing the numerous drafts of this manuscript.

REFERENCES

Abrahamsson, H., Jansson, G. and Martinson, J. (1973) Vagal relaxation of the stomach induced by apomorphine in the cat. *Acta Physiol. Scand.*, **88**, 296–302.

Abrahamsson, H. and Thoren, P. (1973) Vomiting and reflex vagal relaxation of the stomach elicited from heart receptors in the cat. *Acta Physiol. Scand.*, **88**, 433–39.

Ahlman, H. and Dahlstrom, A. (1983) 'Vagal mechanisms controlling serotonin release from the gastrointestinal tract and pyloric motor function', in *Vagal Nerve Function: Behavioural and Methodological Considerations*. (eds J.G. Kral, T.L. Powley and C.Mc.C. Brooks) pp. 119–40. Elsevier, Amsterdam.

Alexander, E., Siddon, R.L. and Loeffer, J.S. (1989) The acute onset of nausea and vomiting following stereotactic radiosurgery: correlation with total dose to the area postrema. *Surg. Neurol.*, **32**, 40–44.

Allan, S.G., Hay, F.G., Leonard, R.C.F. *et al.* (1985) Protective effect of mesna on the gastrointestinal toxicity of *cis*-platinum. *Br. J. Cancer*, **52**, 454 (abstract).

Allan, S.G. and Smyth, J.F. (1986) Small intestinal mucosal toxicity of cisplatinum. Comparison of toxicity with platinum analogues and dexamethasone. *Br. J. Cancer*, **53**, 355–60.

Andrews, P.L.R. (1986a) The non-adrenergic non-cholinergic innervation of the stomach. *Arch. Int. Pharmacodyn*. **280** Suppl., 84–109.

Andrews, P.L.R. (1986b) 'Vagal afferent innervation of the gastrointestinal tract', in *Progress in Brain Research*. Vol. 67 (eds F. Cervero, and J.F.B. Morrison) pp. 65–86. Elsevier, Amsterdam.

Andrews, P.L.R., Bhandari, P., Garland, S. *et al.* (1990a) Does retching have a function?: An experimental study in the ferret. *Pharmacodyn. Ther.* (Life Science Advances), **9**, 135–52.

Andrews, P.L.R. and Bhandari, P. (1992) The 5-hydroxytryptamine$_3$ receptor antagonists as anti-emetics: pre-clinical evaluation and mechanism of action. *Eur. J. Cancer.* S375, S1–6.

Andrews, P.L.R. and Davidson, H.I.M. (1990) Activation of vagal afferent terminals by 5-hydroxytryptamine is mediated by the 5-HT$_3$ receptor in the anesthetised ferret. *J. Physiol.*, **422**, 92P.

Andrews, P.L.R., Davis C.J., Bingham S. *et al.* (1990b) The abdominal visceral innervation and the emetic reflex: pathways, pharmacology and plasticity. *Can. J. Physiol. Pharmacol.*, **68**, 325–45.

Andrews, P.L.R. and Hawthorn, J. (1988) The neurophysiology of vomiting. *Clin. Gastroenterol.*, **2**, 141–68.

Andrews, P.L.R. and Lawes, I.N.C. (1985) Characteristics of the vagally driven non-adrenergic non-cholinergic inhibitory innervation of ferret corpus. *J. Physiol.*, **363**, 1–20.

Andrews, P.L.R., Rapeport, W.G. and Sanger, G.J. (1988) Neuropharmacology of emesis induced by anti-cancer therapy. *Trends in Pharmacological Sciences*, **9**, 334–41.

Barnes, N.M. Ge, J., Jones, W.G. *et al.* (1990) Cisplatin induced emesis: preliminary results indicative of changes in plasma levels of 5-hydroxytryptamine. *Br. J. Cancer*, **62**, 862–64.

Barrett, A., Barrett, A.J. and Powels, R.L. (1979) Total body irradiation and marrow transplantation for acute leukaemia. The Royal Marsden Hospital experience. *Pathol. Biol.* **27**, 357–59.

Beck, P.W. and Handwerker, H.O. (1974) Bradykinin and serotonin effects on various types of cutaneous nerve fibres. *Pflügers Archiv*, **347**, 209–22.

Bermudez, J., Boyle, E.A., Miner, W.D. and Sanger, G.J. (1988) The anti-emetic potential of the 5-hydroxytryptamine receptor antagonist BRL43694. *Br. J. Cancer*, **58**, 644–50.

Bhandari, P. and Andrews, P.L.R. (1991) Preliminary evidence for the involvement of the putative 5-HT$_4$ receptor in zacopride and copper sulphate – induced vomiting in the ferret. *Eur J. pharmacol* **204**, 273–80.

Bhandari, P., Bingham, S. and Andrews, P.L.R. (1992) The neuropharmacology of loperamide induced emesis in the ferret: the role of the area postrema, vagus, opiate, and 5-HT$_3$ receptors. *Neuropharmacology*. **31**, 735–42.

Bhandari, P., Gupta, Y.K., Seth, S.D. and Chugh, A. (1988) Emetic profile of cisplatin in dogs. *Asia Pac. J. Pharmacol.*, **3**, 131–33.

Bhandari, P., Gupta, Y.K. and Seth, S.D. (1989) Effect of diethyldithiocarbamate on cisplatinum induced emesis in dogs. *Asia Pac. J. Pharmacol.*, **3**, 247–50.

Blackshaw, L.A. and Grundy, D. (1991) 5-hydroxytryptamine (5-HT_3) receptor mediated effects on vagal afferent fibres in the upper gastrointestinal tract of the anaesthetized ferret. *J. Physiol.*, **435**, 64P.

Blau, J.N. (1990) The nature of migraine: do we need to invoke slow neurochemical processes? in *Migraine, a Spectrum of Ideas*, Chapter 2, pp. 4–20 (eds M. Sandler, and G. Collins) Oxford Medical Publications, Oxford.

Borison, H.L. (1959) Effect of ablation of medullary emetic chemoreceptor trigger zone on vomiting responses to cerebral intraventricular injection of adrenaline, apomorphine and pilocarpine in the cat. *J. Physiol.*, **147**, 172–77.

Borison, H.L. (1989) Area postrema: chemoreceptor circumventricular organ of the medulla oblongata. *Prog. Neurobiol.*, **32**, 351–90.

Borison, H.L., Brand, E.D. and Orkand, R.K. (1958) Emetic action of nitrogen mustard (mechlorethamine hydrochloride) in dogs and cats. *Am. J. Physiol.*, **192**, 410–16.

Borison, H.L. and McCarthy, L.E. (1983) Neuropharmacology of chemotherapy-induced emesis. *Drugs* **25** (Suppl 1), 8–17.

Borison, H.L., McCarthy, L.E., Douple, E.B. *et al.* (1987) Acute radiation induced vomiting in area postrema ablated cats. *Radiat. Res.*, **109**, 430–39.

Borison, H.L., McCarthy, L.E. and Johnson, J.R. (1987) High dorsal column cordotomy plus subdiaphragmatic vagotomy prevents acute ionizing radiation sickness in cats. *Exp. Neurol.*, **98**, 645–58.

Borison, H.L. and Wang, S.C. (1953) Physiology and pharmacology of vomiting. *Pharmacol. Rev.*, **5**, 193–230.

Bradner, W.T. and Schurig, J.E. (1981) Toxicology screening in small animals. *Cancer Treat. Rev.*, **8**, 93–102.

Brizzee, K.R. (1956) Effect of localised brainstem lesions and supradiaphragmatic vagotomy on X-irradiation emesis in the monkey. *Am. J. Physiol.*, **187**, 567–70.

Brizzee, K.R., Neal, L.M. and Williams, P.M. (1955) The chemoreceptor trigger zone for emesis in the monkey. *Am. J. Physiol.*, **180**, 659–62.

Bronzino, J.D., Morgate, P.J. and Stern, W.C. (1972) EEG synchronization following application of serotonin to the area postrema. *Am. J. Physiol.*, **223**, 376–83.

Burrows, C.F. and Merritt, A.M. (1984) Influence of coronavirus (transmissible gastroenteritis) infection on jejunal myoelectrical activity of the neonatal pig. *Gastroenterology*, **87**, 386–91.

Carl, P.L., Cubeddu, L.X., Lindley, C. *et al.* (1989) Do humoral factors mediate cancer chemotherapy induced emesis? *Drug Metab. Rev.*, **21**, 319–33.

Carmichael, J., Cantwell, B.M.J., Edwards, C.M. *et al.* (1988) Prevention and amelioration of cisplatinum-induced nausea and vomiting by BRL43694, a selective 5-HT_3 receptor antagonist: results of an open dose ranging study. *Br. Med. J.*, **297**, 110–11.

Carpenter, D.O. (1990) Neural mechanisms in emesis. *Can. J. Physiol. Pharmacol.*, **68**, 230–36.

Carpenter, D.O., Briggs, D.B. and Strominger, N. (1983) Responses of neurons of canine area postrema to neurotransmitters and peptides. *Cell. Molec. Neurobiol.*, **3**, 113–26.

Carpenter, D.O., Briggs, D.B. and Strominger, N. (1984) Peptide induced emesis in dogs. *Behav. Br. Res.*, **11**, 277–81.

Carpenter, D.O., Briggs, D.B., Knox, A.P. and Strominger, N. (1988) Excitation of area postrema neurons by transmitters, peptides and cyclic nucleotides. *J. Neurophysiol.*, **59**, 358–69.

Carpenter, D.O., Briggs, D.B., Knox, A.P. and Strominger, N.L. (1986) Radiation-induced emesis in the dog: effect of lesions and drugs. *Radiat. Res.*, **108**, 307–16.

Cassidy, J., Raina, V., Lewis, C. *et al.* (1988) Pharmacokinetics and anti-emetic efficacy of BRL 43694, a new selective 5-HT_3 antagonist. *Br. J. Cancer*, **58**, 651–53.

Cechetto, D.F. and Saper, C.B. (1990) 'Role of the cerebral cortex in autonomic function', in *Central Regulation of Autonomic Functions* (eds A.D. Loewy and K.M. Spyer) pp. 308–23. Oxford University Press, Oxford.

Chaney, S.G. and Kare, M.R. (1966) Emesis in birds. *JAMVA*, **149**, 938–43.

Chen, J-T., Hirai, Y., Hamada, T. *et al.* (1987)

Medical vagotomy: a new effective antiemetic therapy for cisplatin-induced nausea and vomiting. *Acta Obstet. Gynaecol. Jpn.*, **39**, 2231–32.

Cubeddu, L.X., Hoffman, I.S., Fuenmayor, N.T. and Finn, A.L. (1990) Efficacy of ondansetron and the role of serotonin in cisplatin-induced nausea and vomiting. *N. Engl. J. Med.*, **322**, 810–16.

Cunningham, D., Morgan, R.J., Mills, P.R. *et al.* (1985) Functional and structural changes of the human proximal small intestine after cytotoxic therapy. *J. Clin. Pathol.*, **38**, 265–70.

Curry, S.L., Rine, J., Whitney, C.W. *et al.* (1981) The role of prostaglandins in the excessive nausea and vomiting after intra-vascular *cis*-platinum therapy. *Gynaecologic. Oncol.*, **12**, 89–91.

Daunton, N.G. (1990) 'Animal models in motion sickness research', in *Motion and Space Sickness* (ed G.H. Crampton) pp. 88–104. CRC Press, Boca Raton, USA.

Davidson, H.I.M. and Andrews, P.L.R. (1990) Activation of afferent fibres by the cytotoxic drug cisplatinum. *J. Auton. Nerv. Syst.*, **31**, 179.

Davis, C.J. (1988) Neuropharmacological investigations into the mechanisms of emesis caused by cytotoxic drugs and radiation. D.Phil. thesis, University of Oxford.

Davis, C.J., Harding, R.K., Leslie, R.A. and Andrews, P.L.R. (1986) 'The organisation of vomiting as a protective reflex', in *Nausea and Vomiting: Mechanisms and Treatment* (eds C.J. Davis, G.V. Lake-Bakaar, and D.G. Grahame-Smith) pp. 65–75. Springer-Verlag, Berlin.

Davis, C.J., Lake-Bakaar, G.V. and Grahame-Smith, D.G., eds (1986) *Nausea and Vomiting: Mechanisms and Treatment*. Springer Verlag, Berlin.

De Weid, D. (1980) Behavioural actions of neurohypophysiological peptides. *Proc. R. Soc. Lond.* B 210, 183–95.

Dorval, E.D., Mueller, G.P., Eng, R.R. *et al.* (1985) Effect of ionizing radiation on gastric secretion and gastric motility in monkeys. *Gastroenterology*, **89**, 374–80.

Drapanas, T., McDonald, J.C. and Stewart, J.D. (1962) Serotonin release following instillation of hypertonic glucose into the proximal intestine. *Ann. Surg.*, **156**, 528–36.

Dubois, A. Jacobus, J.P., Grissom, M.P. *et al.* (1984) Altered gastric emptying and prevention of radiation-induced vomiting in dogs. *Gastroenterology*, **86**, 444–48.

Dubois, A., Dorval, E.D., Steel, L. *et al.* (1987) Effect of ionizing radiation on prostaglandins and gastric secretion in rhesus monkeys. *Radiat. Res.*, **110**, 289–93.

Edwards, C.M., Carmichael, J., Baylis, P.H. and Harris, A.L. (1989) Arginine vasopressin – a mediator of chemotherapy induced emesis? *Br. J. Cancer*, **59**, 467–70.

Eeckhout, C. (1989) Effect of prokinetics with a different mechanism of action on cisplatin-induced slowing of gastric emptying in the rat. *J. Gastroint. Motil.*, **1**, 52.

Elwell, M.R., Liu, C.T., Spertzel, R.O. and Beisel, W.R. (1975) Mechanism of oral enterotoxin B-induced emesis in the monkey. *Proc. Soc. Exp. Biol. Med.*, **148**, 424–27.

Eversham, T., Gottshamn, M., Uhlich, E. *et al.* (1978) Increased secretion of growth hormone, prolactin, anti-diuretic hormone and cortisol induced by the stress of motion sickness. *Aviat. Space Environ. Med.*, **49**, 53–57.

Feldberg. W. and Sherwood, S.L. (1954) Injections of drugs into the lateral ventricle of the cat. *J. Physiol.*, **123**, 148–67.

Feldman, M., Samson, W.K., and O'Dorisio, T.M. (1988) Apomorphine-induced nausea in humans: release of vasopressin and pancreatic polypeptide. *Gastroenterology*, **95**, 721–26.

Fetting, J.H., McCarthy, L.E., Borison, H.L. and Colvin, M. (1982) Vomiting induced by cyclophosphamide and phosphoramide mustard in cats. *Cancer Treat. Rep.*, **66**, 1625–27.

Fetting, J.H., Wilcox, P.M., Sheidler, V.R. *et al.* (1985) Taste associated with parenteral chemotherapy for breast cancer. *Cancer Treat. Rep.*, **69**, 1249–51.

Fisher, R.D., Rentschler, R.E., Nelson, J.C. *et al.* (1982) Elevation of plasma ADH associated with chemotherapy-induced emesis in man. *Cancer Treat. Rep.*, **66**, 25–29.

Florczyk, A.P., Schurig, J.E. and Bradner, W.T. (1982) Cisplatin-induced emesis in the ferret: A new animal model. *Cancer Treat. Rep.*, **66**, 187–89.

Friedman, O.M., Myles, A. and Colvin, M. (1979) 'Cyclophosphamide and related phosphoramide mustards – current status and future prospects', in *Advances in Cancer Chemotherapy* (ed A. Rosowsky) pp. 143–204. Marcel Dekker, New York.

Gershwin, M.E., Goetzl, E.J. and Steinberg, A.D. (1974) Cyclophosphamide use in practice. *Ann. Int. Med.*, **80**, 531–40.

Grundy, D., Blackshaw, A. and Andrews, P.L.R. (1991) 'Neural correlates of the gastrointestinal motor changes in emesis', in *Brain Gut Interactions* (eds Y. Tache, and D. Wingate) pp. 325–38. CRC Press, Boca Raton, USA.

Grundy, D.G. and Scratcherd, T. (1989) 'Sensory afferents from the gastrointestinal tract', in *Handbook of Physiology*, Section 6, Vol. 1, Part 1. (ed J.D. Wood) pp. 593–620. American Physiological Society, Bethesda, MD, USA.

Gunning, S.J., Hagan, R.M. and Tyers, M.B. (1987) Cisplatin induces biochemical and histological changes in the small intestine of the ferret. *Br. J. Pharmacol.*, **90**, *Proc. Suppl.* P135.

Harding, R.K., McDonald, T.J., Hugenholtz, H. and Kucharczyk, J. (1984) Characteristics of a new emesis producing intestinal factor. *Physiologist*, **27**, 279.

Harding, R.K., Hugenholtz, H., Keany, M. and Kucharczyk, J. (1985) Discrete lesions of the area postrema abolish radiation-induced emesis in the dog. *Neurosci. Lett.*, **53**, 95–100.

Harris, A.L. (1982) Cytotoxic therapy-induced vomiting is mediated via enkephalin pathways. *Lancet*, **1**, 714–16.

Harris, A.L. and Cantwell, B.M.J. (1986) 'Mechanisms and treatment of cytotoxic induced nausea and vomiting', in *Nausea and Vomiting: Mechanisms and Treatment* (eds C.J. Davis, G.V. Lake-Bakaar, and D.G. Grahame-Smith) pp. 78–93. Springer-Verlag, Berlin.

Hatcher, R.A. (1924) The mechanism of vomiting. *Physiol. Rev.*, **4**, 479–504.

Hawthorn, J., Andrews, P.L.R., Ang, V.T.Y. and Jenkins, J.S. (1988) Differential release of vasopressin and oxytocin in response to abdominal vagal afferent stimulation or apomorphine in the ferret. *Brain Res.*, **438**, 193–98.

Hawthorn, J., Ostler, K.J. and Andrews, P.L.R. (1988) The role of the abdominal visceral innervation and 5-hydroxytryptamine-M receptors in vomiting induced by the cytotoxic drugs cyclophosphamide and cisplatin in the ferret. *Q. J. Exp. Physiol.*, **73**, 7–21.

Higgins, G.A., Kilpatrick, G.J., Bunce, K.T. *et al.* (1989) 5-HT_3 receptor antagonists injected into the area postrema inhibit cisplatin induced emesis in the ferret. *Br. J. Pharmacol.*, **97**, 247–55.

Isaacs, B. (1957) The influence of head and body position on the emetic action of apomorphine in man. *Clin. Sci.*, **16**, 215–21.

Kasting, N.W., Mazurek, M.F. and Martin, J.B. (1985) Endotoxin increases vasopressin release independently of known physiological stimuli. *Am. J. Physiol.*, **248**, E420–424.

Kerlin, P. (1989) Postprandial antral hypomotility in patients with idiopathic nausea and vomiting. *Gut*, **30**, 54–59.

Koch, K.L., Summy-Long, J., Bingaman, S. *et al.* (1990) Vasopressin and oxytocin response to illusory self-motion and nausea in man. *J. Clin. Endocrinol. Metab.*, **71**, 1269–75.

Kocmierska-Grodzka, D., Siegienczuk, M. and Szewko, A. (1976) The influence of protease inhibitor on hydroproteolytic activity and serotonin content of rats after fractionated irradiation. *Arch. Immun. Ther. Exp.*, **24**, 259–65.

Kris, M.G., Gralla, R.J., Clark, R.A. *et al.* (1985) Incidence, course, and severity of delayed nausea and vomiting following the administration of high-dose cisplatin. *J. Clin. Oncol.*, **3**, 1379.

Kucharczyk, J. and Harding, R.K. (1990) Regulatory peptides and the onset of nausea and vomiting. *Can. J. Physiol. Pharmacol.*, **68**, 289–93.

Lang, I.M. (1990) Digestive tract motor correlates of nausea and vomiting. *Can. J. Physiol. Pharmacol.*, **68**, 242–53.

Lang, I.M., Sarna, S.K. and Condon, R.E. (1986) Gastrointestinal motor correlates of vomiting in the dog: Quantification and characterization as an independent phenomenon. *Gastroenterology*, **90**, 40–47.

Lang, I.M., Marvig, J., Sarna, S.K. and Condon, R.E. (1986) The gastrointestinal myoelectric correlates of vomiting in the dog. *Am. J. Physiol.*, **251**, G830–838.

Lang, I.M. and Sarna, S.K. (1989) Neural control of initiation and propagation of the retrograde giant contraction associated with vomiting. *Falck Symposium*. **50**, 726–31.

Lefebvre, R.A., Hasrat, J. and Gobert, A. (1992) Influence of N-nitro-L-arginine methyl ester on vagally induced gastric relaxation in the anaesthetised rat. *Br. J. Pharmacol.*, **105**, 315–20.

Leslie, R.A. (1985) Neuroactive substances in the

dorsal vagal complex of the medulla oblongata: nucleus of the tractus solitarius, area postrema and dorsal motor nucleus of the vagus. *Neurochem. Int.*, **7**, 191–211.

Leslie, R.A. (1986) Comparative aspects of the area postrema: fine structural considerations help to determine its function. *Cell. Mol. Neurobiol.*, **6**, 95–120.

Leslie, R.A., Reynolds, D.J.M., Andrews, P.L.R. *et al.* (1990) Evidence for presynaptic 5-hydroxytryptamine 3 recognition sites on vagal afferent terminals in the brainstem of the ferret. *Neurosci.*, **38**, 667–73.

Lindstrom, P.A. and Brizzee, K.R. (1962) Relief of intractable vomiting from surgical lesions in the area postrema. *J. Neurosurg.*, **19**, 228–36.

Magendie, F. (1813) 'Memoire sur le Vomissement', in *A Summary of Physiology* (2nd Edn.) 1824, transl J. Revere (ed E.J. Coale) Baltimore.

Martin, M., Diaz-Rubio, E., Sanchez, A. *et al.* (1990) The natural course of emesis after carboplatin treatment. *Acta Oncologica*, **29**, 593–95.

Matsuki, N., Torii, Y., Ueno, S. *et al.* (1992) *Suncus Murinus* as an experimental animal model for emesis and motion sickness. pp. 323–329. In. Mechanisms and control of emesis. (eds. A.L. Bianchi, L. Grélot, A.D. Miller and G.L. King) Colloque Inserm, J. Libbey, Eurotext, 223.

Matsuoka, O., Tsuchiya, T. and Furukawa, Y. (1962) The effect of X-irradiation on 5-hydroxytryptamine (serotonin) contents in the small intestine of experimental animals. *J. Rad. Res.*, **3–2**, 104–8.

Maxwell, A., Gaffin, S.L. and Wells, M.T. (1986) Radiotherapy, endotoxins and nausea. *Lancet*, **1**, 1148–49.

McCarthy, L.E. and Borison, H.L. (1974) Respiratory mechanics of vomiting in decerebrate cats. *Am. J. Physiol.*, **226**, 738–43.

McCarthy, L.E. and Borison, H.L. (1984) Cisplatin-induced vomiting eliminated by ablation of the area postrema in cats. *Cancer Treat. Rep.*, **68**, 401–4.

Meeroff, J.C., Schreiber, D.S., Trier, J.S. and Blacklow, N.R. (1980) Abnormal gastric motor function in viral gastroenteritis. *Ann. Int. Med.*, **92**, 370–73.

Mehler, W.R. (1983) Observations on the connectivity of the parvicellular reticular formation with respect to a vomiting centre. *Brain, Behav. Evol.*, **23**, 63–80.

Mense, S. (1981) Sensitization of group IV muscle receptors to bradykinin by 5-hydroxytryptamine and prostaglandin E_2. *Brain Res.*, **225**, 95–105.

Michalaowski, A. and Hornsey, S. (1986) Assays of damage to the alimentary tract. *Br. J. Cancer*, **53**, suppl. VII, 1–6.

Miller, A.D. (1990) Respiratory muscle control during vomiting. *Can. J. Physiol. Pharmacol.*, **68**, 237–41.

Miller, A.D. and Wilson, V.J. (1983) 'Vomiting center' reanalyzed: An electrical stimulation study. *Brain Res.* **270**, 154–58.

Money, K.E. and Cheung, B.S. (1983) Another function of the inner ear: Facilitation of the emetic response to poisons. *Aviat. Space Environ. Med.*, **54**, 208–11.

Naitoh, T., Wasserug, R.J. and Leslie, R.A. (1989) The physiology, morphology and ontogeny of emetic behaviour in anuran amphibians. *Physiol. Zool.*, **62**, 819–43.

Neuwelt, E.A. and Barnett, P.A. (1988) 'Blood–brain barrier disruption in the treatment of brain tumours. Animal studies', in *Implications of the Blood–brain Barrier and its Manipulation*, Vol. 2, Clinical Aspects (ed E.A. Neuwelt) Chapter 17A, pp. 107–93. Plenum Medical, New York.

Neuwelt, E.A., Glasberg, M. and Frankel, E. (1983) Neurotoxicity of chemotherapeutic agents after blood–brain barrier modification: Neuropathological studies. *Ann. Neurol.*, **14**, 316–24.

Newson, B., Ahlman, H., Dahlstrom, A. and Nyhus, L.M. (1982) Ultrastructural observations in the rat ileal mucosa of possible epithelial 'taste cells' and submucosal sensory neurons. *Acta Physiol. Scand.*, **114**, 161–64.

Nussey, S.S., Hawthorn, J., Page, S.R. *et al.* (1988) Responses of plasma oxytocin and arginine vasopressin to nausea induced by apomorphine and ipecacuanha. *Clin. Endocrinol.*, **28**, 297–304.

Ogawa, H., Sato, M. and Yamashita, S. (1968) Multiple sensitivity of chorda tympani fibres of the rat and hamster to gustatory and thermal stimuli. *J. Physiol.*, **199**, 223–40.

Ogilvie, G.K., Moore, A.S. and Curtis, C.R. (1989) Evaluation of cisplatin-induced emesis in dogs with malignant neoplasia: 115 cases (1984–1987). *J. Am. Vet. Med. Assoc.*, **195**, 1399–403.

Papp, R.H., Hawkins, H.B. and Share, N.N. (1966) Emesis induced by the intracerebroventricular administration of hydergine mechlorethamine hydrochloride. *J. Pharmacol. Exp. Ther.*, **154**, 333–38.

Pelchat, M.L. and Rozen, P. (1982) The special role of nausea in the acquisition of food dislikes by humans. *Appetite*, **3**, 341–51.

Preziosi, P., Ripanti, G., Navarra, P. *et al.* (1989) Comparison among 5-HT_3 antagonists on cisplatin emesis in pigeons. *Arch. Int. Pharmacodyn. Ther.*, 301–1.

Racke, K. and Schwörer, H. (1991) Regulation of serotonin release from the intestinal mucosa. *Pharmacol. Res.* **23**, 13–25.

Reason, J.T. and Brand, J.J. (1975) *Motion Sickness*, p. 181. Academic Press, London.

Reynolds, D.J.M., Barber, N.A., Grahame-Smith, D.G. and Leslie, R.A. (1991) Cisplatin-evoked induction of c-fos protein in the brainstem of the ferret: the effect of cervical vagotomy and the anti-emetic 5HT_3 receptor antagonist granisteron (BRL 43694). *Brain Res.*, **565**, 231–36.

Roos, I.A., Fairlie, D.P. and Whitehouse, M.W. (1981) A peculiar toxicity manifested by platinum(II) amines in rats: gastric distension after peritoneal administration. *Chem. Biol. Int.*, **35**, 111–17.

Schaeppi, U., Heiman, I.A., Fleischman, R.W. *et al.* (1973) *Cis*-dicholorodiammineplatinum (II) (NSC-119 875) preclinical toxicological evaluation of intravenous injection in dogs, monkeys and mice. *Toxicol. Appl. Pharmacol.*, **25**, 230–41.

Schapiro, H. (1978) Retching responses in the caiman sklerops elicited by telencephalic stimulation: efferent connections. *Exp. Neurol.*, **60**, 244–53.

Schurig, J.E., Florczyk, A.P. and Bradner, W.T. (1984) 'Evaluation of platinum complexes for emetic potential', in *Platinum Coordination Complexes in Cancer Complexes*. (eds M.P. Haker, E.B. Douple, and I.H. Krakoff) pp. 187–99. Martinus Nijhoff, Boston, MA.

Schwartz, J.C., Agid, Y., Bouthenet, M.L. *et al.* (1986) 'Neurochemical investigations into the area postrema', in *Nausea and Vomiting: Mechanics and Treatment*. (eds C.J. Davis, G.V. Lake-Bakaar and D.G. Grahame-Smith) pp. 18–30. Springer-Verlag, Berlin.

Schwörer, H., Racke, K. and Kilbinger, H. (1991) Cisplatin increases the release of 5-hydroxytryptamine (5-HT) from the isolated vascularly perfused small intestine of the guinea pig: Involvement of 5-HT_3 receptors. *Naunyn-Schmiedebergs Arch. Pharmacol.*, **344**, 143–49.

Sem-Jacobsen, C.W. (1968) *Depth Electrographic Stimulation of the Human Brain and Behaviour*. Thomas, Springfield, Ill.

Sicuteri, F., Fan Ciulacci, M., Franci, G. and Dell, B.L. (1965) Serotonin-bradykinin potentiation on pain receptors in man. *Life Sci.*, **4**, 309–16.

Sicuteri, F. (1968) 'Sensitization of nociceptors by 5-hydroxytryptamine in man', in Proceedings of the 3rd International Congress of Pharmacology. (ed R.K.S. Lim) pp. 57–86. Pergamon Press, Oxford.

Smith, G.P. and McHugh, P.R. (1967) Gastric secretory response to amygdaloid or hypothalamic stimulation in monkey. *Am. J. Physiol.*, **213**, 640.

Smith, W.L., Alphin, R.S., Jackson, C.B. and Sancilio, L.F. (1989) The anti-emetic profile of zacopride. *J. Pharm. Pharmacol.*, **41**, 101–105.

Smith, W.L., Callaham, E.M. and Alphin, R.S. (1988) The emetic activity of centrally administered cisplatinum in cats and its antagonism by zacopride. *J. Pharm. Pharmacol.*, **40**, 142–43.

Stern, R.M., Koch, K.L., Stewart, W.R. and Lindblad, I.M. (1987) Spectral analysis of tachygastria recorded during motion sickness. *Gastroenterology*, **92**, 92–97.

Stewart, J.J. (1983) Effects of emetic and cathartic agents on the gastrointestinal tract and the treatment of toxic ingestion. *J. Toxicol. Clin. Toxicol.*, **20**, 199–253.

Sugiyama, H., Chow, K.L. and Dragstedt, L.R. (1961) Study of emetic receptor sites for staphylococcal enterotoxin in monkeys. *Proceedings of the Society for Experimental Biology and Medicine*, **108**, 92–95.

Talley, N.J., Phillips, S.F. and Hadda, A. (1989) Effect of selective 5HT_3 antagonist (GR38032F) on small intestinal transit and release of gastrointestinal peptides. *Dig. Dis. Sci.*, **34**, 1511–15.

Thomford, N.R. and Sirinek, K.R. (1975) Intravenous vasopressin in patients with portal hypertension. *J. Surg. Res.*, **18**, 113–17.

Thompson, P.I., Bingham, S., Andrews, P.L.R. *et al.* (1992) Morphine-6-glucuronide: a metabolite of morphine with greater emetic potency than morphine in the ferret. *Br. J. Pharmacol.*, **106**, 3–8.

Tiersch, T.R. and Griffith, J.S. (1988) Apomorphine-induced vomiting in rainbow trout (*Salmo gairdneri*). *Comp. Biochem. Physiol.*, **91**A, 721–25.

Treisman, M. (1977) Motion sickness: an evolutionary hypothesis. *Science*, **197**, 493–95.

Tsurui, K., Kosakai, Y., Horie, T. and Awazu, S. (1990) Vitamin A protects the small intestine from methotrexate-induced damage in rats. *J. Pharm. Exp. Ther.* **253**, 1278–84.

Ueno, Y. (1979) 'Toxicological evaluation of trichothecene mycotoxins', in *Natural Toxins.* (eds D. Eaker, and T. Wadstrom) pp. 633–71. Proc. Int. Symp. Anim. Plant Microb. Toxins, Uppsala. Pergamon Press, Elmsford, New York.

Ueno, Y. (1983) 'Disturbances of the central nervous system', in *Development in Food Science.* Vol. 4; Trichothecenes – Chemical, Biological and Toxicological Aspects. (ed Y. Ueno) pp. 135–46. Elsevier, Amsterdam.

Ueno, S., Matsuki, N. and Saito, H. (1987) Suncus murinus: A new experimental model in emesis research. *Life Sci.*, **41**, 513–18.

Verbalis, J.G., Richardson, D.W. and Stricker, E.M. (1987) Vasopressin release in response to nausea producing agents and cholecystokinin in monkeys. *Am. J. Physiol.*, **252**, R749–753.

Von Hoff, D.D., Schilsky, R., Reichert, C.M. *et al.* (1979) Toxic effects of *cis*-dichlorodiammine-platinum (II) in man. *Cancer Treat. Rep.*, **63**, 1527–31.

Wang, S.C. and Borison, H.L. (1950) The Vomiting Center. A critical experimental analysis. *Arch. Neurol. Psych.*, **63**, 928–41.

Wang, S.C. and Borison, H.L. (1951) The vomiting center: Its destruction by radon implanatation in dog medulla oblongata. *Am. J. Physiol.*, **166**, 712–17.

Wang, S.C. and Borison, H.L. (1952) A new concept of organization of the central emetic mechanism: Recent studies on the sites of action of apomorphine, copper sulfate and cardiac glycosides. *Gastroenterology*, **22**, 1–12.

Wang, S.C., Renzi, A.A. and Chinn, H.I. (1958) Mechanism of emesis following X-irradiation. *Am. J. Physiol.*, **193**, 335–39.

Wengrower, D., Zaltzman, S., Karmeli, F. and Goldin, E. (1991) Idiopathic gastroparesis in patients with unexplained nausea and vomiting. *Dig. Dis. Sci.* **36**, 1255–58.

Yamada, K., Ushio, Y. and Hayakawa, T. (1988) 'Effect of steroids on the blood–brain barrier', in *Implications of the Blood–brain Barrier and its Manipulation*, Vol. 2, Clinical Aspects. (ed E.A. Neuwelt) Chapter 15, pp. 53–76. Plenum Medical, New York.

8

Radiotherapy-induced emesis

R.K. HARDING, R.W. YOUNG and G.H. ANNO

8.1 INTRODUCTION

Both humans and certain laboratory animals are very sensitive to the emetic stimulation provided by exposure to ionizing irradiation (Harding, 1988; Anno *et al.*, 1989; King, 1990).

In this chapter we review the status of vomiting as seen in the context of radiotherapy. We shall discuss data derived from animal experiments in order to provide some interpretation and understanding of the probable underlying mechanisms. We shall also include some novel approaches to the presentation and calculation of data gathered in certain accident and other situations, which bear on projections of the ED_{50} for radiation-induced nausea and vomiting in man, and on the timing and character of other prodromal symptoms which may be observed in a wide range of exposure conditions.

We discuss how radiation may damage cells and tissues and also consider similarities and differences between radiation- and chemotherapy-induced vomiting. Finally, we will discuss radioprotective compounds as well as combination therapies involving ionizing irradiation and cytostatic agents.

8.2 IONIZING IRRADIATION

When attempting to understand the radiotherapeutic effects of ionizing radiation, it is helpful to consider that radiation is essentially a toxin, not unlike chemotherapy compounds. There are many different chemotherapy compounds and each is employed for its ability to treat particular types of metastatic disease, or particular tissues or sites. Similarly, different types and sources of ionizing irradiation are employed in radiotherapy and these are chosen for their ability to treat certain diseases or sites. Each of these radiation types can be described as 'ionizing', but each varies fundamentally in features such as energy and form (i.e. gamma-photons versus electrons [$^{-}$e]). These features dictate factors such as the depth of penetration and the amount of ionizing energy transferred to the biomolecules transited or impacted by the radiation (reviewed in Hall, 1988).

There are some fundamental differences in the nature, mechanisms and actions of chemo- versus radiation therapies. The 'ionizing' action of radiotherapy, for example, is virtually instantaneous. There is no need, as there is with chemotherapy compounds, for such actions as cleavage or conversion, delivery (from some circulating volume), cellular uptake, metabolism, etc. In addition, there are no 'kinetics' with ionizing irradiation; no 'curve' ascending to a maximal dose and no 'washout'. Once the radiation source is returned to its shielded position (as is the case for the gamma-emitting isotopes of cobalt [^{60}Co] or

Emesis in Anti-cancer Therapy
Mechanisms and treatment
Published in 1993 by Chapman & Hall, London
ISBN 0 412 37250 9

caesium [^{137}Cs]), or the generator is turned off (X-ray sources, Linear Accelerators [producing high-energy ^{-}e beams]), the direct effects of irradiation cease in the tissues. The prodromal symptoms (nausea, vomiting, anorexia, malaise) seen after exposure to radiation are part of a cascade of effects set in motion by the radiation exposure. As might be expected, it is generally true that the latency period prior to the onset of vomiting following irradiation is shorter than that in patients treated with chemotherapy compounds.

8.3 RADIATION LETHALITY

8.3.1 CELL DEATH

In general, proliferating cell populations are the most at risk from the lethal effects of ionizing irradiation. Radiation-damaged proliferating cells fail to produce viable daughters, with a consequent reduction in the mass of proliferating tissue. Other cells will certainly be damaged, but the amount of radiation energy deposited is not usually sufficient to cause substantial acute changes in somatic functions (exceptions include the demonstrable changes in absorption kinetics across enterocytes of the irradiated small bowel). Somatic functions are more likely to be affected as a consequence of the recovery and repair process in irradiated tissues.

8.3.1.1 Radiation and the cell cycle

We know a great deal about the lethal effects of radiation on cells and tissues (Hall, 1988; Haskell, 1990). Radiosensitivity is typically defined in terms of the dose necessary to reduce clonogens to 37% of the initial population. This is typically expressed on the exponential portion of a radiation dose–cell survival curve. The D_{37} or the D_0 value, for most oxygenated mammalian cells, is between 110 and 240 cGy (Suit, 1973). The LD_{50} for man (assuming no medical intervention) has recently been placed at a dose of approximately 290 cGy delivered to the bone marrow (Levin *et al.*, 1992).

Mammalian cells are most radiosensitive during the mitotic phase of the cell cycle. Radiosensitivity decreases as the cells progress through G_1 and S phases. Sensitivity increases in G_2. The relatively low radiosensitivity of the main 'growth' phases reflects the considerable capacity for repair of sub-lethal radiation-induced damage; this is indicated by the 'shoulder' characteristic of post-radiation cell survival curves (Elkind *et al.*, 1963).

8.3.1.2 Different sensitivities

There are particular tissues which are more at risk from the effects of ionizing irradiation than others. The most life-threatening effects are seen through damage to the bone marrow (van Bekkum, 1991). Pancytopenia and, in particular, myeloid depression, is an important feature which limits the radiation dose, and indeed that of radiomimetic compounds such as cyclophosphamide. Most radiotherapy is delivered in multiple, relatively low dose treatments, confined as much as possible to defined regions of the body. There are two main reasons for this. One is to optimize tumour kill and this aspect will be further discussed below. The second reason is to reduce both the morbidity and the mortality resulting from radiation exposure and damage to healthy tissues.

As with any toxin, marked individual sensitivities are obvious between tissues. There are also obvious differences within tissues. Cell death can occur quickly and in the absence of a failure at mitosis. Apoptosis, or 'active cell death' (ACD) has been invoked (Potten, 1977), to explain the selective and rapid death seen following irradiation of certain cells near the bases of the intestinal crypt, in hair follicles, and in other tissues. ACD has recently been characterized as an inducible process in certain hormonally dependent tissues (Bursch *et al.*, 1990). It will be interesting to find out if ACD processes are involved in the well-known rapid and low dose kill of peripheral lymphocytes (interphase death), seen following irradiation.

As is the case with chemotherapy, the radiosensitivity of a tumour is not necessarily a predictor of cure. This is primarily due to the location and the distribution of malignant cells and the increasing limitations imposed by an escalating dose (in terms of morbidity), in achieving complete eradication.

8.3.2 RADIOPROTECTIVE COMPOUNDS

A enormous effort has been expended over the last 40 years to find agents which will reduce the damaging effects of radiation in cells and tissues. The most widely known radioprotective compound is the aminothiol WR-2721. Yuhas (1980) suggested a role for this compound as an adjunct to cytostatic therapies. Grdina and Sigdestad (1989) have listed other possible uses for these compounds. There is no evidence to suggest that radio-protective compounds will reduce the incidence of radiation-induced vomiting. The temporal relationships between radiation, the majority of cell death episodes and vomiting, do not prove the hypothesis that cell death is involved as a major source of acute emetic stimulus.

Furthermore, experiments in animals (reviewed in Cairnie, 1983) anticipated the observations in patients (Glover *et al.*, 1986), which showed that WR-2721 itself caused nausea and vomiting. Most of the emphasis in the study of radioprotection has moved to the investigation of combinations of agents which achieve some protection while presenting reduced toxicity (Weiss *et al.*, 1990). Further work in this area focuses less on protection and more on enhanced recovery (Klimberg *et al.*, 1990; MacVittie *et al.*, 1991).

8.3.3 RADIATION-INDUCED INFLAMMATION

Buell and Harding (1989) have described accumulation of neutrophils in the rat intestinal mucosa in the acute period following exposure to 10 Gy. This and other data (Harding *et al.*, 1990; 1992) are consistent with a post-irradiation inflammatory response. This inflammatory reaction is important for several reasons. First, local gastro-intestinal mucosal irritation is a potent emetic stimulus (Andrews *et al.*, 1988), and inflammation may constitute the 'irritant' emetic stimulus following irradiation. Secondly, inflammation can lead to further tissue damage and exacerbate the destruction due to radiation-induced cell death alone. Therefore, multiple fraction radiotherapy may also be considered in terms of a series of inflammatory insults. Repair of damage due to inflammation and the inflammatory reaction itself, may contribute to the strictures and adhesions which complicate the long-term post-irradiation period in patients (Buell and Harding, 1989). Finally, the post-irradiation inflammatory reaction would complicate the recovery of tissues, and would contribute to the histopathologies seen in the days following irradiation. We know that the new 5-HT_3 antagonists are effective anti-emetics in the acute post-irradiation period. Vomiting in the first day may be viewed as a pathophysiological effect. Delayed vomiting is perhaps more related to histopathology and may involve additional mechanisms. We know that the 5-HT_3 antagonist ondansetron (Zofran) is less effective in preventing emesis on days two and three following irradiation, than it is on day one (Priestman, 1989). We need to know more about vomiting throughout the post-irradiation period. We also need to know more about the post-irradiation inflammatory response, its role in tissue damage and repair, and its potential role in emesis.

8.4 RADIOTHERAPY

8.4.1 RADIO-VERSUS CHEMOTHERAPY

Certain alkylating chemotherapy compounds are said to be 'radiomimetic'. This relates to their mechanism of cell killing. Nitrogen mustard compounds such as mechlorethamine and its derivatives, produce breaks in molecules, including DNA. Both ionizing irradiation and alkylating chemotherapeutic compounds produce breaks and cross-linking in DNA. This interferes with DNA replication and RNA transcription.

Resistance to a chemotherapeutic compound or other drugs may develop through changes in metabolism or altered cellular uptake. These features do not affect radiation damage and, consequently, the standard log-normal distribution of cell killing versus dose is less affected. In addition, radiotherapy can be localized and more site-specific than systemic chemotherapy. Radiation sources are designed so that the size of the irradiation field can be adjusted and tailored to each need.

8.4.2 RADIATION COMBINED WITH OTHER MODALITIES

As mentioned above, fractionated radiotherapy improves the kill of tumours. Some synchronization does occur in recovering and repairing irradiated tissues. This may be exploited through the appropriate timing of subsequent irradiation. There is an increasing use of radiotherapy, in combination with chemotherapy, surgery and immunotherapy. Combination therapies often result in improved tumour kill (Haskell, 1990). Biological response modifiers (i.e. cytokines) can encourage division and enhance the radiation kill. Radiation can help to overcome or to exploit drug resistance which may develop in tissues treated with cytostatic chemicals. Alternatively, chemotherapy may serve as a useful adjunct to radiotherapy, to achieve a curative kill of dispersed or resistant malignant units.

Immunotherapies that use cell-specific antibodies bound to either chemotherapy compounds or radiation-emitters (Scott and Dillehay, 1990), photodynamic therapies as well as other modalities, are part of developing technologies which will provide further local and specific treatment. It may be speculated that a reduction in prodromal symptoms, such as vomiting, will be observed, since toxicity will be confined to a smaller population of cells. However, we do not yet know the possible systemic emetic potential of the carriers, the active agents or the process. It will be interesting to follow the results of this work with reference to emesis, method, tissue type and location. Will the incidence of emesis, for example, be greater in treatments targeted at tissues in the gut wall, than for those affecting lung or skin?

8.4.2.1 Bone marrow transplantation

A good example of a therapy that combines radiation and chemotherapeutic compounds is the eradication of malignant haematopoietic tissue prior to bone marrow transplantation. Typically, patients are treated with cyclophosphamide and with antibiotics, prior to total body irradiation (TBI). The dose and dose rate of radiation chosen for these therapies is usually the maximum which can be tolerated without evoking serious gastro-intestinal (GI) symptoms and without incurring significant medium- and long-term morbidity and mortality from radiation-induced pneumonitis, or morbidity from radiation enteritis. Vomiting in TBI patients has been particularly troublesome, due both to the coincident use of potent emetogenic chemotherapeutic agents and the high radiation dose (8–11 Gy). A wide range of anti-emetic therapies have been employed with variable success. Recent experience with serotonin 5-HT_3 receptor antagonist anti-emetics (Hewitt *et al.*, 1991; Hunter *et al.*, 1991), indicates that considerable improvement will be realized in controlling this difficult and debilitating symptom.

8.5 POST-IRRADIATION SYMPTOMS

It is instructive to look at the range of symptoms and effects which can occur following exposure to a wide range of doses of ionizing irradiation. This information can be drawn from clinical experience, from accident and other data, as well as from extrapolation from animal experimentation (Anno *et al.*, 1989). Most observers are aware that vomiting is an important post-irradiation symptom. There are other effects, such as post-irradiation fatigue and weakness which are also widely reported in the literature, but which are less understood and more difficult to quantify than radiation-induced vomiting. The work of Anno *et al.* (1989) also highlights the involvement of other GI symptoms, such as dysmotility and diarrhoea, in both early and later responses to radiation exposure. These effects occur at lower doses and with greater frequency than would be surmised by many observers.

8.5.1 FATIGUE AND WEAKNESS

A feeling of severe fatigue (Court Brown, 1953; Lushbaugh, 1969), exercise intolerance (Lushbaugh, 1973) and muscle fatigue (Rubin and Casarett, 1968) have long been observed in a wide range of radiotherapy patients. Fatigue is perhaps the most common and bothersome of the post-irradiation symptoms. It is also one of the least understood. Ricks (1972) measured diminished exercise capacity after irradiation and related this observation to increased pulmonary impedance. Other correlations of fatigue and observed effects include increased creatinuria (Kurohara, 1961), depressed ATP levels (Bigatello, 1987) and microvascular changes (Griem, 1989). Figure 8.1 shows that radiation-induced fatigue and weakness are prevalent effects which are present at relatively low doses. It is also evident from these reports that both the dose rate and the accumulated dose are important factors in the appearance of these symptoms.

The sense of tiredness and lack of energy after cytostatic therapy have recently been reported to exceed or equal patient concerns about nausea and vomiting (Cooper, 1991). Fatigue is not limited to radiotherapy patients who have underlying illness, but has also been observed in radiation accident victims (Thoma and Wald, 1959; Bond, 1965; Vodopick and Andrews, 1980; Guskova, 1989). Asthenia and decreased work capacity were reported to persist for up to six months in three out of four Chernobyl victims who received doses of from 4 to 6 Gy. Figure 8.2 represents the fatigue and weakness information accumulated by Anno *et al.* (1989) and is a compilation of results from radiotherapy, accident and other radiation exposures. These results show a direct relationship between total dose and latency; the higher the dose, the shorter the period prior to the onset of radiation-induced fatigue and weakness. Severity also is related to dose. As can be seen, these effects are remarkably persistent and there is a transient improvement at the end of the first week post-exposure.

Fatigue and weakness are commonly reported and often persistent side-effects of treatments which cause haematopoietic depression. King and Nail (1987) and Piper *et al.* (1989) have described fatigue associated with cancer treatment as a continuing scale ranging from tiredness to exhaustion. They have reported that fatigue can be seen in 65–100% of radiotherapy patients and that in many cases the effects can persist for months.

Quality of life for the patient undergoing radiation and other therapies for metastatic disease is a prominent concern. Most effort has been centred on the amelioration of vomiting; an immediate and relatively easy to quantify effect. Recent advances in anti-emetic therapy have resulted in significant improvements in controlling this difficult

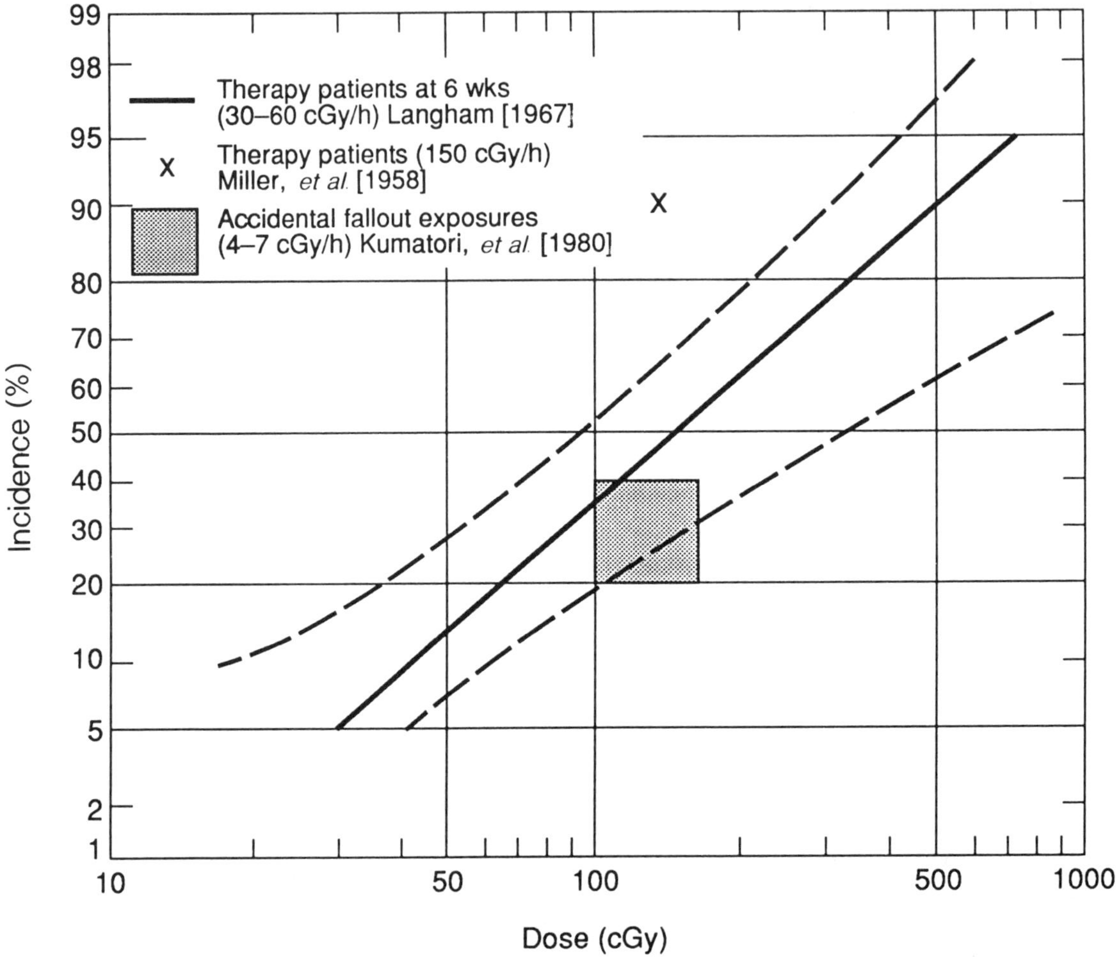

Figure 8.1 Incidence of fatigue and weakness: Dose rate effect. The solid line represents the log-normal plot of the data from Langham (1967), the dotted lines are the confidence limits. These data show a clear dose relationship versus the incidence of fatigue and weakness. The data of Miller *et al.* (1958) and Kumatori *et al.* (1980) are plotted separately. Note that the incidence of fatigue and weakness is highest in the higher dose-rate radiotherapy exposures of Miller *et al.* and lowest in the the low dose-rate group (Kumatori *et al.*).

symptom. Currently, there are renewed efforts in several countries to attempt to identify and to quantify those symptoms which patients find most difficult to endure. The clinical experience presented here indicates the seriousness and the scope of radiation-induced fatigue and weakness. It is to be hoped that more attention and resources can be focused on these effects to achieve a better understanding and reduction of these debilitating aspects of cancer treatment.

8.5.2 ANIMAL MODELS OF EMESIS

Considerable effort has been expended in animal research in order to determine the

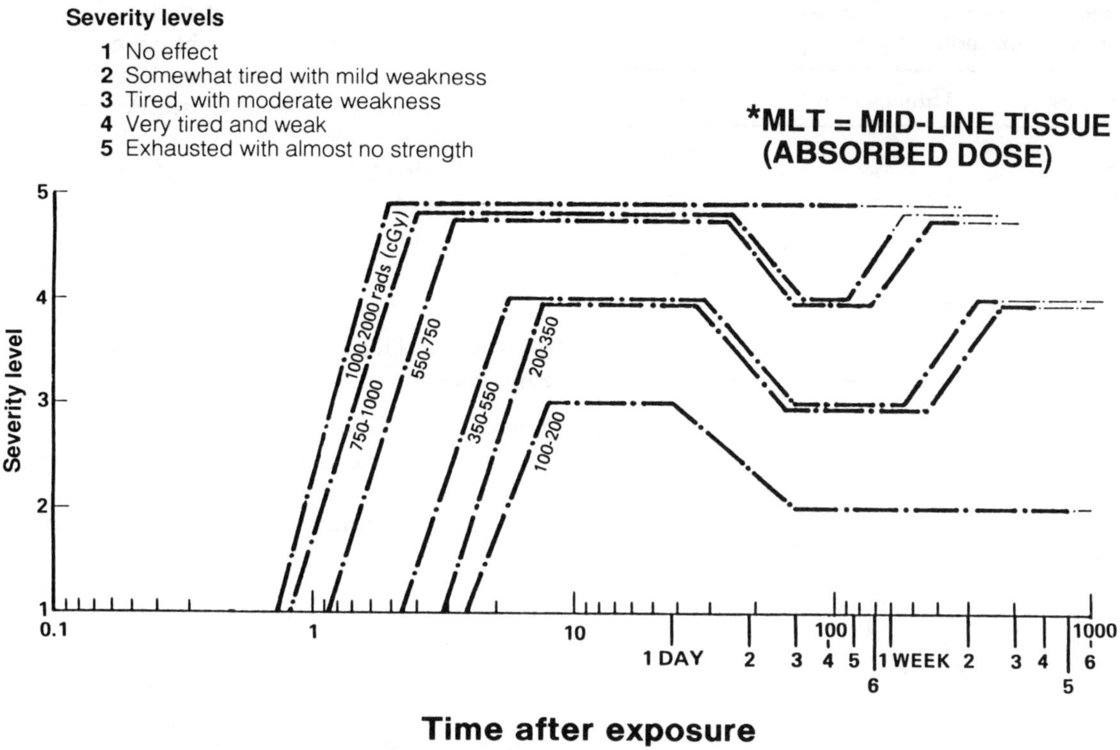

Figure 8.2 Severity levels of fatigue and weakness versus dose and time. These data are developed from the information accumulated by Anno *et al.* (1989). Note the Severity levels scale 1–5. Time is expressed on a log scale of hours and is annotated also in days and weeks. Radiation doses (cGy) are presented on the individual plots. These data confirm a direct relationship between total dose, latency and severity of effects.

radiation dose-response curves for effects such as lethality and vomiting. Dose-response curves for lethality (Morris and Jones, 1989) are typically steeper than those for vomiting (King, 1988). The variance in response for lethality is less, therefore, than that for vomiting. In addition, the median dose (LD_{50} and ED_{50}) can have broad confidence limits when a relatively small number of animals in a sample are exposed over a range of doses. Table 8.1 offers a comparison of the latency and ED_{50} for radiation-induced vomiting in man and other responsive species, and is derived from the summaries presented by Harding (1988) and King (1990). It is not clear which of these species is most relevant to man?

8.5.3 EMESIS IN MAN

We have little direct knowledge of the ED_{50} for radiation-induced vomiting in man. Fortunately, there have been relatively few radiation accidents. Those accidents which have occurred have been very chaotic, and it has been difficult to reconstruct doses and exposure conditions and to relate these directly to the recorded symptoms. Anno *et al.* (1989) have

Table 8.1 Species differences in latency and ED_{50} for radiation-induced vomiting

Species	Latency (min)	ED_{50} (cGy)
Ferret	15	100
Dog	92	230
Rhesus	45	450
Cat	258	>2000
Man	60–90	<200

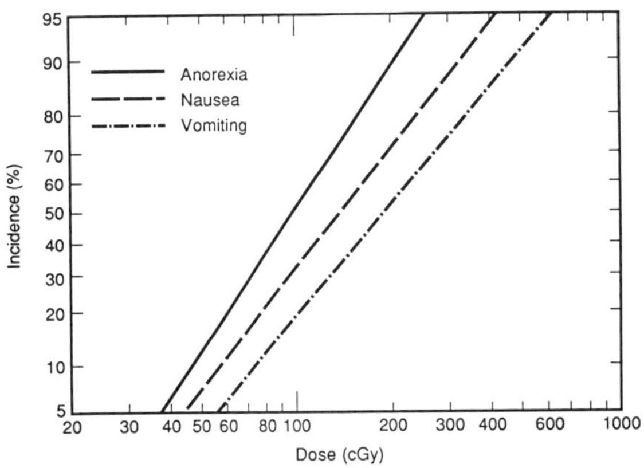

Figure 8.3 Relationship of prodromal symptoms (percentage incidence of anorexia, nausea and vomiting) and radiation dose (cGy). Probit analysis of the data of Langham (1967) and Lushbaugh (1969 and 1973), presented in a log-normal plot.

recently completed a broad survey of the available literature and knowledge, encompassing results from nuclear accident victims, certain radiotherapy data, and information from records of atomic bomb survivors. Figure 8.3 is a composite analysis, based on data from Langham (1967). These results show that the ED_{50} for radiation-induced vomiting in man is probably less than 2 Gy (this assumes prompt, essentially whole-body irradiation). Severity (number and duration of emetic episodes; degree of debilitation [analogous to effects on quality of life]) is directly related to the dose. Radiation-induced vomiting was an important triage symptom utilized by clinical personnel attempting to identify those persons injured at Chernobyl who might have received a significant radiation exposure. Results from this experience (USSR, 1986) support the reported calculations of Anno *et al.* (1989). Figure 8.4 is also taken from the data of Anno *et al.* (1989) and represents a 3-D plot indicating that the latency, prior to the onset of emesis, is inversely related to the dose.

8.5.4 VOMITING IN RADIOTHERAPY PATIENTS

It is often difficult to generalize expected results concerning the incidence and severity of nausea and vomiting between different radiotherapy clinics who are treating similar diseases. There are usually differences both in the treatment design among clinics (as with the differences in conditioning therapy and radiation dose and delivery prior to bone marrow transplant), age and sex of the patients, region of the body irradiated, and concurrent medications. Local practice also varies widely in the application of anti-emetic therapies. In some cases this is analogous to the situation with various cytostatic treatment regimes, where particular anti-emetic protocols have evolved to treat the emesis resulting from different cytotoxic agents. However, this cannot be the only answer since there are fewer qualitative differences in the radiation sources employed in radiotherapy than there are in the chemicals used in chemotherapy. Part of the explanation for the wide range of anti-emetic treatments in radiotherapy practice must reside with other features of the illness, other concurrent treatments, the absolute dose, and the region of the body involved in the radiation field.

8.5.4.1 Incidence and severity

In general, nausea and vomiting in radiotherapy practice is reported to be less severe than that seen with more aggressive chemo-

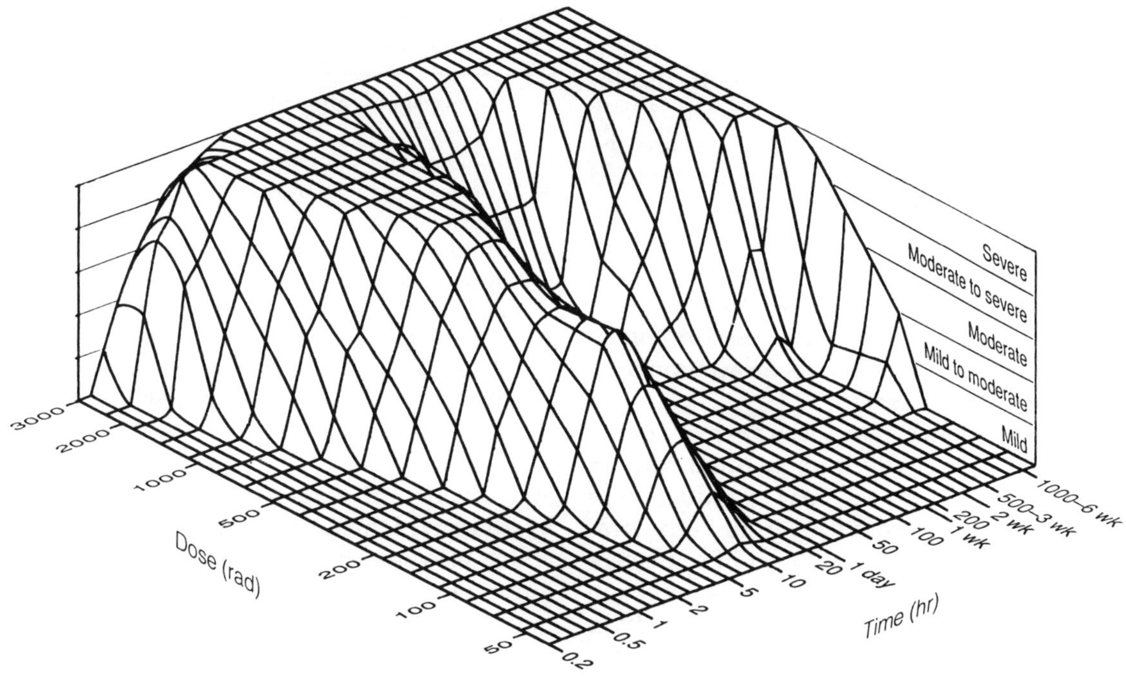

Figure 8.4 3-D plot of the relationship of radiation dose (in rads or cGy), time (log plot of hours post-exposure, annotated in days and weeks) and severity of 'Upper gastro-intestinal symptoms' (primarily those related to nausea and vomiting). Developed from the data accumulated in Anno *et al.* (1989).

therapy treatments (Priestman, 1988). Typically, when it occurs, vomiting first appears in the second hour post-irradiation. The threshold for vomiting, following irradiation of a large volume, is approximately 1 Gy. The incidence of emesis is highest in the several hours following irradiation (Lushbaugh *et al.*, 1967; Barnes, 1984).

As can be seen in Figures 8.3 and 8.4 above, the incidence of emesis increases with the dose of radiation. However, in man, there is no ED_{100} for radiation-induced vomiting. Even with the most emetogenic radiotherapy, only about 80–90% of patients can be expected to vomit in the absence of anti-emetic therapy (Barrett, 1982). The expected incidence of vomiting can be much less in other regimes employing lower doses of radiation. This fact is important when one is trying to establish the efficacy of a particular anti-emetic compound. A drug may be reported to be 65% effective; this is less impressive, however, if the anticipated incidence of emesis in the patient population was only 50%. See Pater and Wilan (1984) for a discussion of the design of clinical trials of anti-emetic drugs.

8.5.4.1.1 Regions particularly sensitive to radiation

Most radiation therapy protocols require multiple, moderate dose fractions, delivered to discrete regions of the body. As discussed previously, one reason for this is to increase the efficiency of kill of metastatic cells. A second and important reason is the reduction of morbidity and debilitating side-effects, including nausea and vomiting (Barrett, 1982). Two other features of radiotherapy are the dose rate and the region of the body exposed to the radiation beam. Most radiotherapies utilize dose rates of between 1 and 50 cGy/minute. Interestingly, these rates have little effect on the dose which causes emesis. Thus, in one low dose rate series, emesis occurred when a dose of 2–3 Gy had been accumulated (Westbrook *et al.*, 1987).

It is well known that the upper abdomen is the most sensitive site, in man and in other responsive species, for the induction of radiation-induced vomiting. Half-body irradiation is a technique employed in some centres for the palliation of pain and the reduction of disseminated metastases (Salazar *et al.*, 1978; Danjoux *et al.*, 1979). This technique requires high dose (8 Gy) single fraction irradiation of either the upper or lower half-body. Irradiation of the upper half-body results in about double the incidence of emesis. Interestingly, this result was not affected if the head was excluded from the radiation field (Danjoux *et al.*, 1979). These examples of irradiation provide a relatively clearer indication in man of the emetic effects of ionizing irradiation alone. It should be noted that TBI patients are typically treated with emetogenic chemotherapy compounds and antibiotics prior to irradiation and bone marrow infusion and other elements afterwards. Table 8.2 shows a compilation of some characteristics of radiation-induced vomiting in man.

Table 8.2 Characteristics of radiation-induced vomiting in man

- Low threshold, about 1Gy
- ED_{50} = <2 Gy
- No ED_{100}
- Dose rate less important than actual accumulated dose (@ >2 cGy/min)
- Vomiting usually seen in the second hour following accumulation of emetic dose
- Emetic episodes last for several hours
- Emesis typically less severe than with some cytotoxics
- Upper abdomen = most emetic radiation site

8.5.4.2 Factors affecting emesis

Although it is intuitively obvious to most radiotherapists, it is not generally stated that the 'condition' of the patient during irradiation (position, frequency of movement) has an impact on the emetic profile. Westbrook *et al.* (1987) described a decrease in the frequency and severity of emesis when patients were irradiated in a more comfortable position which also required less movement. The additive effects of motion on the incidence of radiation-induced vomiting is also seen in the animal literature. Mattsson and Yochmowitz (1980) reported that coincident oscillation reduced by 42% the ED_{50} for radiation-induced emesis in the rhesus monkey.

8.6 MECHANISMS OF RADIATION-INDUCED VOMITING

8.6.1 INTRODUCTION

Ultimately, studies in animals and reviews of other data are intended to assist in the understanding and reduction of the emetic response in patients subjected to radiotherapy. There is no clear answer to the question concerning the 'most appropriate animal model'. If one looks solely at the ED_{50} dose for radiation-induced vomiting and the latency period to the first vomit, then the dog is the most appropriate model for man (Table 8.1, above). However, does similar sensitivity and emetic pattern imply similar mechanisms? These questions have important implications for the transfer of data between species concerning the efficacy of new anti-emetic compounds.

8.6.2 CURRENT CONCEPTS

The most current information concerning the mechanisms of vomiting is discussed elsewhere in this book and only a summary will be presented here. First, it is important to state that the vomiting response initiated by exposure to ionizing irradiation probably serves no useful purpose. Davis *et al.* (1986) have described vomiting in terms of an hierarchically-organized, toxin defence system, in which the irradiated individual responds in a stereotypic manner to a perceived toxin. Chapter 6 describes central nervous system structures and their organization in terms of controlling the emetic process. Particular importance is placed on the area postrema and underlying medullary sites. It is also important to consider visceral afferent stimulation as carrying and mediating at least part of the emetic stimulus.

8.6.3 5-HT_3

There are many parallels in the mechanisms of emesis induced by chemotherapeutic compounds and ionizing irradiation. Indeed, the proposals of Andrews *et al.* (1988) include a prominent role for cytotoxics, radiation, and orally ingested toxins, causing emesis by inducing the release of modulators such as serotonin (5-HT) or substance P. These authors envision a predominant role for 5-HT, acting at 5-HT_3 receptors on visceral (vagal) afferents. This peripheral sensory system is thought to relay the message to medullary structures to initiate the vomiting response.

Andrews *et al.* (1990) have described how visceral deafferentation effectively reduces or eliminates emesis induced by various chemotherapy compounds or ionizing radiation in the ferret. However, Andrews and Hawthorn (1987) and Andrews *et al.* (1990) also present data which indicate an extra-abdominal site in the ferret which mediates vomiting induced by exposure to high doses of ionizing irradiation. Harding (1988) has summarized the apparently conflicting data in the animal literature; this indicates that in some animals, and for only some stimuli, the chemoreceptor area postrema was the emetic stimulus site, while in others visceral afferent section was required to block emesis. Harding *et al.* (1985) have confirmed that area postrema ablation eliminates emesis in the dog as a result of exposure to 6–7 Gy. However, Harding (1988) also describes experiments where area postrema-ablated dogs (with proved visceral afferent function) vomited in response to 15 Gy.

8.6.4 EMETIC PATHWAYS

Figure 8.5 is a cartoon representation showing vomiting in terms of a reservoir and siphon. This siphon empties the reservoir when the content reaches a certain critical level. The arrows indicate that the reservoir may be filled from various sources and at different rates. In this vomiting analogy, the sources include chemoreceptors either in the area postrema or other circumventricular organs, visceral afferents, vestibular stimuli (motion), learned aversions (mediated by taste, olfaction or sight) and other central nervous system-mediated stimuli. The bold arrow represents the fact that the model envisions that for each emetic species and each emetic stimulus, there will be a **predominant emetic pathway**. The evidence presented in section 8.6.3 above suggests that in the ferret, low doses of ionizing irradiation mediate emesis primarily through the visceral afferents. However, a less sensitive mechanism (perhaps the area postrema) is also a contributor (Andrews *et al.*, 1990). In the dog, it appears that the area postrema is the more sensitive site but a visceral mechanism is also present (Harding, 1988). The work of Mattsson and Yochmowitz (1980) and the observations of Westbrook *et al.* (1987) show that motion can be a contributory emetic stimulus, in addition to that provided by radiation. Thus there exist **parallel** as well as **predominant** emetic mechanisms.

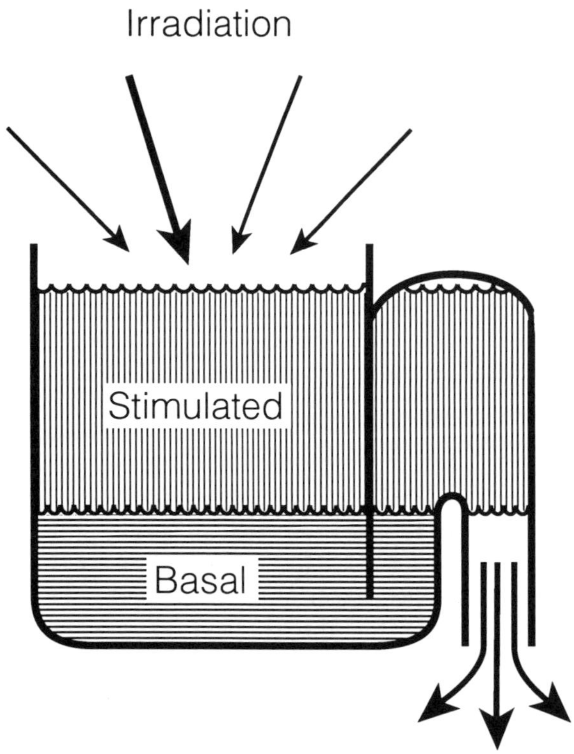

Figure 8.5 Siphon analogy of radiation-induced vomiting. The analogy envisions various sources of emetic stimuli filling a 'reservoir', which upon reaching an appropriate level 'empties' through the act of vomiting. 'Sources' of stimuli implies parallel emetic mechanisms and pathways. The thick input arrow implies a predominant pathway.

There are three important implications of the concept of predominant/parallel pathways in the consideration of the efficacy of anti-emetic therapies. First, the existence of parallel pathways may explain the partial effectiveness of certain drugs that in themselves would not ordinarily be expected to be relevant anti-emetic treatments. Secondly, the existence of parallel pathways may explain some cases where highly specific anti-emetics fail to provide complete treatment. Thirdly, the identification of predominant pathways provides the opportunity to develop more specific drugs, to provide better therapeutic results, and to incur fewer side-effects due to extraneous effects.

8.6.4.1 Application and relevance in man

There is little direct evidence which indicates where man fits into all of this. No-one has attempted, and no-one would suggest, area postrema ablation prior to a course of radiotherapy. No-one has published a retrospective assessment of the incidence of vomiting in persons who were vagotomized (for example, in the treatment of peptic ulcer disease) and who subsequently were candidates for radio- or chemotherapy. In any event, it is not clear what would be learned from this, since gastric tone is known to return following vagotomy and there are other indications of plasticity and recovery of visceral afferent function. Thus we must question whether the possible anti-emetic effects of acute vagotomy would be obtained in the longer term.

The new 5-HT_3 receptor antagonist anti-emetics offer another opportunity to compare and contrast results in the ferret, dog and man. Emesis in the ferret exposed to low doses of radiation can be completely inhibited by the 5-HT_3 antagonists granisetron or ondansetron (Andrews *et al.*, 1990). Vomiting in the dog exposed to 7 Gy can be substantially reduced by prior exposure, or by post-irradiation treatment with granisetron (Harding *et al.*, 1988). Both granisetron (Hunter *et al.*, 1991) and ondansetron (Priestman, 1989; Hewitt *et al.*, 1991) have been shown to substantially reduce vomiting seen in irradiated patients. Complete blockade of radiation-induced vomiting was not observed in any of the clinical studies. This perhaps provides further evidence that the dog is the more relevant model for the study of radiation-induced vomiting in man.

The availability of 5-HT_3 receptor antagonist anti-emetics is increasing as approval for their clinical use is obtained in a growing number of countries. There remains an overriding need for good quality follow-on trials to evaluate the evolving clinical experience and to identify the most appropriate uses and dose regimes for these compounds. Ultimately, this information will provide the best indication of the appropriate animal model and, more importantly, will facilitate the rational use of these new compounds.

8.7 FUTURE DEVELOPMENTS

The new 5-HT_3 receptor antagonist anti-emetics represent a substantial improvement over current therapies and will undoubtedly result in improved symptom management and reduced drug-induced side-effects in radiotherapy. There is, however, some room for improvement. Doses of some drugs will need to be optimized and we will need to learn more about potentially confounding effects at other receptors. We will need to learn more about the stimulation effects which result in the purported release of serotonin in the irradiated gastro-intestinal tract. What cells are the source(s); where are the nerve endings which receive the stimulus; can we reduce the source, as well as the transmission of the emetic stimulus?

Some changes in ferret GI mast cells have been observed immediately following irradiation (Harding *et al.*, 1992). It will be interesting to learn if dexamethasone increases the anti-emetic effectiveness of 5-HT_3 antagonists in irradiated patients. Dexamethasone has been shown to be a useful adjunctive anti-emetic therapy, particularly when it is given on the day prior to chemotherapy (Cunningham *et al.*, 1989). If dexamethasone is affecting the mast cell populations, and hence a source of 5-HT stimulation, we would have both a further explanation for the mechanism of radiation-induced vomiting and an improved method to control this unpleasant and debilitating symptom.

It is important that we learn more about the effects of radiation in the days following treatment. What is different about vomiting after the first day and what anti-emetic strategies should we adopt? It is also important to note that animal research has been of little help here, since most experiments are terminated within hours of irradiation. Well designed clinical trials will be important in answering these and other questions.

Furthermore, well designed clinical trials and informed and careful surveys of patient responses and opinions will be important in the continuing attempt to reduce morbidity and to improve the quality of life for the radiotherapy patient. It is clear that vomiting is not the only symptom which affects patients: we know, for example, relatively little about the follow-on effects such as diarrhoea, anorexia, inflammation, fatigue and weakness. Research efforts are warranted in these and other areas and will be required before we can truly understand and control the bulk of the symptoms which accompany, follow on from and compromise radiotherapy.

REFERENCES

Andrews, P.L.R. and Hawthorn, J. (1987) Evidence for an extra-abdominal site of action for the 5-HT_3 receptor antagonist BRL24924 in the inhibition of radiation-evoked emesis in the ferret. *Neuropharmacol.*, **9**, 1367–70.

Andrews, P.L.R. and Rapeport, W.G. and Sanger, G.J. (1988) Neuropharmacology of emesis induced by anti-cancer therapy. *Trends Pharmacol. Sci.*, **9**, 334–41.

Andrews, P.L.R., *et al.* (1990) The abdominal visceral innervation and the emetic reflex: pathways, pharmacology and plasticity. *Can. J. Physiol. Pharmacol.*, **68**, 325–45.

Anno, G.H., Baum, S.J., Withers, H.R. and Young, R.W. (1989) Symptomatology of acute radiation effects in humans after exposure to doses of 0.5–30 Gy. *Health Phys.*, **56**, 821–38.

Barnes, J.H. (1984) The physiology and pharmacology of emesis. *Mol. Aspects Med.*, **7**, 397–508.

Barrett, A. (1982) Total body irradiation (TBI) before bone marrow transplantation in leukaemia: a cooperative study from the European Group for Bone Marrow Transplantation. *Br. J. Radiol.*, **55**, 562–57.

Bigatello, L. *et al.* (1987) Phosphorus and ATP depletion in blood tissue following whole-body irradiation. *Surg. Forum* **38**, 8–10.

Bond, V.P., Fliedner, J.O. and Archambeau, M. (1965) *Mammalian Radiation Lethality: A Disturbance in Cellular Kinetics*, Academic Press, New York.

Buell, M.G. and Harding, R.K. (1989) Pro-inflammatory effects of local irradiation on the rat gastrointestinal tract. *Dig. Dis. Sci.*, **34**, 390–99.

Bursch, W., Kleine, L. and Tenniswood, M. (1990) The biochemistry of apoptosis. *Biochem. Cell Biol.*, **68**, 1071–74.

Cairnie, A.B. (1983) Adverse effects of the radioprotector WR-2721. *Radiat. Res.*, **94**, 221–26.

Cooper, S. (1991) The impact of cytotoxic chemotherapy – patient's and medical profession's perspective. ECCO 6 Satellite Symposium. *Caring for the Cancer Patient: Managing Emesis Now – An Interactive Workshop*, pp. 38–41.

Court Brown, W.M. (1953) Symptomatic disturbance after single therapeutic dose of X-rays. *Br. J. Med.*, **1**, 802–805.

Cunningham, D., Turner, A., Hawthorn, J. and Rosin, R.D. (1989) Ondansetron with and without dexamethasone to treat chemotherapy-induced emesis. *Lancet* **1**, 1323.

Danjoux, C.E., Rider, W.D. and Fitzpatrick, P.J. (1979) The acute radiation syndrome. A memorial to William Michael Court Brown. *Clin. Radiol.*, **30**, 581–84.

Davis, C.J., Harding, R.K., Leslie, R.A. and Andrews, P.L.R. (1986) 'The organization of vomiting as a protective reflex', in *Nausea and Vomiting: Mechanisms and Treatment* (eds. C.J. Davis, G.V. Lake-Bakaar, D.G. Grahame-Smith) pp. 65–75. Springer-Verlag, Berlin.

Elkind, M.M., Han, A. and Voltz, K.W. (1963) Radiation response of mammalian cells grown in culture. IV. Dose dependence of division delay and postirradiation growth of surviving and nonsurviving Chinese hamster cells. *J. Natl. Cancer Inst.*, **30**, 705–21.

Glover, D. *et al.* (1986) Phase I/II trials of WR-2721 and cisplatinum. *Int. J. Radiat. Oncol. Biol. Phys.*, **12**, 1509–12.

Greim, M.L. (1989) 'Early responses of blood vessels to radiation', in *Prediction of Response to Radiation Therapy*, Part 1: The Physical and Biological Basis, (ed B.R. Paliwal) American Institute of Physics, New York.

Guskova, A.K. *et al.* (1989) Acute effects of radiation exposure following the Chernobyl accident: Immediate results of radiation sickness and outcome of treatment. *Medical Aspects of the Chernobyl Accident*, IAEA-TECDOC – 516, International Atomic Energy Agency, Vienna, pp. 233–56.

Hall, E.J. (1988) *Radiobiology for the Radiologist*, 3rd edn. J.B. Lippincott, Philadelphia.

Haskell, C.M. (1990) *Cancer Treatment*, 3rd edn. W.B. Saunders, Philadelphia.

Harding, R.K., Hugenholtz, H., Keaney, M. and Kucharczyk, J. (1985) Discrete lesions of the area postrema abolish radiation-induced emesis in the dog. *Neurosci. Lett.*, **53**, 95–100.

Harding, R.K. (1988) Prodromal effects of radiation: pathways, models and protection by antiemetics. *Pharmacol. Ther.*, **39**, 335–45.

Harding, R.K., Leach, K.E. and Prud'homme-Lalonde, L (1988) Effects of BRL 43694 on emesis in the dog induced by ionizing irradiation. *Physiologist*, **31**, A126.

Harding, R.K., Leach, K.E., Prud'homme-Lalonde, L. and Ferrarotto, C.L. (1991) Release of inflammatory mediators from irradiated gastrointestinal tissues. *Gastroenterology*, **98**, A285.

Harding, R.K., Morris, G.P., Prud'homme-Lalonde, L. and Leach, K.E. (1992) Acute effects of 5 Gy ionizing irradiation on mast cell populations in the ferret jejunum. *Gastroenterology*, **102**, A635.

Hewitt, M., Cornish, J., Pamphilon, D. and Oakhill, A. (1991) Effective emetic control during conditioning of children for bone marrow transplantation using ondansetron, a 5-HT_3 antagonist. *Bone Marrow Transplant*, **7**, 431–33.

Hunter, A.E. *et al.* (1991) Granisetron, a selective 5-HT_3 receptor antagonist, for the prevention of radiation-induced emesis during total body irradiation. *Bone Marrow Transplant*, **7**, 439–41.

King, G.L. (1988) Characterization of radiation-induced emesis in the ferret. *Radiat. Res.*, **114**, 599–612.

King, G.L. (1990) Animal models in the study of vomiting. *Can. J. Physiol. Pharmacol.*, **68**, 260–68.

King, K.B. and Nail, L.M. (1987) Fatigue. *Sem. Oncol. Nursing*, **3**, 257–61.

Klimberg, V.S. *et al.* (1990) Prophylactic glutamine protects the intestinal mucosa from radiation injury. *Cancer*, **66**, 62–68.

Kumatori, T. *et al.* (1980) Follow-up studies over a 25-year period in the Japanese fisherman exposed to radioactive fallout in 1954, in *The Medical Basis of Radiation Accident Preparedness*, (eds K.F. Hubner, and S.A. Fry) pp. 35–54. Elsevier, New York.

Kurohara, S.S., Rubin, P. and Hempelmann, L.H. (1961) Creatinuria and fatigue in patients undergoing radiotherapy. *Radiology* **77**, 804–12.

Langham, W.H. (1967) Radiobiological factors in manned space flight. National Academy of Sciences, National Research Council Publication 1487, Washington, DC.

Levin, S.G., Young, R.W. and Stohler, R.L. (1992) Estimates of the median human lethal radiation dose, computed from data on occupants and architecture, of two reinforced concrete structures in Nagasaki Japan. *Health Phys*. **63**, 522–31.

Lushbaugh, C.C., Comas, F. and Hofstra, R. (1967) Clinical studies of radiation effects in man: A preliminary report of a retrospective search for dose-relationships in the prodromal syndrome. *Radiat. Res.*, **7**(Suppl), 398–412.

Lushbaugh, C.C. (1969) Reflections on some recent progress in human radiobiology, *Adv. Radiat. Biol.*, **3**, 277–315.

Lushbaugh, C.C. (1973) Human radiation tolerance, in *Bioastronautics Data Book*. Parker, Jr., J. and West, V.R. (eds) National Aeronautics and Space Administration, Washington, DC, NASA-S-30006, pp. 421–522.

MacVittie, T.J. *et al.* (1991) The relative biological effectiveness of mixed fission-neutron-gamma radiation on the hematopoietic syndrome in the canine: effect of therapy on survival. *Radiat. Res.*, **128**, S29–S36.

Mattsson, J.L. and Yochmowitz, M.G. (1980) Radiation-induced emesis in monkeys. *Radiat. Res.*, **82**, 191–99.

Miller, L.S., Fletcher, G.H. and Gerstner, H.B. (1958) Radiobiologic observations on cancer patients treated with whole-body X-radiation. *Radiat. Res.*, **8**, 150–65.

Morris, M.D. and Jones, T.D. (1989) Hematopoietic death of unprotected man from photon irradiations: statistical modelling from animal experiments. *Int. J. Radiat. Biol.*, **55**, 445–61.

Pater, J.L. and Wilan, A.R. (1984) Methodological issues in trials of antiemetics. *J. Clin. Oncol.*, **2**, 484–87.

Piper, F.P. *et al.*, Recent advances in the management of radiotherapy-related side-effects. *Oncol. Nurs. Forum*, **16** (Suppl) 27–34.

Potten, C.S. (1977) Extreme sensitivity of some intestinal crypt cells to X- and gamma irradiation. *Nature* 269, 518–21.

Priestman, T. (1988) Radiation-induced emesis. *Clinician*, **6**, 40–43.

Priestman, T. (1989) Clinical studies with ondansetron in the control of radiation-induced emesis. *Eur. J. Cancer Clin. Oncol.*, **25** (Suppl 1), S29–S33.

Ricks, R.C., Lushbaugh, C.C., McDow, E. and Frome, E. (1972) Pulmonary impedance power spectral analysis: a facile means of detecting radiation-induced GI distress and performance decrement in man. National Symposium on Natural and Manmade Radiation in Space, (ed E.A. Warman) NASA TM X-2440, National Aeronautics and Space Administration, Washington, DC, pp. 238–48.

Rubin, P. and Casarett, G.W. (1968) *Clinical Radiation Pathology*. 1st edn. W.B. Saunders, Philadelphia.

Salazar, P.M. *et al.* (1978) Systemic half-body radiotherapy: response and toxicity. *Int. J. Radiat. Oncol. Biol. Phys.*, **4**, 937–50.

Scott, B.R. and Dillhay, L.E. (1990) A model for haematopoietic death in man from irradiation of bone marrow during immunotherapy. *Br. J. Radiol.*, **63**, 862–70.

Suit, H.D. (1973) in *Textbook of Radiotherapy*, 2nd edition, (ed G.H. Fletcher) Lea & Febiger, Philadelphia.

Thoma, G.E., Jr. and Wald, N. (1959) The diagnosis and management of accidental radiation injury. *J. Occup. Med.*, **1**, 421–47.

USSR Committee on the Utilisation of Atomic Energy. (1986) The accident at the Chernobyl nuclear power plant and its consequences. Report to the International Atomic Energy Agency, Vienna.

van Bekkum, D.W. (1991) Radiation sensitivity of the hematopoietic stem cell. *Radiat. Res.*, **128**, S4–S8.

Vodopick, H. and Andrews, G.A. (1980) The University of Tennessee Comparative Animal Research laboratory accident in 1971, in *The Medical Basis for Radiation Accident Preparedness.* (eds K.F. Hubner and S.A. Fry) pp. 141–50. Elsevier, New York.

Weiss, J.F. *et al.* (1990) Advances in radioprotection through the use of combined agent regimes. *Int. J. Radiat. Biol.*, **57**, 709–22.

Westbrook, C., Glaholm, J. and Barrett, A. (1987) Vomiting associated with whole body irradiation. *Clin. Radiol.*, **38**, 263–66.

Yuhas, J.M. (1980) A more general role for WR-2721 in cancer therapy. *Br. J. Cancer*, **41**, 832–34.

9
The pharmacology of anti-emetic agents

G.J. SANGER

9.1 INTRODUCTION

The importance of developing effective anti-emetic treatments is left in no doubt by the graphic descriptions of the prolonged nausea and vomiting which may be evoked by cytotoxic therapy (Scogna and Smalley, 1979; Lazlo, 1983; Dodds, 1986; Warren, 1988; Hogan, 1990) and by the patient perception that nausea and vomiting are the worst of all the side-effects evoked by cytotoxic therapy (Coates *et al.*, 1983). This type of emesis can be classified as 'acute' (covering the first 24–48 hours after cytotoxic treatment), 'delayed' (occurring during the days following the acute response) and 'anticipatory' (emesis which can occur in anticipation of a subsequent course of treatment if there has been poor anti-emetic treatment during the first course). The emetogenic potential of a cytotoxic therapy may, therefore, be 'severe' if a prolonged acute response almost always occurs and this is followed by delayed and anticipatory emesis in a proportion of these patients (e.g. cisplatin or cyclophosphamide; Fetting *et al.*, 1982; Kris *et al.*, 1985). The terms 'severe', 'moderate' and 'mild' emesis are used purely for the convenience of description and are not based on exhaustive clinical data (Craig and Powell, 1987).

The discovery of new anti-emetic drugs has inevitably lagged behind the introduction of the new anti-cancer treatments, some of which evoke severe nausea and vomiting (Joss *et al.*, 1990). Indeed, until the use of high dose metoclopramide, high dose dexamethasone and, in particular, the selective 5-HT_3 receptor antagonists, improvements in anti-emetic therapy have long depended on introducing new compounds which were derived by making small changes in the properties of drugs already available. 'Cocktails' of anti-emetic drugs were varied according to established criteria (De Vita *et al.*, 1975). Often this has been done to increase the degree of sedation or to reduce the side-effects of an anti-emetic drug (e.g. diphenhydramine used to control the extrapyramidal reactions sometimes evoked by dopamine D_2 receptor antagonists). More recently, drug 'cocktails' have been designed to treat the different phases of cytotoxic-induced emesis such as anticipatory vomiting and the acute and delayed phases of severe emesis. For recent reviews on the types of anti-emetic drugs commonly in use and for an assessment of their efficacy see Craig and Powell (1987); Gralla (1989); Grunberg (1989); Harding (1989); Morrow (1989); Hogan (1990); Marin *et al.* (1990) and Tortorice and O'Connell (1990).

Emesis in Anti-cancer Therapy
Mechanisms and treatment
Published in 1993 by Champman & Hall, London
ISBN 0 412 37250 9

If new and better types of anti-emetic treatment are to be developed, it is first necessary to understand the mechanisms and sites of action for the existing drugs. The importance of this approach has been illustrated by the introduction of 5-HT_3 receptor antagonists as powerful anti-emetic agents. The anti-emetic properties of this new class of drug were identified by a combination of clinical observations and knowledge of the basic pharmacology of metoclopramide (Miner *et al.*, 1987; see also below). Research into the mechanisms of action of anti-emetic drugs is also leading to a growing acceptance that appropriate animal models can reliably predict at least the acute human response to both anti-emetic and emetic drugs. As such, new anti-cancer therapies with the potential to cause vomiting (e.g. carboplatin; Martin *et al.*, 1990) can be evaluated for their emetic potential before entering clinical use; this is in addition to the use of such models to predict the anti-emetic activity of therapeutic drugs.

9.2 REDUCTION OF EMESIS WITHOUT THE USE OF DRUGS

Apart from psychological counselling and the reduction of anxiety (Chapter 10) it has been claimed that cytostatic-induced emesis can be reduced by the following measures: altering the amount and type of pre-therapy food allowed (Peters, 1989), considering the influence that circadian rhythms will have on the sensitivity to emesis (there is less emesis if cisplatin is administered during the early evening: Hrushesky and Roemeling, 1986; Headley, 1987) or by administering cisplatin over a longer period of time (Jordan *et al.*, 1985). Each of these modifications to the treatment regimen are sub-optimal methods of reducing emesis, but are worthy of consideration if optimal anti-emetic therapy is not available.

As a consequence of renal wasting, the use of cisplatin can lead to hypomagnesaemia. Since this condition is known to cause dysphagia and oesophageal spasms, Ballmer and Reinhart (1989) considered the value of concomitantly administering intravenous magnesium sulphate. When this idea was tested in patients, there was, however, no additional benefit over that already provided by a sub-optimal anti-emetic therapy. Nevertheless, since only two of the patients were subsequently shown to be hypomagnesaemic, the trial needs to be repeated. If the hypothesis is correct, replacement of magnesium could be of some benefit in a small number of patients.

Recent attention has been given to the ability of acupuncture to reduce emesis evoked by different stimuli. For cytotoxic therapy-induced emesis, electroacupuncture at the P_6 point ('wrist') considerably reduced cisplatin-evoked emesis in patients receiving metoclopramide and prednisolone but who had previously experienced a severe and persistent emetic response with cisplatin. By contrast, randomized cross-over with a dummy treatment was without effect (Dundee *et al.*, 1989). Although successful, this type of treatment was considered, by the authors, to be time consuming for both medical and nursing staff. In addition, the treatment had a short duration of action. A similar conclusion was also reached by Aglietti *et al.* (1990), who combined acupuncture with metoclopramide, dexamethasone and diphenhydramine. Prolongation of the anti-emetic action of P_6 acupuncture was achieved by combining with subsequent pressure at the acupuncture point (acupressure) every two hours (Dundee and Yang, 1990); acupressure alone may be less effective than acupuncture (Stannard, 1989). The mechanisms by which acupuncture and acupressure reduce cytostatic-induced emesis are not known. However, it has been suggested that at least part of the mechanism may involve an emotional expectation-placebo type of response (Dundee *et al.*, 1989; Dundee and Yang, 1990).

Other non-drug methods used to control the degree of emesis include hypnosis for anticipatory vomiting (Redd *et al.*, 1982), progressive muscle relaxation at the beginning of chemotherapy (Cotanch and Strum, 1987), moderate aerobic exercise (Winningham and MacVicar, 1988) and maintaining a positive fluid intake during therapy (Jordan, 1989). Creation of conditioned taste aversion to candy, given prior to chemotherapy instead of a normal meal, has been used to minimize cytotoxic therapy-induced food aversion (Broberg and Bernstein, 1987).

9.3 REDUCTION OF EMESIS WITH THE USE OF NATURAL PRODUCTS

Cisplatin-induced emesis in animals has been successfully prevented by feverfew (Rudd and Naylor, 1990) and the ginger extract 6-gingerol (Yamahara *et al.*, 1989a). For the feverfew extract, the anti-emetic action was preceded by mild emesis. Its mechanism of action may be related to the ability of this substance to reduce 5-HT release from blood platelets. For the ginger extract, further experiments suggest that it can antagonize the actions of 5-HT in a model normally used for assaying the 5-HT_3 receptor (Yamahara *et al.*, 1989b). However, it is not known whether this antagonism was selective or non-selective for the receptor. There have been no reports of the use of either feverfew or gingerol in cancer patients receiving therapy. However, against post-operative emesis, preliminary studies with ginger root suggest efficacy comparable to that of metoclopramide and greater than placebo (Bone *et al.*, 1990).

There has been one report on the evaluation of intravenous ethanol as an anti-emetic in patients being treated with cisplatin but who had obtained unsatisfactory anti-emetic control with high dose metoclopramide. The mistaken rationale for the study was based on the observation that patients with a history of chronic alcohol intake experience less cytotoxic-induced emesis. However, in this study, the intravenous ethanol proved inferior to metoclopramide as an anti-emetic (Spiess *et al.*, 1987).

9.4 REDUCTION OF EMESIS WITH THE USE OF PHARMACEUTICAL AGENTS

9.4.1 ANTI-CHOLINERGIC DRUGS AS AN ADJUNCT TO ANTI-EMETIC THERAPY

Anti-cholinergic drugs are not generally thought to be effective against cytotoxic-induced emesis (Hogan, 1990). In one study, transdermal scopolamine failed to reduce cisplatin-evoked emesis (Longo *et al.*, 1975). However, in another study, transdermal scopolamine reduced (albeit in a limited manner) emesis evoked by cisplatin in children (Sawicka and Sallan, 1977; Winter and Hart, 1987 [critical assessment]). Similarly, in Japan, injection of 0.5 mg atropine sulphate and 50 mg hexamethonium bromide ('medical vagotomy') reduced cisplatin-evoked emesis (Chen *et al.*, 1987). Transdermal scopolamine patches have also been shown to improve the anti-emetic activity of a combination of metoclopramide and dexamethasone (Meyer *et al.*, 1987), but to have no effect in combination with metoclopramide alone (Malone *et al.*, 1990). In ferrets, atropine reduced the emesis evoked by cyclophosphamide or by total body X-radiation (Roylance *et al.*, 1989).

These studies support the existence of a central cholinergic pathway in the emetic reflex (Beleslin *et al.*, 1989) but do not indicate that this pathway plays a major role in the mechanisms of cytotoxic therapy-induced emesis. Nevertheless, where anti-emetic treatment is clearly sub-optimal the addition of an anti-cholinergic agent to the anti-emetic 'cocktail' could produce a further reduction in emesis. For metoclopramide, Graham and Burgess (1989) have suggested that at the high doses used to reduce cisplatin-evoked emesis, this drug could at least partly inhibit cholinesterase activity. If correct, this suggestion would provide a rational explanation for the ability of scopolamine to improve on the anti-emetic activity of metoclopramide in some trials but not in others.

9.4.2 HISTAMINE H_1 RECEPTOR ANTAGONISTS AS AN ADJUNCT TO ANTI-EMETIC THERAPY

Antagonists of histamine H_1 receptors (e.g. diphenhydramine) are often also effective muscarinic receptor antagonists. However, they are used in cancer therapy only to prevent the extrapyramidal side-effects that can occur in response to D_2 receptor antagonists. These drugs have no significant or consistent ability to reduce cytotoxic-induced emesis themselves (Craig and Powell, 1987), but can cause mild sedation.

9.4.3 BENZODIAZEPINES AS AN ADJUNCT TO ANTI-EMETIC THERAPY

Benzodiazepines such as lorazepam, diazepam or flunitrazepam are frequently used in conjunction with other anti-emetic agents. Their primary mode of action results from a combination of amnesia and sedation. The latter can reduce the incidence of emesis and the former often prevents the patient recalling the experience of emesis or even of receiving chemotherapy (Laszlo *et al.*, 1985; Olynyk *et al.*, 1989). This profile of action makes the benzodiazepines particularly useful in treating anticipatory nausea and vomiting (Maher, 1981), as an adjunct therapy for those patients likely to suffer from severe emesis evoked by high-doses of cisplatin, and as an additional treatment for patients who cannot tolerate some of the side-effects of dopamine D_2 receptor antagonists.

The major side-effect of the benzodiazepines is of course sedation. In addition, the combination of the amnesia with the hydration procedures associated with cisplatin therapy can lead to an equally high incidence of urinary incontinence (Laszlo *et al.*, 1985).

9.5 THE ANTI-EMETIC PROPERTIES OF SPECIFIC DRUGS

9.5.1 ANTI-EMETIC ACTIVITIES OF CORTICOSTEROIDS

9.5.1.1 Discovery and usage

It has long been believed that high doses of corticosteroids can inhibit cytotoxic-induced emesis. The first indication arose from a pilot study by Baker *et al.* (1979), in which 10 mg dexamethasone was shown to reduce the vomiting evoked by a range of different cytotoxic drugs. The mechanism of action was unknown, but it was suggested that the associated euphoria could play a role. Subsequently, high doses of dexamethasone were shown to greatly reduce cisplatin-evoked emesis (Aapro *et al.*, 1981).

Most studies with corticosteroids have been performed using dexamethasone and, to a lesser extent, prednisolone and methylprednisolone. Because of the disparity of studies between dexamethasone and the other corticosteroids, it is difficult to make proper comparisons. However, on the basis of current evidence, there is no reason to suppose that large differences in efficacy exist between the three corticosteroids (Cersomimo and Karp, 1986). In general, high doses of corticosteroids will reduce mild-to-moderately-severe cytotoxic-induced emesis, with an efficacy equivalent or superior to that of dopamine D_2 receptor antagonists. Against high dose cisplatin, however, metoclopramide may have a superior anti-emetic efficacy when tested as a single agent (Donovitz *et al.*, 1984; Fustaci *et al.*, 1986).

When combined with metoclopramide or prochlorperazine, high doses of dexamethasone usually improve both the acute anti-emetic efficacy (Cersomimo and Karp, 1986) and the ability to reduce the delayed emesis associated with high doses of cisplatin (Gralla, 1989). As such, a high dose of dexamethasone is now often used as part of a 'cocktail' anti-emetic therapy (e.g. with dopamine D_2 receptor antagonists), so that each agent exerts a beneficial action through several different mechanisms, presumably by summating together.

9.5.1.2 Mechanisms of action

The mechanisms by which dexamethasone inhibit cytotoxic-induced emesis are not clearly understood and several possible mechanisms exist as follows:

9.5.1.2.1 The involvement of prostanoids

At least part of the mechanism by which dexamethasone reduces emesis involves the ability of steroids to reduce prostanoid turnover by inhibiting arachidonic acid release. It has long been known that emesis can be evoked by certain prostaglandins (Brenner *et al.*, 1975; Eiler *et al.*, 1979). Furthermore, since the actions of prostanoids can act in synergy with the actions of other substances (e.g. in pain sensitivity; Ferreira, 1972), a dual emetic action may operate, with the prostanoids exerting both a direct and indirect (increasing the emetic sensitivity to other substances) emetic action. In animals, prostanoid turnover can be increased by doxorubicin (rats: Robinson and Giri, 1987), by total body irradiation (mice: Eisen and Walker, 1978; monkeys: Dubois *et al.*, 1987) or by local radiation (guinea-pig: Steel *et al.*, 1983). In cancer patients, cisplatin did not increase blood plasma concentrations of prostaglandins (Curry *et al.*, 1981), but since many prostanoids are substantially metabolized on passage through the lungs the results of this study must be treated with caution.

Evidence that the prostanoids released by cytotoxic therapy are involved in the mechanisms of nausea and vomiting is provided by the ability of ibuprofen to prevent emesis evoked by pelvic irradiation in cancer patients. In this study, the severity of nausea was also reduced, but was not abolished (Stryker *et al.*, 1979). Similarly, preliminary experiments with indomethacin resulted in a substantial reduction of radiation-evoked emesis in dogs (Carpenter *et al.*, 1986).

9.5.1.2.2 Other mechanisms

Because steroids reduce prostanoid turnover by inhibiting the release of arachidonic acid from cell membranes, they will also inhibit the turnover of other substances which are derived from arachidonic acid metabolism. The abilities of these other substances (e.g. lipoxygenase products) to evoke emesis is unknown. Nevertheless, lipid peroxides of arachidonic acid have been implicated in the mechanisms of cerebral oedema following brain ischaemia (Shimizu and Wolfe, 1990). If these substances also contribute to the cerebral oedema that can be caused by radiation and cytotoxic agents, then they could cause emesis as a result of the raised intracranial pressure. The ability of dexamethasone to inhibit this type of oedema may therefore be an important mechanism by which delayed emesis is controlled by corticosteroid administration (Young, 1986). Inhibition by dexamethasone of oedema within the area postrema may also inhibit emesis caused by stereotactic radiosurgery to this region (Alexander *et al.*, 1989).

Among other possible actions of corticosteroids, it has been suggested that these agents could actually decrease the amount of available 5-HT by activating tryptophan pyrrolase, shunting the metabolism of tryptophan away from the 5-HT synthetic pathways (Andrews *et al.*, 1988). Since 5-HT may play an important role in the mechanisms of cytotoxic-induced vomiting (see section 9.6.4 on 5-HT_3 receptor antagonists), any mechanism which reduced the available 5-HT would contribute to a reduction of this type of vomiting.

9.5.1.2.3 *Inhibition of adrenal secretions*

The ability of dexamethasone to suppress adrenal secretion, when given at a high dose (20 mg) over five consecutive days, could lead to adrenal failure and emesis when the dexamethasone is suddenly withdrawn. Such a mechanism of action would contribute to the delayed emesis which can follow therapy with cisplatin (Alberola *et al.*, 1986). However, in a study to investigate this possibility, dexamethasone given as a single dose of 10 mg caused only a short-lived reduction of serum cortisol concentration. The short-term use of this dose of dexamethasone was, therefore, justified. Nevertheless, caution must still be exercised in patients with an advanced stage of the disease or where endogenous steroid secretion is severely reduced by, for example, hepatic or adrenal metastasis (Aasebo and Slordal, 1990).

9.5.2 ANTI-EMETIC ACTIVITY OF DOPAMINE D_2 RECEPTOR ANTAGONISTS

9.5.2.1 Discovery and usage

There are three structural classes of dopamine D_2 receptor antagonists: the phenothiazines, the butyrophenones and the substituted benzamides. In general, each of these classes of drug reduce, but do not abolish the mild-to-moderately-severe type of nausea and vomiting evoked by cytotoxic therapy. Furthermore, these agents do not consistently reduce cisplatin-evoked emesis, although there are some very notable exceptions to this generalization (see below). The limited efficacy of the dopamine D_2 receptor antagonists restricts their use as single agent therapies. These drugs are, therefore, often used as part of a combination anti-emetic therapy.

The phenothiazines were the first class of drug used to inhibit cytotoxic drug-induced emesis (Moertal *et al.*, 1963) having been developed for their anti-histamine and sedative actions (Edmonds-Seal and Prys-Roberts, 1970; Wampler, 1983). The original compound was chlorpromazine, for which anti-emetic activity was demonstrated against apomorphine-induced emesis in animals (Boyd *et al.*, 1953) and then against vomiting induced in patients by cytotoxic therapy or severe uraemia (Friend and Cummins, 1953). Subsequently, prochlorperazine, thiethylperazine and perphenazine have become more commonly used. These drugs are available as multiple preparations, including slow-release formulations, which gives them a practical advantage over many other currently available anti-emetic agents (Hogan, 1990).

Among the phenothiazines, some studies with high intravenous doses of prochlorperazine suggest that this agent could prevent cisplatin-evoked emesis in cancer patients, when administered as a single anti-emetic agent (Carr *et al.*, 1987) or in combination with dexamethasone (Akhtar *et al.*, 1990). Further studies with high doses of prochlorperazine and with the other phenothiazines must now be carried out to establish whether this is a genuine property of prochlorperazine and/or the phenothiazines in general. Of particular concern must be the absence of any clear mechanism by which prochlorperazine can exert this activity, whereas most other dopamine D_2 receptor antagonists do not (see below).

The butyrophenones include haloperidol, droperidol and the butyrophenone derivative, domperidone. Haloperidol and droperidol were originally developed for their sedative and tranquillizer properties (Janssen *et al.*, 1963; Yelnosky *et al.*, 1964; Edmonds-Seal and Prys-Roberts, 1970), but were subsequently used as anti-emetic agents in an attempt to improve on the efficacy of the phenothiazines. Indeed, the combination of D_2 receptor block and strong sedation is considered by some to be an improvement (see below). By contrast, domperidone does not normally cross the blood–brain barrier and is, therefore, relatively free of the sedation and extrapyramidal side-effects which are associated with other dopamine D_2 receptor antagonists (Brogden *et al.*, 1982). However, in high intravenous doses, domperidone has been associated with cardiac arrhythmia and even death (Roussak *et al.*, 1984; Osborne *et al.*, 1985). As a consequence, the intravenous formulation of domperidone is no longer available.

The substituted benzamides include metoclopramide, alizapride and clebopride. The discovery of metoclopramide arose from an attempt to improve on the properties of the local anaesthetic procainamide. However, in 1964, the ability of metoclopramide to block apomorphine-induced emesis in animals was described and subsequently, its ability to stimulate gastro-intestinal motility (Sanger and King, 1988). Metoclopramide has since found clinical use as a treatment of reflux oesophagitis and dyspepsia, in addition to its use as an anti-emetic drug. Other substituted benzamides were then introduced (Sanger and King, 1988). However, of these compounds, only metoclopramide has consistently been shown to reduce emesis evoked by high doses of cisplatin. This action of metoclopramide occurred only at high intravenous doses and directly led to the development of the selective 5-HT_3 receptor antagonists as a new and more effective class of anti-emetic agent (see section 9.5.4).

9.5.2.2 Pharmacology

Table 9.1 summarizes the affinities of the more commonly used dopamine D_2 receptor antagonists for the D_2 receptor, the α_1-adrenoceptor, the histamine H_1 receptor, the muscarinic receptor and the 5-HT_3 receptor. Much of these data were obtained in the laboratories of S.J. Peroutka and colleagues. Some of the dopamine D_2 receptor antagonists have also been examined for their ability to inhibit prostanoid synthesis (Krupp and Wesp, 1975). This property occurs with very high concentrations of some compounds (e.g. chlorpromazine), but not with others (e.g. haloperidol); it will not be discussed further in relation to this class of anti-emetic agent, since the concentrations are too high to be of clinical relevance.

The major anti-emetic activity of D_2 receptor antagonists is, of course, due to their ability to antagonize at this receptor (Ison and Peroutka, 1986). With regard to the mechanisms of emesis, the D_2 receptor is located within the area postrema on post-synaptic neuronal tissue and possibly on the vascular tissue (Stefanini and Clement-Cormier, 1981; Harding *et al.*, 1987; Chugh *et al.*, 1988).

Antagonism at the D_2 receptor within this important area of the brain also results in an increase in blood plasma prolactin concentration. While this has little or no clinical significance during acute use, prolonged antagonism at the D_2 receptor can lead to side-effects such as galactorrhoea. Since domperidone does not normally cross the blood–brain barrier, there is only a minimal potential of this drug to cause extrapyramidal side-effects. By contrast, dopamine D_2 receptor antagonists which cross the blood–brain barrier can cause extrapyramidal side-effects (e.g. dystonic reactions) by antagonism at the receptor located within the mesolimbic systems. This can be of particular significance for the very young or the very old (Perrot *et al.*, 1982) where the blood–brain barrier is either poorly developed or no longer sufficiently effective. As a consequence, it is not uncommon to administer drugs such as diphenhydramine or benzotropine in conjunction with dopamine D_2 receptor antagonists, to minimize or control the occurrence of extrapyramidal reactions. In dogs, diphenhydramine does not interfere with the ability of metoclopramide to reduce cisplatin-evoked emesis (Smith *et al.*, 1985).

Table 9.1 The affinities of dopamine D_2 receptor antagonists for dopamine D_2 and D_3 receptors, α_1-adrenoceptors, histamine H_1, muscarinic (M) and 5-HT_3 receptors in rat brain tissue

Affinity data is given as K_i values (nM), with a multiple of the mean D_2 receptor affinity given in parenthesis. The data compiled in this table has been obtained from Peroutka and Snyder (1982), Ison and Peroutka (1986), Lobbezoo *et al.* (1985), Hamik and Peroutka (1989), Nelson and Thomas (1989) and Sokoloff *et al.* (1990)

	D_2	D_3	α_1	H_1	M	5-HT_3
Thiethylperazine	1.1	–	17 (×15)	–	–	–
Prochlorperazine	6.8, 7.3, 15, 4.7*	35* (×7.4)	200 (×21)	100 (×11)	2100 (×225)	1800 (×193)
Chlorpromazine	18, 21, 25, 2.8*	6.1* (×2.2)	8.8 (×0.4)	28 (×1.4)	130 (×6)	1900 (×91)
Haloperidol	1.3–1.4, 0.5*	9.8* (×22)	14 (×10)	16 000 (×1185)	>10 000 (×>7400)	–
Droperidol	1.9–2.4	–	1.3 (×0.6)	2500 (×1179)	>10 000 (×>4650)	4200 (×1953)
Domperidone	0.9, 11, 12, 0.3*	9.5* (×32)	74 (×32)		–	3900, >10,000 (×>1250)
Metoclopramide	33.6, 160, 240	–	>10 000 (×>69)	>1000 (×>85)	>10 000 (×>85)	120–160 (×1.2)

* Data from rat brain receptor clone expressed in CHO cells.

See also: Laville and Margarit (1982) and Roberts (1982) for a functional analysis of alizapride and clebopride against the D_2 receptor. Both these agents are also poorly effective against cisplatin–evoked emesis and are, therefore, predicted to have low affinity for the 5-HT_3 receptor.

As Table 9.1 clearly demonstrates, the dopamine D_2 receptor antagonists are not generally selective for the D_2 receptor. Of particular significance is the ability of some antagonists to block at the α_1-adrenoceptor and at the histamine H_1 receptor. Antagonism of the α_1-adrenoceptor can cause sedation and orthostatic hypotension (Yelnosky *et al.*, 1964; Peroutka *et al.*, 1977; U'Pritchard *et al.*, 1978). Sedation and somnolence is also caused by antagonism at histamine H_1 receptors. From Table 9.1, it can be seen that chlorpromazine and droperidol have an affinity for the α_1-adrenoceptor which is equal or greater than that for the D_2 receptor. In addition, chlorpromazine has an equally high affinity for the H_1 receptor and an appreciable affinity for the muscarinic receptor. Both chlorpromazine and droperidol are associated with an incidence of sedation and orthostatic hypotension which is far higher than for other members of their class, such as prochlorperazine or haloperidol (Ison and Peroutka, 1986). As already described, antagonism at the muscarinic receptor or the histamine H_1 receptor does not have any consistent anti-emetic benefit in cancer patients. In contrast to chlorpromazine and droperidol, dopamine D_2 receptor antagonists which have a relatively low affinity for the α_1 and H_1 receptors are likely to occupy only a small number of these receptors at the clinical dose required to block at the D_2 receptor. These drugs, therefore, cause some sedation but not to the same extent as chlorpromazine and droperidol.

Orthostatic hypotension is clearly a disadvantageous property, limiting the use of those D_2 receptor antagonists which cause this side-effect. Of particular concern are older patients who may have cardiopulmonary disease (Kelley *et al.*, 1986). However, the side-effect of sedation can sometimes be an advantage for those patients in which D_2 receptor antagonism is not a wholly effective anti-emetic treatment. For example, sedation has been regarded as a positive advantage for patients undergoing total body irradiation, who experience severe nausea and vomiting but cannot move away from the source of radiation. Nevertheless, in an ideal situation and for patients receiving therapy with a low emetogenic potential, sedation caused by the purposeful antagonism of these different receptors does not greatly improve on the degree of anti-emetic control and cannot be accepted as a satisfactory form of anti-emetic treatment (Martin-Timenez and Diaz-Rubio, 1986).

Among the substituted benzamides, the anti-emetic activity of conventional doses of alizapride and metoclopramide are similar. However, in contrast to metoclopramide, alizapride is more often associated with severe hypotensive side-effects (Joss *et al.*, 1985; Saller and Hallenbrecht, 1985; Bleiberg *et al.*, 1988). While the mechanism of this action is not known and is not readily detected in animal studies (Laville and Margarit, 1982; Perrot *et al.*, 1982), the above analysis would suggest that the affinity of alizapride for the α_1-adrenoceptor (and for other receptors associated with hypotension) should be checked.

Apart from metoclopramide, none of the commonly used anti-emetic drugs have any meaningful affinity for the 5-HT_3 receptor (see also Table 9.1). Since antagonism at this receptor is the most effective single means of reducing or abolishing severe emesis (see below), it is, therefore, not unexpected that agents which lack the ability to antagonize at the 5-HT_3 receptor will generally be poorly effective against cisplatin-evoked emesis. Similarly, it is predicted that those dopamine D_2 receptor antagonists which have not yet been tested for an affinity for the 5-HT_3 receptor, but which do not readily reduce cisplatin-evoked emesis (e.g. alizapride; Basurto *et al.*, 1988), will have a low affinity for this receptor.

9.5.2.3 Relationships between dopamine and mechanisms of emesis

In dogs and ferrets, intravenous injection of stable dopamine D_2 receptor agonists such as apomorphine evoke only one or two episodes of vomiting. Even intracerebroventricular injection of apomorphine in dogs evokes only five or six episodes of vomiting (Harding *et al.*, 1987). This small number of emetic episodes evoked by a single administration of apomorphine clearly does not mimic the sustained nausea and vomiting evoked by cytotoxic agents. Furthermore, if endogenous turnover is increased using amphetamine then nausea and vomiting is rarely, if ever, evoked (Barnes, 1984). How then, can dopamine play a role in cytotoxic drug-induced vomiting?

Within the peripheral nervous system, there are no known studies which have sought to demonstrate a cytotoxic-induced increase in the turnover of dopamine. Nevertheless, in ferrets, cisplatin treatment increased dopamine levels in the caudate nucleus and tended to increase dopamine in the area postrema (Barnes *et al.*, 1987). In rats, whole body X-irradiation reduced the amount of dopamine present in the corpus striatum (Stepanovic and Nikolic, 1979). It is, therefore, potentially possible for cytotoxic therapy to modify endogenous dopamine turnover at least within the CNS and perhaps in a manner that differs from amphetamine. However, if cytotoxic drugs do increase dopamine turnover then it is clearly not an essential mechanism of cytotoxic drug- or radiation-induced emesis. Thus, dopamine D_2 receptor antagonism, by itself, is only a partially effective means of preventing mild-to-moderately-severe emesis and has only minimal ability to reduce severe emesis. Curiously, there is some evidence to suggest that the mechanism of apomorphine-induced gastric retropulsion may be at least partly mediated by 5-HT acting within the peripheral nervous system (Miolan *et al.*, 1984). Since apomorphine-induced vomiting is not blocked by 5-HT_3 receptor antagonism (Miner *et al.*, 1987; Bermudez *et al.*, 1988; Smith *et al.*, 1989), the receptor which may mediate this response to apomorphine is unlikely to be of the 5-HT_3 type.

9.5.3 ANTI-EMETIC ACTIVITY OF CANNABINOIDS

9.5.3.1 Discovery and use

The therapeutic use of cannabinoids derives from ancient Mediterranean, Chinese, Arab and Indian cultures. In both Germany and England in the nineteenth century, cannabis was well known as an anti-emetic agent (Mechoulam and Feigenbaum, 1987).

The realization that the active principle of cannabis (delta-9-tetrahydrocannabinol; THC) reduced the nausea and vomiting evoked by cytotoxic therapy occurred in 1975, following anecdotal reports from smokers of marijuana (Sallen *et al.*, 1975). Large scale clinical trials quickly followed, leading to both the registration of THC as a clinical drug and to the synthesis and registration of the THC-derivatives nabilone and levonantradol.

All of the cannabinoid drugs act as effective anti-emetic agents against mild-to-moderate cytotoxic drug-induced emesis, with only weak activity reported against the severe type of emesis evoked by cisplatin (Vincent *et al.*, 1983). Their anti-emetic actions are not restricted to cytotoxic therapy-induced emesis, since nabilone reduces emesis evoked in cats by apomorphine or deslanoside, but not by nicotine (McCarthy and Borison, 1977; 1981). Nabilone may also be effective against the emesis evoked by bronchial bacterial infection in AIDS patients (Green *et al.*, 1989). However, for many patients, the side-effects of the existing cannabinoids (sedation, somnolence, anxiety, dysphoria, increased heart rate, orthostatic hypotension, mental confusion, hallucinations) severely restrict their use.

Attempts are currently being made to limit the side-effects of cannabinoids, either by developing inhalation techniques (Vinciguerra *et al.*, 1988) or by synthesizing new derivatives where it is hoped that the psychotropic properties can be separated from the anti-emetic properties. To some extent this has been achieved with levonantradol (Barnes, 1984), but a more recent attempt is illustrated by the compound HU-211 (7-hydroxy-delta-6-tetrahydrocannabinol, dimethylheptyl homolog), which exhibits anti-emetic properties in pigeons but is claimed to be devoid of psychotropic activity (Feigenbaum *et al.*, 1989). The recent cloning of a cannabinoid receptor should now further facilitate the task of separating out the 'wanted' activities of the cannabinoids from the 'unwanted'. Nevertheless, the actual wisdom of pursuing increased anti-emetic selectivity for an agent which is only effective against mild-to-moderate cytotoxic therapy-induced emesis seems doubtful, unless such drugs could find use in other types of emesis outside the oncology clinic.

9.5.3.2 Pharmacology

There is a considerable body of knowledge available on the many different pharmacological actions of the cannabinoids. However, it is still not known which of these many actions are involved in reducing emesis. It is to be hoped that further research with those cannabinoid derivatives claimed to have specificity as anti-emetic agents (see above) will provide valuable information.

The extensive actions of the cannabinoids within the CNS make it difficult to separate out the sites of true anti-emetic activity (Butler *et al.*, 1976). Nevertheless, one of the most striking observations is the ability of the opioid antagonist naloxone to inhibit the anti-emetic activity of nabilone in cats (McCarthy and Borison, 1977). This observation, coupled with the ability of nabilone to inhibit emesis evoked by drugs acting within the central nervous system, led London *et al.* (1979) to propose that the cannabinoids exert their anti-emetic activity predominantly by inhibiting the output from the so-called vomiting centre within the medulla oblongata. Whether the cannabinoids exert this action by acting directly or indirectly at the opiate receptors is not currently known.

In paediatric patients receiving cyclophosphamide or cisplatin, continuous intravenous infusion of the opioid antagonist naloxone caused a dose-related increase in the nausea, vomiting and aversion (Kobrinsky *et al.*, 1988). While the ethics of such a study may seem dubious, the data provided does suggest that endogenous opioids provide at least some reduction in the overall severity of cytotoxic-induced emesis. If cannabinoids exert their anti-emetic activity at least partly by activating an opioid-dependent system, their limited anti-emetic efficacy against severe emesis suggests that in these patients, an endogenous opioid system must be operating at or near maximal efficacy.

An additional action of cannabinoids (or their metabolites; see Burnstein *et al.*, 1988) which could contribute to their anti-emetic activity, includes the ability to inhibit prostanoid synthesis (Krupp and Wesp, 1975; Burnstein, 1976). (See also section 9.5.1 on corticosteroids.)

9.5.4 ANTI-EMETIC ACTIVITY OF SELECTIVE 5-HT_3 RECEPTOR ANTAGONISTS

9.5.4.1 Discovery and usage

The process of the discovery that moderate and severe cytotoxic-induced emesis could be prevented or greatly reduced by selective 5-HT_3 receptor antagonism has been previously described (Miner *et al.*, 1987; Andrews *et al.*, 1988; Sanger and King, 1988; King and Sanger, 1989; Sanger, 1990; Barnes *et al.*, 1991a). In essence, the story began with studies by Gylys *et al.* (1979), who found that high intravenous doses of metoclopramide gave better protection against cisplatin-evoked emesis in dogs compared with prochlorperazine. Gralla *et al.* (1981) also gave high intravenous doses of metoclopramide to cancer patients in an attempt to control cisplatin-evoked emesis. In these initial studies, metoclopramide was said to prevent cisplatin-evoked emesis. However, most clinicians would now claim that high doses of metoclopramide greatly reduce but do not completely prevent cisplatin-evoked emesis, so that combination therapy with a corticosteroid may be required, coupled with diphenhydramine or a benzodiazepine to control any extrapyramidal side-effects (see section 9.5.2 on dopamine D_2 receptor antagonists).

As described earlier, attempts to mimic the findings of Gralla and colleagues by increasing the doses of other dopamine D_2 receptor antagonists were generally unsuccessful. It was proposed that metoclopramide might reduce cisplatin-evoked emesis by a mechanism which did not involve D_2 receptor antagonism (McRitchie *et al.*, 1984). The proposal was followed by research into the mechanism of action. At that time, animal models of cytotoxic-induced emesis were poorly understood. Nevertheless, for a variety of reasons, we chose to study emesis in the ferret (Florczyk *et al.*, 1982), which has since become accepted as one of the species of choice for predicting the anti-emetic activities of drugs given to cancer patients (Andrews *et al.*, 1990). Early in 1986, it was suggested that cisplatin-evoked emesis in ferrets may be reduced by 5-HT_3 receptor antagonism (Miner *et al.*, 1986). However, because the compound used in this study (BRL 24924), antagonized at the 5-HT_3 receptor and stimulated gut motility via a second 5-HT receptor (5-HT_4), the possibility that at least part of the anti-emetic activity was due to stimulation of gastro-intestinal motility could not be excluded. However unlikely the possibility (Miner *et al.*, [critical commentary] 1987; Sanger and King, 1988), this mechanism of action was still being actively considered at the time (see, for example, Alphin *et al.*, 1986). It was, therefore, necessary to prove this new hypothesis by testing the first selective 5-HT_3 receptor antagonist (MDL 72222), a compound which does not directly stimulate gut motility. Our published findings (Miner and Sanger, 1986) then opened the door to many other studies with 5-HT_3 receptor antagonists (Sanger, 1990) including near simultaneous reports on the anti-emetic activity of MDL 72222 in dogs (Berga *et al.*, 1986) and ICS 205–930 in ferrets (Costall *et al.*, 1986).

The eventual clinical usage of selective 5-HT_3 receptor antagonists remains to be established. However, it is already clear that these antagonists are probably the most effective single anti-emetic agents known. For example, against cisplatin (>50 mg/m^2), ondansetron 8 mg i.v. followed by a continuous infusion of 1 mg h^{-1} for 24 hours, was superior to high dose metoclopramide (3 mg kg^{-1} i.v., followed by a continuous infusion of 4 mg kg^{-1} for 8 hours), when assessments were made of side-effect profile and the acute phases of nausea and vomiting (De Mulder *et al.*, 1990). Similarly, a single injection of granisetron 40 µg kg^{-1} i.v. against patients receiving cisplatin >49 mg/m^2, was as effective against nausea and vomiting as a high dose of metoclopram-ide (3 mg kg^{-1} i.v., followed by a continuous infusion of 4 mg kg^{-1} for 8 hours) plus dexamethasone (12 mg i.v.). However, granisetron had a superior side-effect profile and a more convenient usage (Chevallier, 1990). Perhaps more startling, however, is the observation that granisetron can arrest cisplatin-evoked emesis even after it has begun. This finding was first reported using granisetron in ferrets (Bermudez *et al.*, 1988) and then again in cancer patients (Cassidy *et al.*, 1988; Cupissol *et al.*, 1990).

While 5-HT_3 receptor antagonism demonstrates high anti-emetic efficacy against acute and severe nausea and vomiting, there is some evidence to suggest that such agents may be less effective against the less severe delayed nausea and vomiting which occurs in some patients several days after dosing with cisplatin. For example, in the trial with ondansetron described above (De Mulder *et al.*, 1990), the superior profile over metoclopramide during the first 24 hours was lost during the delayed phase. It is likely that further studies on the control of delayed vomiting will now be necessary, so that combination anti-emetic therapy can be tested. In particular, it has been found that dexamethasone is capable of controlling emesis in those patients who have failed with ondansetron (Cunningham *et al.*, 1989; Smith *et al.*, 1990). A combination of 5-HT_3 receptor antagonism plus corticosteroid might, therefore, be required for the control of delayed emesis.

Direct comparisons between the efficacy of different 5-HT_3 receptor antagonists have yet to be undertaken in the clinical setting. Clearly, there are differences in the current dosing regimes for ondansetron and granisetron (see above, for example), although the optimal dose of ondansetron could still be in doubt (Anonymous, 1990). It is, however, too soon to predict whether other differences in clinical efficacy will become apparent. At present, a subjective analysis would suggest that if there are differences, these will be difficult to detect (Jones and Cunningham, this volume). Nevertheless, as with all new drugs, long-term post-marketing surveillance is required and important differences in efficacy and side-effect profile could still become apparent. A recent survey of the clinical anti-emetic activities of ondansetron, granisetron, ICS 205–930, MDL 72222, MDL 73147EF, batanopride and LAS 30451 can be found in the proceedings of the Perugia International Cancer Conference III; Supportive therapy: Challenges for the '90s (1990).

In general, the selective 5-HT_3 receptor antagonists seem to be a remarkably safe class of compound. Many of the antagonists currently being evaluated in the clinic are highly selective for the 5-HT_3 receptor (see section that follows) and presumably for this reason, side-effects are minimal. For the selective antagonists, the side-effects which are detected include a low incidence of mild constipation and mild headache (Jones and Cunningham, this volume).

9.5.4.2 Pharmacology

Of the 5-HT receptors, the 5-HT_3 receptor is unique. It is coupled not to an intracellular second messenger system via a G-protein, but to a ligand-gated ion channel, permeable to monovalent cations (K^+, Na^+). As such, 5-HT_3 receptor-mediated responses are characterized by a fast onset of action and rapid desensitization (Peters and Lambert, 1989). Some experiments suggest that subtypes of the 5-HT_3 receptor exist or that the same receptor exists in more than one conformation (Derkach *et al.*, 1989). Species differences can also occur in the sensitivity of the 5-HT_3 receptor to antagonists (Lattimer *et al.*, 1989; Butler *et al.*, 1990). However, these important findings still require further analysis (e.g. structural determination of the receptor) before it can be concluded that more than one 5-HT_3 receptor exists.

Table 9.2 lists a number of 5-HT_3 receptor antagonists which have been demonstrated to have anti-emetic properties and which have been at least partially characterized using functional assays of antagonism. Their ability to antagonize the 5-HT_3 receptor is demonstrated *in vivo* by the inhibition of the 5-HT-evoked Bezold-Jarisch reflex in anaesthetized rats. This vago-vagal reflex is activated by stimulation of sensory afferent nerve terminals in and around the heart, leading to a rapid and transient bradycardia. It is a reflex that exists in man (Mark, 1983). It can also be activated via lung sensory neurons to affect respiratory rate (Mott and Paintal, 1953) and has close connections with the mechanisms of nausea and the pathways via which cytotoxic therapy evokes emesis (Sanger, 1990). Drugs which block this reflex correlate well with an

Table 9.2 A comparison of the potencies and affinities of 5-HT_3 receptor antagonists

Data obtained using 5-HT as the agonist, although in some cases only data using 2-methyl-5HT is available (marked with an asterisk). References appear in parenthesis. Compounds not listed here, but which have been shown to inhibit cytotoxic-emesis in animals for which there is minimal data to indicate 5-HT_3 receptor antagonism or for which antagonism has been demonstrated using different assays to those listed below, include RG 12915 (Davis and Martin, 1990; Fitzpatrick *et al.*, 1990), Y-25130 (Fukuda *et al.*, 1990), DA 6215 (Sagrada *et al.*, 1990), LAS 30451 (Martin, 1990), and L-683–877 (Tattersall *et al.*, 1990).
NB: numerals in brackets denote references below.

	Inhibition of the Bezold-Jarisch effect in rats (ID_{50} µg kg^{-1} i.v.)	Antagonism of contraction in guinea-pig ileum (pA_2)	Antagonism of tachycardia in rabbit heart (pA_2)	Antagonism of depolarization in rabbit vagus (pA_2)	References of anti-emetic efficacy
Metoclopramide	188(7), 503(8)	Non-competitive(2)	7.2(6)	7.3(7), 7.6(12)	Gylys *et al.*, 1979 Florczyk *et al.*, 1982 Smith *et al.*, 1985 Costall *et al.*, 1986 Miner *et al.*, 1987
MDL72222	39(5), 42(7), 35(8)	Non-competitive(5)	9.3(5), 8.9(2)	7.9(2), 8.0(7)	Miner and Sanger, 1986; Berga *et al.*, 1986; Lucot, 1989
ICS 205–930	0.4(2), 0.4(7) 1.4(8), 3(9)	7.9(2), 8.3(7)	10.6(2)	10.2(2), 10.2(7)	Costall *et al.*, 1986; 1987b; Lucot, 1989

Granisetron (BRL 43694)	0.7(3)	8.1(3)	10.7(3)	10.86(12)	Bermudez *et al.*, 1988 Harding *et al.*, 1988; Bhandari *et al.*, 1989
Ondansetron (GR 38032F)	3.6(8), 2(9)	7.3(1)	10.1(3)	9.4(1)	Costall *et al.*, 1987 Stables *et al.*, 1987 Higgins *et al.*, 1989
Zacopride	0.12(7), 0.5(8) 0.4(9)	8.5(7)	–	10.1(7)	Costall *et al.*, 1987; Smith *et al.*, 1988 King *et al.*, 1988; Smith *et al.*, 1989
Batanopride (BMY 25801)	70(4)	–	–	–	Gylys *et al.*, 1988
LY277359	0.9(9)	8.8*(9)	–	–	Cohen *et al.*, 1990
Pancopride	0.56(10)	–	–	–	Fernández *et al.*, 1990
AS-5370	0.13*(11)	–	–	–	Ito *et al.*, 1990
MDL 73147	–	Non-competitive	–	9.8(13)	
YM060	0.04(14)	–	–	–	Kamato *et al.*, 1991

References: (1) Butler *et al.*, 1988 (2) Donatsch *et al.*, 1984 (3) Sanger and Nelson, 1989 (4) Gylys *et al.*, 1988 (5) Fozard, 1984 (b) Fozard and Mobarok Ali, 1978 (7) Smith *et al.*, 1988 (8) Sanger, 1990 (9) Cohen *et al.*, 1990 (10) Fernandez *et al.*, 1990 (11) Yoshida *et al.*, 1990 (12) Elliot *et al.*, 1990 (13) Fozard, 1989 (14) Honda *et al.*, 1991.

ability to inhibit cytotoxic-induced emesis. Antagonism at the 5-HT_3 receptor can also be assessed *in vitro* by measuring the ability to inhibit various 5-HT-evoked functional responses (e.g. contraction of guinea-pig ileum; tachycardia of rabbit heart; depolarization of rabbit vagus). These techniques are used for modelling the 5-HT_3 receptor, but their physiological significance is not clear. For convenience, a comparison of receptor binding affinities has not been included in Table 9.2, since many different radioligands have been used with different laboratories adopting different methods to express antagonist potency or affinity.

A significant feature of Table 9.2 is that, unless specified, data have been collected only from those experiments where 5-HT was used to activate the 5-HT_3 receptor. There has been an understandable trend in some laboratories to substitute 5-HT with the more selective 5-HT_3 receptor agonist 2-methyl-5-HT. However, recent evidence suggests that 2-methyl-5-HT acts as only a partial agonist at the 5-HT_3 receptor (Cramer *et al.*, 1990; Newberry *et al.*, 1991; Sepulveda *et al.*, 1991) which could lead to an over-estimate of the potency and affinity of 5-HT_3 receptor antagonists assessed using this agonist.

Two features of 5-HT_3 receptor antagonists are particularly prominent. Firstly, Table 9.2 shows that many are highly potent antagonists in those animal species studied (see exceptions, below). Fortunately, this also seems to be true in man, at least so far as emesis is concerned. However, in one species (pigeon) some of these selective antagonists behave as partial agonists and evoke vomiting (Preziosi *et al.*, 1989). Secondly, most of the compounds tested in Table 9.2 are also highly selective for the 5-HT_3 receptor, with little or no meaningful affinity for all other 5-HT receptors, adrenoceptors, dopamine receptors, opiate receptors, etc. (Van Wijngaarden *et al.*, 1990 and the references quoted in Table 9.2). However, this general concept of selectivity is not true for all compounds. It is particularly untrue of zacopride, a mixture of two enantiomers with different affinities for the 5-HT_3 receptor (Waeber *et al.*, 1990). When these enantiomers were assessed functionally, the S-enantiomer was found to activate the Bezold–Jarisch reflex in ferrets, whereas it was the R-enantiomer which acted as the antagonist (Middlefell and Price, 1991). Activation of the 5-HT_3 receptor by S-zacopride may, at least partly, explain why oral doses of the racemate actually evoke emesis in ferrets (King, 1990; Sanger, 1990; Sancilio *et al.*, 1991), although the ability of zacopride to activate 5-HT_4 receptors (Villalon *et al.*, 1991) could also contribute to the mechanisms of emesis (Bhandari and Andrews, 1991). Activation of 5-HT_4 receptors by zacopride will also increase out motility, a possible mechanism for the diarrhoea evoked by zacopride in ferrets (King, 1990). Finally zacopride can cause sedation in ferrets (King and Landauer, 1990).

A compound which may also promote the occurrence of emesis is Y–25130, which prevents cisplatin-evoked emesis when given intravenously. However, in contrast to those dogs which did not receive the antagonist and vomited in response to cisplatin, dogs which received cisplatin and Y–25130 tended to vomit when presented with food 18 hr after cisplatin (Fukuda *et al.*, 1991).

Another exception to the concept of high selectivity is batanopride. In contrast to other 5-HT_3 receptor antagonists, this compound markedly reduces systolic blood pressure in man (Smaldone *et al.*, 1990), but the mechanism of this action is unknown. Finally, it has been shown that high concentrations (approx. 10^{-6} M or greater) of ICS 205–930 antagonize at the 5-HT_4 receptor (Clarke *et al.*, 1989). However, in view of the high concentration required to interact with the 5-HT_4 receptor, it is unlikely that this finding has clinical significance.

9.5.4.3 Relationship between 5-HT and mechanisms of emesis

In animal studies, using several different species, sectioning of the abdominal vagus nerve reduces or prevents emesis evoked by a variety of different cytotoxic drugs or by total body irradiation. For those animals in which vagal nerve section only reduces and does not prevent emesis, sectioning of the splanchnic nerves in combination with the vagus does prevent emesis. In these circumstances, the ability of the vagus to 'sense' and 'drive' the act of emesis seems to be supported by other visceral afferent fibres. By contrast, vomiting evoked by agents which act directly within the central nervous system (e.g. apomorphine) are not prevented by vagotomy. This difference in vagal dependence is matched by the ability of 5-HT_3 receptor antagonists to block only those forms of emesis which depend on the vagus nerve. It has therefore been concluded that cytotoxic-induced emesis is mediated predominantly via the vagus nerve (Andrews *et al.*, 1990). As described in Chapters 5 and 10, this nerve is well placed to signal the onset of nausea and vomiting, since it innervates both the area postrema and, more importantly, the *nucleus tractus solitarius*. The area postrema is the region that has historically been known as the 'chemoreceptor trigger zone' and is not protected by the blood–brain barrier. The *nucleus tractus solitarius* forms part of the 'vomiting centre' and as such, has some protection by the blood–brain barrier.

The vagus nerve has 5-HT_3 receptors situated all along its length. They are located on the nerve terminals within the gut wall (Andrews and Davidson, 1990), on the afferent nerve axons, on the cell bodies within the nodose ganglion (Wallis, 1990) and on the nerve terminals contained within the *nucleus tractus solitarius* and the area postrema (Leslie *et al.*, 1990). In ferrets, those 5-HT_3 receptors located within the area postrema do not seem to be involved in cisplatin-evoked emesis (Reynolds *et al.*, 1991). Experiments in which immunoreactive c-*fos* protein (a product of c-*fos* gene activation brought about by neurotransmitter receptor interaction) has been detected in cisplatin-treated ferrets, shows that both the *nucleus tractus solitarius* and the area postrema are metabolically active during this procedure. However, when emesis is prevented using granisetron, only the c-*fos* protein generation with the NTS disappears (Reynolds *et al.*, 1991). Neuronal activity within the area postrema may, therefore, be due either to the action of a second emetogenic substance released by cisplatin or to a direct action of cisplatin itself.

The function of the 5-HT_3 receptors on the nerve axons must be questioned on the grounds that these are only detected when the protective nerve sheath is removed. Since it is unlikely that these receptors will be activated by 5-HT it can be assumed that they are 'in transit' from the nodose ganglion to the peripheral and central nerve terminals of the vagus. Antagonism of 5-HT_3 receptors within the nodose ganglion is a theoretical mechanism by which emesis can be reduced (Jacobs and Comroe, 1971). However, activation of this site must depend on maintaining a raised concentration of circulating 5-HT. Since 5-HT is quickly broken down within the liver, this method of activating 5-HT_3 receptors seems an unlikely mechanism by which cytotoxic therapy causes prolonged emesis (see below). Furthermore, experiments in which blood from a cat treated with cisplatin is circulated into a recipient cat, suggests that a circulating emetic agent is not involved in the mechanisms of cisplatin-induced emesis (Carl *et al.*, 1989). Antagonists at the 5-HT_3 receptor could, therefore, prevent cytotoxic-induced emesis by acting at either the abdominal vagal terminal or the terminal within the *nucleus tractus solitarius*.

9.5.4.3.1 Site of 5-HT$_3$ receptor antagonism

The question of which vagal terminal is most relevant to the mechanisms of cytotoxic-induced vomiting has been previously discussed by Andrews *et al.* (1988; 1990) and Sanger (1990). It was concluded that although the evidence was still subjective, it pointed towards a predominant importance of the abdominal terminals, although it is likely that the central terminal will also have some role to play.

Firstly, it has long been appreciated that although radiation to almost all parts of the body can cause emesis, the most sensitive site is the upper abdomen in humans (Gestener, 1960) and in cats (Borison, 1957). Indeed, radiation applied directly onto the floor of the fourth ventricle (stereotactic radiosurgery) evokes emesis only when given at very high doses (Alexander *et al.*, 1989). This type of emesis can be prevented by pretreatment with dexamethasone and droperidol, suggesting that emesis was evoked not by a 5-HT$_3$ receptor-related mechanism, but by local oedema.

Secondly, conflicting data exists on the emetic or anti-emetic activities of 5-HT and 5-HT$_3$ receptor antagonists when these substances are administered into the area postrema or the fourth ventricle. In dogs, cisplatin-evoked emesis was not prevented by granisetron or ICS 205–903 given into the fourth ventricle (Gupta *et al.*, 1988; Fukui *et al.*, 1991), whereas similar experiments with zacopride in cats (Smith *et al.*, 1988) and AS-5370 in ferrets (Ito *et al.*, 1990) were effective. In ferrets ondansetron 1.0 μg injected directly into the area postrema (or, as Andrews *et al.* point out [1990] it could have been the *nucleus tractus solitarius*) immediately after the first cisplatin-evoked emetic episode, caused only a short-lived reduction in the number of retches and vomits. By contrast, when ondansetron was given by intraperitoneal injection, cisplatin-evoked emesis was prevented for up to three hours (Higgins *et al.*, 1989). If the ondansetron had actually reached the nucleus tractus solitarius (as suggested by Andrews *et al.*, 1990), this difference in time course of anti-emetic activity argues strongly in favour of a predominantly peripheral site of action. However, to be sure of the actual site of injection, this important experiment needs to be repeated.

A central site of action is suggested by the experiments of Robertson *et al.* (1990) and Gidda *et al.* (1991), who found that quaternary LY 277359 (a 5-HT$_3$ receptor antagonist with little or no ability to cross the blood–brain barrier in rats) did not block cisplatin-evoked emesis in dogs. However, in similar experiments in ferrets, quaternary ICS 205–930 or quaternary LY 277359 did block emesis (Buchheit *et al.*, 1990; Gidda *et al.*, 1991). These experiments are, therefore, inconclusive and at variance with the ability of vagotomy to prevent cisplatin-evoked emesis in both species (Andrews *et al.*, 1990; Fukui *et al.*, 1991). Whatever the mechanism, the experiments could also suggest a species-dependence on the ratio of 'central' versus 'peripheral' activity of the 5-HT$_3$ receptor. The question of which species is most like man must now be debated. However, the inability of Alexander *et al.* (1989) to evoke emesis by directly-applied radiation to the lower brain stem (except at extremely high doses; see earlier discussion) would suggest that the mechanism of cytotoxic-evoked emesis in humans would be more like the ferret than the dog.

Finally, an abdominal site of action is supported by the evidence obtained using 5-HT receptor agonists. When given into the fourth ventricle of the cat, 5-HT is noticeable as being one of the few substances which actually does not evoke emesis (Feldberg and Sherwood, 1954). Similarly, injection of the 5-HT$_3$ receptor agonist, 2-methyl-5-HT, into the ferret area postrema (or *nucleus tractus solitarius*), evoked only signs of 'nausea' (salivation, searching, licking of lips, backwards walking, some retching) and sedation (Higgins *et al.*, 1989). Furthermore, intravenous 2-methyl-5-HT (up to 0.2 mg kg^{-1}) also failed to evoke emesis in the dog and ferret (Monkovic and Gylys, 1990). By contrast, S-zacopride, 2-methyl-5-HT 10 µg kg^{-1} p.o. and phenylbiguanide 10 µg kg^{-1} p.o. each evoked emesis in ferrets by a mechanism sensitive to antagonism by ICS 205–930 (Sancilio *et al.*, 1991). Cytotoxic-induced emesis may, therefore, be caused predominantly by the generation of a high concentration of 5-HT within the gastro-intestinal mucosa activating 5-HT_3 receptors on the vagal nerve terminals. By contrast, intravenously or centrally administered 5-HT does not appear to evoke emesis.

The administration of a therapeutic dose of a 5-HT uptake inhibitor does not mimic the prolonged and severe emesis which is evoked by cisplatin. Thus, fluoxetine is associated with only nausea in 24–40% of subjects (Benfield *et al.*, 1986). However, it is not clear if higher doses of fluoxetine could evoke more severe symptoms. In ferrets, fluoxetine does not cause emesis and actually tends to reduce cisplatin-evoked vomiting (Costall *et al.*, 1988). Infusion of the 5-HT precursor 5-hydroxytryptophan (5-HTP) evokes nausea and vomiting for 1–2 hours and always in conjunction with a marked stimulation of gut motility (Davidson *et al.*, 1957; Chadwick *et al.*, 1977; Magnussen and Nielsen Kudsk, 1979).

9.5.4.3.2 Evidence for increased 5-HT turnover

Whatever the major site of 5-HT_3 receptor antagonists, it is clear that acute cytotoxic-induced emesis must depend on a continuously renewable mechanism (e.g. turnover of 5-HT). This is illustrated by the ability of granisetron to stop on-going emesis within seconds after intravenous administration (Bermudez *et al.*, 1988). This result would not have been possible if a long-lasting mechanism had been switched on by the cytotoxic therapy. The reduction of emesis in ferrets by 5-HT depletion with para-chlorophenylalanine supports this concept (Barnes *et al.*, 1988).

Experiments which seek to demonstrate an increase in the turnover of 5-HT after cytotoxic treatment have had only limited success. Within the gastro-intestinal tract, the effects of X-radiation on the 5-HT content of the intestinal tract may be highly variable (Pentillä and Kormano, 1971), although, in general, irradiation of rats decreases the intestinal 5-HT content (Matsuoka *et al.*, 1962; Kocmierska-Grodzka, 1976). In one study, 400 rad whole body irradiation immediately reduced the 5-HT content of rat duodenum, with the content of other regions of the gut falling one day after irradiation. The time taken for the 5-HT content to recover then varied according to the region (Pentilla *et al.*, 1975). It could be argued that the significance of these experiments is questionable, because the rat does not vomit. Alternatively, this could be seen as an advantage, since the very absence of vomiting means that in contrast to those species which vomit, 5-HT will not be released from the gut by the mechanical movement of the gut which occurs during vomiting.

Within the central nervous system, local exposure to a high-dose of radiation caused an immediate increase in the total amount of 5-HT metabolites (5-hydroxyindoles), but only within the rat brainstem (Attman *et al.*, 1970). However, in terms of emetic mechanisms, the significance of this finding must be weighed against the observation that in man, only very high doses of radiation evoke emesis when applied directly to the floor of the fourth ventricle (Alexander *et al.*, 1989). Since the mechanism of this emesis is probably related to the generation of a local oedema it seems unlikely that this procedure generated a sufficiently high turnover of 5-HT in order to trigger emesis. Alternatively, 5-HT turnover may be increased, but the brainstem is not a major site at which emesis can be evoked by 5-HT_3 receptor activation (see above).

Gunning *et al.*, (1987) found raised levels of 5-HT and 5-hydroxyindole in the gastric mucosa of ferrets pre-treated with cisplatin. Endo *et al.* (1990) found increased levels of 5-HT in the ileum mucosa of ferrets pre-treated for two days with cisplatin; the 5-HT content of the stomach was unaffected. However, since the ferrets in both of these studies had presumably vomited and retched in response to the cisplatin, these experiments must be treated with caution. Thus, mechanical movement of the gut will release 5-HT from enterochromaffin cells (Bennett *et al.*, 1966). Cubeddu *et al.*, (1990) measured the 5-hydroxyindole content of the urine of patients treated with cisplatin. However, in this trial, there was a reasonably good correlation between the occurrence of raised 5-hydroxyindole and emesis. The released 5-HT could, therefore, be due to either the cisplatin or to the act of emesis. Similarly, Barnes *et al.* (1991b) measured changes in blood plasma 5-HT concentrations in patients receiving cisplatin and found only an inconsistent increase in 5-HT and only after the patients are assumed to have vomited.

To try and overcome some of the technical problems associated with measuring a meaningful increase in 5-HT turnover *in vivo*, Racké and Schwörer (1991) measured 5-HT release from the vascularly perfused guinea-pig isolated ileum. These authors found that 5-HT and 5-hydroxyindole release was increased by intra-arterial perfusion of cisplatin. Tetrodotoxin prevented this action of cisplatin. Cisplatin may, therefore, have an indirect ability to release 5-HT from gut enterochromaffin cells via activation of a neuronal pathway. These experiments also lend credibility to the conclusions drawn from those experiments in which 5-HT turnover has been measured *in vivo*. However, the surprising observation was that ondansetron antagonized this ability of cisplatin to increase 5-HT turnover. If this is confirmed, it suggests that 5-HT_3 receptor antagonists prevent cytotoxic-induced emesis by antagonizing the action of 5-HT at the 5-HT_3 receptor and also by inhibiting the release of 5-HT from the gut. It should, nevertheless, be noted that in ferrets, ondansetron (dose and efficacy not specified) did not affect the level of 5-HT evoked by cisplatin in the ileum mucosa (Endo *et al.*, 1990).

9.5.4.3.3 Proposed mechanism of action of 5-HT_3 receptor antagonists

One of the properties of the 5-HT_3 receptor is to both activate and sensitize unmyelinated afferent neurons to the actions of other substances (King and Sanger, 1989) probably by increasing membrane cation permeability (Reisner and Hamprecht, 1988). Since cytotoxic therapy is known to increase the turnover of different toxins and potential emetogenic substances, the severity of the resulting emesis could be due to the interactions between several different substances, only one of which is 5-HT. Removal of the sensitizing properties of 5-HT_3 receptor activation would, therefore, lead to a reduction of the emetic effects of both 5-HT and non–5-HT substances. Thus, the severity of cisplatin-evoked emesis may be due to different substances acting in synergy at the abdominal vagus nerve terminal, but all are blocked or greatly reduced by 5-HT_3 receptor antagonism. Perhaps long-lasting emesis evoked by cytotoxic therapy is due to a continuous release of 5-HT or to a relatively transient release of 5-HT, causing a long-lasting sensitization of vagal nerve endings to the emetogenic actions of other substances. In studies on the algesic properties of 5-HT, sensitization to the actions of other algesic substances can last for days (Sicuteri, 1968).

9.6 INTERACTIONS BETWEEN ANTI-EMETIC AND CYTOTOXIC DRUG ACTIVITY

Chlorpromazine 15 mg kg^{-1} i.p. and caffeine 100 mg kg^{-1} s.c. enhance cytotoxicity of alkylating agents in some, but not all rodent transplantation tumours and in a human melanoma xenograft system in mice (Osieka *et al.*, 1986). The mechanism of action may be related to increased drug retention within the tumour cells, to fixation of DNA damage, and/or to a non-specific cytotoxicity. However, tumour cytotoxicity with semustine was not enhanced in patients with disseminated malignant carcinoma treated with chlorpromazine and caffeine (Cohen *et al.*, 1980). The failure to measure a positive benefit of the two agents in this trial may be due to an insufficient number of patients tested for the detection of a small enhancement of cytotoxicity (Osieka *et al.*, 1986). In some animal models, chlorpromazine alone may act as a radiosensitizer, enhancing cytotoxicity and leading to suggestions that the combination of this anti-emetic with radiation should lead to a re-evaluation of the dose of radiation given (Harding, 1989).

There have been several studies using metoclopramide, which, in general, demonstrate a potentially beneficial action of this compound. Kjellén *et al.* (1987; 1989) reasoned that metoclopramide might enhance anti-tumour activity since structurally related compounds (nicotinamide, benzamide, 3-aminobenzamide) inhibit the chromatin-bound enzyme adenosine diphosphate ribosyl transferase (ADPRT). This enzyme is activated by DNA-damaging agents and may play a role in DNA repair. The hypothesis was tested against a squamous cell carcinoma of the H and N xenografted nude mice. Metoclopramide 2 mg kg^{-1} i.p. was given at the same time as cisplatin and again 24 and 48 hours later. Compared with mice not given metoclopramide, cisplatin anti-tumour activity was doubled; there were no other increases in cisplatin cytotoxicity. Later work by the same authors demonstrated a similar activity of metoclopramide with ionizing radiation (Lybak *et al.*, 1990). In another study, with high concentrations of metoclopramide (0.5 and 5 μg ml^{-1}) and chlorpromazine (0.01 μg and 0.1 μg ml^{-1}), epirubicin cytotoxic activity was enhanced when tested against Chinese hamster fibroblasts, without any intrinsic cytotoxic activity; droperidol 0.1 μg ml^{-1} was cytotoxic (Henriksson *et al.*, 1989). The mechanism of enhancement was not related to a further increase in oxygen radical formation and inhibition of ADPRT activity was a suggested mechanism. Finally, metoclopramidate 3, 10 or 15 mg kg^{-1} i.p. itself dose-dependently inhibited neuroblastoma tumour growth after grafting of the cultured mouse tumour cells into nude mice (Busse *et al.*, 1990).

Inhibition of tumour growth by chemical xenogenization with 5-(3,3-dimethyl-1-triazeno)-imidazole-4-carboxamine (DTIC) is a highly emetogenic treatment. Fortunately, when tested in mice, this method of treatment is not reduced by dexamethasone or by metoclopramide plus orphenadrine hydrochloride plus diazepam (Ballerini *et al.*, 1989). However, prolonged treatment with steroids could suppress the immune system and enhance tumour metastasis (Haid, 1981).

Preliminary findings with deta-9-tetrahydro cannabinol suggests that cannabinoids could suppress the growth of certain tumours in animals (Harris, 1976).

Finally, of the selective 5-HT_3 receptor antagonists, both granisetron and ondansetron have been tested for their potential to affect drug cytotoxicity. Goddard *et al.* (1990) found no evidence that granisetron could antagonize the anti-tumour properties of cisplatin. Hall *et al.* (1991) found no evidence that ondansetron affected the cytotoxicity of cisplatin in cultured human hepatoma cells.

9.7 FUTURE DEVELOPMENTS

The final impact of the selective 5-HT_3 receptor antagonists is not yet certain. These drugs will, almost certainly, change the way anti-emetic treatment is given to cancer patients. As such, the future may see less use of the anti-emetic drugs which are generally associated with low efficacy and side-effects (dopamine receptor antagonists, cannabinoids, muscarinic receptor antagonists). Anticipatory vomiting may also become less common, as severe emesis evoked by drugs such as cisplatin will be better controlled. Likewise, the incidence of delayed emesis could be reduced if the acute phase is well controlled although there is some suggestion that the two events may not be connected.

Once the 5-HT_3 receptor antagonists are fully established in clinical practical, efforts will focus on the 'residual' emesis which is not prevented by 5-HT_3 receptor antagonism. Drug combinations are already undergoing tests (e.g. dexamethasone with ondansetron). However, because the 5-HT_3 receptor antagonists have such a high efficacy, it will require large scale clinical trials in order to properly assess whether any additional anti-emetic benefit is truly reproducible and meaningful. As a consequence, future developments in anti-emetic therapy, arising from clinical practice, could be difficult and slow. Nevertheless, the 5-HT_3 receptor antagonists have left one legacy to basic science–animal models which can at long last be used to predict the human response. Experiments are already underway to define the plasticity of the emetic neuronal pathways, in which the lesioning of one pathway leads to the uncovering or creation of another (Andrews *et al.*, 1990). Out of such work new types of anti-emetic therapy could arise.

As a result of better anti-emetic control, the future will also see increasing attention given to some of the other symptoms of cytotoxic therapy, such as conditioned taste aversion (Strohl, 1983) diarrhoea and the flu-like symptoms associated with the 'biological response modifiers' (interferon, etc.) that are used to treat cancer (Haeuber, 1989). Drugs currently being used to treat emesis may be effective inhibitors of one or more of these associated symptoms, but in all probability, their study will create a 'new' pharmacology.

REFERENCES

Aapro, M.S. and Alberts, D.S. (1981) High-dose dexamethasone for prevention of cisplatin-induced vomiting. *Cancer Chemother. Pharmacol.*, **7**, 11–14.

Aasebo, U. and Slordal, L. (1990) Transient reduction in serum cortisol levels after dexamethasone antiemetic therapy in cancer patients undergoing chemotherapy. *Acta Oncol.*, **29**, 314–16.

Aglietti, L., Roila, F., Tonato, M. *et al.* (1990) A pilot study of metoclopramide, dexamethasone, diphenhydramine and acupuncture in women treated with cisplatin. *Cancer Chemother. Pharmacol.*, **26**, 239–40.

Akhtar, S.S., Akhter, Z., Bhat, M.A. and Mohammed, G. (1990) High dose prochlorperazine infusion for cisplatin (P) induced emesis: Double-blind randomized cross-over comparison with high dose metoclopramide. *Br. J. Cancer*, **62**, 484–85.

Alberola, V., Garcia, J., Lluch, A. *et al.* (1986) Relationship between adrenal failure and delayed emesis in patients receiving dexamethasone to prevent gastrointestinal toxicity of high-dose cisplatin. *Cancer Chemother.*, **18**, (suppl 1), A2.

Alexander, E., Siddon, R.L. and Loeffler, J.S. (1989) The acute onset of nausea and vomiting following stereotactic radiosurgery: correlation with total dose to area postrema. *Surg. Neurol.*, **32**, 40–44.

Alphin, R.S., Proakis, A.G., Leonard, C.A. *et al.* (1986) Antagonism of cisplatin-evoked emesis by metoclopramide and dazopride through enhancement of gastric motility. *Dig. Dis. Sci.*, **31**, 524–29.

Andrews, P.L.R., Rapeport, W.G. and Sanger, G.J. (1988) Neuropharmacology of emesis induced by anti-cancer therapy. *Trends Pharmacol. Sci.*, **9**, 334–41.

Andrews, P.L.R. and Davidson, H.I.M. (1990) Activation of vagal afferent terminals by 5-hydroxytryptamine is mediated by the 5-HT_3 receptor in the anaesthetised ferret. *J. Physiol.*, **422**, 92P.

Andrews, P.L.R., Davis, C.J., Bingham, S. *et al.* (1990) The abdominal visceral innervation and the emetic reflex: pathways, pharmacology and plasticity. *Can. J. Physiol. Pharmacol.*, **68**, 325–45.

Anonymous (1990) Zophren. *La Revue Prescrire*, **10**, 285–86.

Altman, K.I., Gerber, G.B. and Okada, S. (1970) Radiation biochemistry. Vol. II. Tissues and Body Fluids. Academic Press, London.

Baker, J.J., Lokey, J.L., Price, N.A. *et al.* (1979) Nabilone as an anti-emetic (use of high dose dexamethasone). *N. Engl. J. Med.*, **301**, 728.

Ballerini, P., Franchi, A., Fuschiotti, P. *et al.* (1989) Two antiemetic regiments do not impair chemical xenogenization induced in vivo by 5-(3,3-dimethyl-1-triazeno)-imidazole-4-carboxamide. *Cancer Chemother. Pharmacol.*, **24**, 359–62.

Ballmer, P.E. and Reinhart, W.H. (1989) Does parenteral magnesium sulphate have an anti-emetic effect during chemotherapy with *cis*-platinum? *Cancer Chemother. Pharmacol.*, **24**, 109–12.

Barnes, J.H. (1984) The physiology and pharmacology of emesis. *Mol. Aspects Med.*, **7**, 397–508.

Barnes, J.M., Barnes, N.M., Costall, B. *et al.* (1988) Reserpine, para-chlorophenylalanine and fenfluramine antagonise cisplatin-induced emesis in the ferret. *Neuropharmacol.* **27**, 783–90.

Barnes, J.M., Barnes, N.M., Costall, B., and Naylor, R. J. *et al.* (1991a). Development of 5-HT_3 receptor antagonists as anti-emetics. *Pharmaceutical J.*, **246**, 112–14.

Barnes, N.M., Barry, J.M., Costall, B. *et al.* (1987) Antagonism by para-chlorophenylalanine of cisplatin-induced emesis. *Br. J. Pharmacol.*, **92**, 649P.

Barnes, N.M., Ge, J., Jones, W.G. *et al.* (1991b) Changes in plasma 5-HT levels during cisplatin treatment in man. *Br. J. Clin. Pharmacol.*, **31**, 235P.

Basurto, C., Roila, F., Del Favero, A. *et al.* (1988) A prospective randomized double-blind crossover study comparing the antiemetic activity of alizapride and metoclopramide in patients receiving cisplatin chemotherapy. *Cancer Invest.*, **6**, 475–79.

Beleslin, D.B., Strbac, M., Jovanovic-Micic, D. *et al.* (1989) Area postrema: cholinergic and noradrenergic regulation of emesis. A new concept. *Arch. Int. Physiol. Biochim.*, **97**, 107–15.

Benfield, P., Heel, R.C. and Lewis, S.P. (1986) Fluoxetine. A review of its pharmacodynamic and pharmacokinetic properties and therapeutic efficacy in depressive illness. *Drugs*, **32**, 481–508.

Bennett, A., Bucknell, A. and Dean, A.C.B. (1966) The release of 5-hydroxytryptamine from the rat stomach *in vitro*. *J. Physiol.*, **182**, 57–65.

Berga, P., Bon, J., Llenas, J. *et al.* (1986) Relacion entre los efectos antiemeticos de metoclopramida (MTC) y clebopride (CLB) y el antagonismo de los receptores de 5-HT. *Rev. Farmacol. Clin. Exp.*, **3**, 139.

Bermudez, J., Boyle, E.A., Miner, W.D. and Sanger, G.J. (1988) The anti-emetic potential of the 5-hydroxytryptamine$_3$ receptor antagonist BRL 43694. *Br. J. Cancer*, **58**, 644–50.

Bhandari, P., Andrews, P.L.R. (1991) Preliminary evidence for the involvement of the putative 5-hydroxytryptamine 4 receptor in zacopride and copper sulphate-induced vomiting in the ferret. *Eur. J. Pharmacol.* **204**, 273–80.

Bhandari, P., Gupta, Y.K. and Seth, S.D. (1989) BRL 43694, a new 5-HT_3 receptor antagonist, prevents cisplatin-induced emesis in dogs. *Meth. Find. Exp. Clin. Pharmacol.*, **11**, 361–63.

Bleiberg, H., Gerard, B., Dalesio, O. *et al.* (1988) Activity of a new anti-emetic agent: alizapride. *Cancer Chemother. Pharmacol.*, **22**, 316–63.

Bone, M.E., Wilkinson, D.J., Young, J.R. and Charlton, S. (1990) Ginger root – a new antiemetic. The effects of ginger root on postoperative nausea and vomiting after major gynaecological surgery. *Anaesthesia*, **45**, 669–71.

Borison, H.K. (1957) Site of emetic action of X-radiation in the cat. *J. Comp. Neurol.*, **197**, 439–553.

Brenner, W.E., Dingfelder, J.R. and Stavrousky, L.G. (1975) The efficacy and safety of intramuscularly administered 15(S)15 methylprostaglandin E_2 methyl ester for induction of artificial abortion. *Am. J. Obstet. Gynecol.*, **123**, 19–31.

Broberg, D.J. and Bernstein, I.L. (1987) Candy as a scapegoat in the prevention of food aversions in children receiving chemotherapy. *Cancer*, **60**, 2344–47.

Brogden, R.N., Carmine, A.A., Creel, R.C. *et al.* (1982) Domperidone. A review of its pharmacological activity, pharmacokinetics and therapeutic efficacy in the symptomatic treatment of chronic dyspepsia and as an antiemetic. *Drugs*, **24**, 360–400.

Buchheit, K.H., Büscher, H.H. and Gamse, R. (1990) The antiemetic profile of the 5-HT_3 receptor antagonist, ICS 205–930, and its quaternary derivative. Proc. Second IUPHAR Mtg on Serotonin, Basle, P148, pp. 111.

Burstein, S.H. (1976) 'Prostaglandins and cannabis. IV: A biochemical basis for therapeutic applications', in *The Therapeutic Potential of Marijuana*. (ed S. Cohen, and R.C. Stillman) pp. 19–33. Plenum Press, New York.

Burstein, S.H., Hull, K., Hunter, S.A. and Latham, V. (1988) Cannabinoids and pain responses: A possible role for prostaglandins. *FASEB J.*, **2**, 3022–26.

Busse, E., Bartsch, O., Schneider, A. and Kornhuber, B. (1990) Influence of metoclopramide and bromocriptine upon the growth of human and murine neuroblastoma cells. *Oncology*, **47**, 199–205.

Butler, A., Hill, J.M., Ireland, S.J. *et al.* (1988) Pharmacological properties of GR 38032F, a novel antagonist at 5-HT_3 receptors. *Br. J. Pharmacol.*, **94**, 397–412.

Butler, A., Elswood, C.J., Burridge, J. *et al.* (1990) The pharmacological characterization of 5-HT_3 receptors in three isolated preparations derived from guinea-pig tissues. *Br. J. Pharmacol.*, **101**, 591–98.

Butler, J.R., Peek, L.A., Regelson, W. *et al.* (1976) Treatment effects of delta-9-THC in an advanced cancer population, in *The Therapeutic Potential of Marijuana*. (eds S. Cohen, and R.C. Stillman) pp. 313–28. Plenum Press, New York.

Carl, P.L., Cubeddu, L.X., Lindley, C. *et al.* (1989) Do humoral factors mediate cancer chemotherapy-induced emesis? *Drug Metab. Rev.*, **21**, 319–33.

Carpenter, D.O., Briggs, D.B., Knox, A.P. and Strominger, N.L. (1986) Radiation-induced emesis in the dog: Effects of lesions and drugs. *Radiat. Res.*, **108**, 307–16.

Carr, B.I., Blayney, D.W., Goldberg, D.A. *et al.* (1987) High doses of prochlorperazine for cisplatin-induced emesis. *Cancer*, **60**, 2165–69.

Cassidy, J., Raina, V., Lewis, C. *et al.* (1988) Pharmacokinetics and anti-emetic efficacy of BRL 43694, a new selective 5-HT_3 antagonist. *Br. J. Cancer*, **58**, 651–53.

Cersosimo, R.J. and Karp, D.D. (1986) Adrenal corticosteroids as antiemetics during cancer chemotherapy. *Pharmacotherapy*, **6**, 118–27.

Chadwick, D., Hallett, M., Harris, R. *et al.* (1977) Clinical, biochemical and physiological features distinguishing myoclonus responsive to 5-hydroxytryptophan, tryptophan with a monoamine oxidase inhibitor and clonazepam. *Brain*, **100**, 455–87.

Chen, J-T., Hirai, Y., Hamada, T. *et al.* (1987) Medical vagotomy: a new effective antiemetic therapy for cisplatin-induced nausea and vomiting. *Acta Obstet. Gynaecol. Jpn.*, **39**, 2231–32.

Chevallier, B. (1990) Efficacy and safety of granisetron compared with high-dose metoclopramide plus dexamethasone in patients receiving high-dose cisplatin in a single-blind study. *Eur. J. Cancer*, **26** (Suppl 1): S33–S36.

Chugh, A., Gupta, Y.K., Bhandari, P. and Seth, S.D. (1988) Characterization of dopamine receptor subtypes in chemoreceptor trigger zone involved in emesis in dogs. *Asia Pac. J. Pharmacol.*, **3**, 135–39.

Clarke, D.E., Craig, D.A. and Fozard, J.R. (1989) The 5-HT_4 receptor: naughty but nice. *Trends Pharmacol. Sci.*, **10**, 385–86.

Cohen, M.H., Schoenfeld, D. and Wolter, J. (1980) Randomized trial of chlorpromazine, caffeine and methyl-CCNU in disseminated melanoma. *Cancer Treat. Rep.*, **64**, 151–53.

Cohen, M.L., Bloomquist, W., Gidda, J.S. and Lacefield, W. (1990) LY 277359 maleate: A potent and selective 5-HT_3 receptor antagonist without gastroprokinetic activity. *J. Pharm. Exp. Ther.*, **254**, 350–55.

Coates, A., Abraham, S., Kaye, S.B. *et al.* (1983) On the receiving end: Patient perception of the side-effects of cancer chemotherapy. *Eur. J. Cancer Clin. Oncol.*, **19**, 203–208.

Costall, B., Domeney, A.M., Naylor, R.J. and Tattersall, F.D. (1986) 5-Hydroxytryptamine M-receptor antagonism to prevent cisplatin-induced emesis. *Neuropharmacol.*, **25**, 959.

Costall, B., Domeney, A.M., Gunning, S.J. *et al.* (1987) GR 38032F: A potent and novel inhibitor of cisplatin-induced emesis in the ferret. *Br. J. Pharmacol.*, **90** Proc. Suppl: 90P.

Costall, B., Naylor, R.J. and Tattersall, F.D. (1988) Tranylcypromide and 5-hydroxy-L-tryptophan antagonise cisplatin-induced emesis in the ferret. *Br. J. Pharmacol.*, **95**, 866P.

Cotanch, P.H. and Strum, S. (1987) Progressive muscle relaxation as antiemetic therapy for cancer patients. *Oncol. Nurs. Forum.*, **14**, 33–37.

Craig, J.B. and Powell, B.L. (1987) The management of nausea and vomiting in clinical oncology. *Am. J. Med. Sci.*, **293**, 34–44.

Cramer, W., van Drimmelen, M., Long, S. and Tulp, M. (1990) Bufotenin: actions of 5-HT_3 receptors. *Eur. J. Pharmacol.*, **183**, 2148–49.

Cubeddu, L.X., Hoffmann, I.S., Fuenmayor, N.T. and Finn, A.L. (1990) Efficacy of ondansetron (GR 38032F) and the role of serotonin in cisplatin-induced nausea and vomiting. *N. Engl. J. Med.*, **322**, 810–16.

Cunningham, D., Turner, A., Hawthorn, J. and Rosin, R.D. (1989) Ondansetron with and without dexamethasone to treatment chemotherapy-induced emesis. *Lancet*, **2**, 1323.

Cupissol, D.R., Serrou, B. and Caubel, M. (1990) The efficacy of granistron as a prophylactic antiemetic and intervention agent in high-dose cisplatin-induced emesis. *Eur. J. Cancer*, **26** (Suppl. 1): 523–27.

Curry, S.L., Rine, J., Whitney, C.W. *et al.* (1981) The role of prostaglandins in the excessive nausea and vomiting after intravascular *cis*-platinum therapy. *Gynecol. Oncol.*, **12**, 89–91.

Davidson, J., Sjoerdsma, A., Loomis, L.N. and Udenfriend, S. (1957) Studies with the serotonin precursor, 5-hydroxytryptophan, in experimental animals and man. *J. Clin. Invest.*, **36**, 1594–99.

Davis, M.A. and Martin, G.E. (1990) Patent antagonism of the von Bezold-Jarisch effect by the novel 5-HT_3 antagonist RG 12915. *FASEB J.*, **4**, A475.

Derkach, V., Surprenant, A. and North, R.A. (1989) 5-HT_3 receptors are membrane ion channels. *Nature*, **339**, 706–709.

De Mulder, P.H.M., Seynaeve, C., Vermorken, J.B. *et al.* (1990) Ondansetron compared with high-dose metoclopramide in prophylaxis of acute and delayed cisplatin-induced nausea and vomiting. *Annals Int. Med.*, **113**, 834–40.

De Vita, V.T., Young, R.C. and Canellos, G.P. (1975) Combination versus single agent chemotherapy. A review of the basis for selection of drug treatment of cancer. *Cancer*, **35**, 98–110.

Dodds, L. (1986) Cancer chemotherapy-induced nausea and vomiting. *Pharm. J.*, **10**, 588–90.

Donovitz, G.S., O'Quinn, A.G. and Smith, M.L. (1984) Antiemetic efficacy of high-dose corticosteroids and droperidol in cisplatin-induced emesis: A controlled trial with droperidol and metoclopramide. *Gynecol. Oncol.*, **18**, 320–25.

Donatsch, P., Engel, G., Richardson, B.P. and Stadler, P. (1984) ICS 205–930, A highly selective and potent antagonist at peripheral neuronal 5-hydroxytryptamine (5-HT) receptors. *Br. J. Pharmacol.*, **81**, 34P.

Dubois, A., Dorval, E.T., Steel, L. *et al.* (1987) Effect of ionizing radiation on prostaglandins and gastric secretion in rhesus monkeys. *Radiat. Res.*, **110**, 289–93.

Dundee, J.W., Ghaly, R.G., Fitzpatrick, K.T.J. *et al.* (1989) Acupuncture prophylaxis of cancer chemotherapy-induced sickness. *J. Roy. Soc. Med.*, **82**, 268–71.

Dundee, J.W. and Yang, J. (1990) Prolongation of the antiemetic action of P6 acupuncture by acupressure in patients having cancer chemotherapy. *J. Roy. Soc. Med.*, **83**, 360–62.

Edmonds-Seal, J. and Prys-Roberts, C. (1970) Pharmacology of drugs used in neuroleptanalgesia. *Br. J. Anaesth.*, **42**, 207–16.

Eiler, H. and Paddleforth, R. (1979) Induction of intestinal evacuation or vomition (or both) in the dog by prostaglandin $F_{2\alpha}$ injection: clinical potential. *Am. J. Vet. Res.*, **40**, 1731–33.

Eisen, V. and Walker, D.I. (1978) Effect of ionizing radiation on prostaglandin 15-OH-dehydrogenase (PGDH). *Br. J. Pharmacol.*, **62**, 461P.

Elliott, P., Seemungal, B.M. and Wallis, D.I. (1990) Antagonism of the effects of 5-hydroxytryptamine on the rabbit isolated vagus nerve by BRL 43694 and metoclopramide. *Naunyn-Schmiedeberg's Arch. Pharmacol.*, **341**, 503–509.

Endo, T., Minami, M., Monma, Y. *et al.* (1990) Effect of GR 38032F on cisplatin- and cyclophosphamide-induced emesis in the ferret. *Biogenic Amines*, **7**, 525–33.

Feigenbaum, J.J., Richmond, S.A., Weissman, Y. and Mechoulam, R. (1989) Inhibition of cisplatin-induced emesis in the pigeon by a non-psychotropic synthetic cannabinoid. *Eur. J. Pharmacol.*, **169**, 159–65.

Feldberg, W. and Sherwood, S.L. (1954) Injections of drugs into the lateral ventricle of the cat. *J. Physiol.*, **123**, 148–67.

Fernandez, A.G., Puig, J., Bou, J. *et al.* (1990) Pancopride: A novel 5-HT_3 antagonist with potent antiemetic action. *Eur. J. Pharmacol.*, **183**, 1214.

Ferreira, S.H. (1972) Prostaglandins, aspirin-like drugs and analgesia. *Nature*, **240**, 200.

Fetting, J.H., Grochow, L.B., Folstein, M.F. *et al.* (1982) The course of nausea and vomiting after high-dose cyclophosphamide. *Cancer Treat. Rep.*, **66**, 1487–93.

Fitzpatrick, L.R., Lambert, R.M., Pendley, C.E. *et al.* (1990) RG 12915, A potent 5-hydroxytryptamine$_3$ antagonist that is an orally effective inhibitor of cytotoxic drug-induced emesis in the ferret and dog. *J. Pharmacol. Exp. Ther.*, **254**, 450–55.

Florczyk, A.P., Schurig, J.E. and Bradner, W.T. (1982) Cisplatin-induced emesis in the ferret: a new animal model. *Cancer Treat. Rep.*, **66**, 187–89.

Fozard, J.R. (1984) MDL 72222, A potent and highly selective antagonist at neuronal 5-hydroxytryptamine receptors. *Naunyn-Schmiedeberg's Arch. Pharmacol.*, **326**, 36–44.

Fozard, J.R. (1989) 'Agonists and antagonists at 5-HT$_3$ receptors', in *Cardiovascular Pharmacology of 5-hydroxytryptamine.* (ed P.R. Saxena *et al.*) pp. 101–15, Kluwer, Dordrecht.

Fozard, J.R. and Mobarok Ali, A.T.M. (1978) Blockade of neuronal tryptamine receptors by metoclopramide. *Eur. J. Pharmacol.*, **49**, 109–112.

Friend, D.G. and Cummings, J.F. (1953) New antiemetic drug: Preliminary report. *J. Am. Med. Assoc.*, **153**, 480–81.

Fukuda, T., Setoguchi, M., Inaba, K. *et al.* (1991) The antiemetic profile of Y-25130, a new selective 5-HT$_3$ receptor antagonist. *Eur. J. Pharmacol.*, **196**, 299–305.

Fukuda, T., Inaba, K., Shoji, H. *et al.* (1990) The antiemetic profile of Y-25130, a new 5-HT$_3$ receptor antagonist. *Jap. J. Pharmacol.*, **52**, 339P.

Fukui, H., Imai, K. Chikaato, M. *et al.* (1991) Visceral afferent fibres and peripheral 5-HT$_3$ receptors mediate cisplatin-induced emesis in dogs. *Jap. J. Pharmacol.*, **55** Suppl 1, 152p.

Frustaci, S., Grattoni, E., Tumulo, S. *et al.* (1986) Randomized crossover antiemetic study in cisplatin-treated patients. Comparison between high-dose iv metoclopramide and high-dose IV dexamethasone. *Cancer Chemother. Pharmacol.*, **17**, 75–79.

Gestener, H.B. (1960) Reaction to short-term radiation in man. *Ann. Rev. Med.*, **11**, 289–302.

Gidda, J.S., Evans, D.C., Krushinski, J.U. and Robertson, D.W. (1991) Differential effects of quaterized 5-HT$_3$ antagonists. Proc. 'Serotonin 1991. 5-Hydroxytryptamine-CNS receptors and brain function'. Birmingham, UK (Abstract pp. 135 and 165)

Graham, S.G. and Burgess, A.M. (1989) Metoclopramide inhibits plasma cholinesterase. *Can. J. Anaesth.*, **36**, 728–35.

Goddard, P.M., Jones, M., Pollard, L.A. *et al.* (1990) The 5-HT$_3$ antagonist, BRL 43694, does not compromise the efficacy of cisplatin in tumour-bearing mice. *Cancer Chemother. Pharmacol.*, **25**, 377–79.

Gralla, R.J. (1989) An outline of anti-emetic treatment. *Eur. J. Cancer. Clin. Oncol.*, **25** (Suppl 1): S7–S11.

Gralla, R.J., Hri, L.M., Pisko, S.E. *et al.* (1981) Antiemetic efficacy of high dose metoclopramide: Randomized trials with placebo and prochlorperazine in patients with chemotherapy-induced nausea and vomiting. *N. Engl. J. Med.*, **305**, 905–909.

Green, S.T., Nathwani, D., Goldberg, D.J. and Kennedy, D.H. (1989) Nabilone as effective therapy for intractable nausea and vomiting in AIDS. *Br. J. Clin. Pharmacol.*, **28**, 494–95.

Grunberg, S.M. (1989) Advances in the management of nausea and vomiting induced by non-cisplatin containing chemotherapeutic regimes. *Blood Rev.*, **3**, 216–21.

Gunning, S.J., Hagan, R.M. and Tyers, M.B. (1987) Cisplatin induces biochemical and histological changes in the small intestine of the ferret. *Br. J. Pharmacol.*, **90**, 135P.

Gupta, Y.K., Bhandari, P., Dhar, A. and Seth, S.D. (1988) Effect of BRL 43694, a novel 5-HT-M receptor antagonist, on cisplatin-induced emesis in dogs and gastric stasis in rats. Symposium on Nausea and Vomiting: A multidisciplinary perspective. Ottawa, Canada; Abstract 16, 30.

Gylys, J.A., Doran, K.M. and Buyniski, J.P. (1979) Antagonism of cisplatin induced emesis in the dog. *Res. Commun. Chem. Pathol. Pharmacol.*, **23**, 61–68.

Gylys, J.A., Wright, R.N., Nicolosia, W.D. *et al.* (1988) BMY 25801, an anti-emetic agent free of D2 dopamine receptor antagonist properties. *J. Pharmacol. Exp. Ther.*, **244**, 830–37.

Haeuber, D. (1989) Recent advances in the management of biotherapy-related side-effects: Flu-like syndrome. *Oncol. Nurs. Forum*, **16** (Suppl): 35–41.

Haid, M. (1981) Steroid antiemesis may be harmful. *N. Engl. J. Med.*, **304**, 1237.

Hall, T.J., Cambridge, G. and James, P.R. (1991) Development of a co-culture system with induced HEPG2 cells and K562 cells for examining drug metabolism *in vitro*. Studies with cyclophosphamide, ondansetron and cisplatin. *Res. Commun. Chem. Pathol. Pharmacol.*, **72**, 161–68.

Hamik, A. and Peroutka, S.J. (1989) Differential interactions of traditional and novel antiemetics with dopamine D_2 and 5-hydroxytryptamine$_3$ receptors. *Cancer Chemother. Pharmacol.*, **24**, 307–310.

Harding, R.K. (1989) Prodromal effects of radiation: Pathways, models and protection by antiemetics. *Pharmacol., Ther.*, **39**, 335–45.

Harding, R.K., Hugenholtz, H., Kucharczyk, J. and Lemoine, J. (1987) Central mechanisms for apomorphine. induced emesis in the dog. *Eur. J. Pharmacol.*, **144**, 61–65.

Harding, R.K., Leach, K.E. and Prud'homme-Lalonde, L. (1988) Effect of BRL 43694 on emesis in the dog induced by ionizing irradiation. *Pharmacologist*, **30**, A126.

Harris, L.S. (1976) 'Analgesic and antitumour potential of the cannabinoids', in *The Therapeutic Potential of Marijuana*. (eds S. Cohen and R.C. Stillman), pp. 299–312. Plenum Press, New York.

Headley, J.A. (1987) The influence of administration time on chemotherapy-induced nausea and vomiting. *Oncol. Nurs. Forum.*, **14**, 43–47.

Henriksson, R. and Grankvist, K. (1989) Epirubicin cytotoxicity but not oxygen radical formation is enhanced by four different anti-emetics. *Med. Oncol. Tumor Pharmacother.*, **6**, 175–78.

Higgins, G.A., Kilpatrick, G.J., Bunce, K.T. *et al.* (1989) 5-HT$_3$ receptor antagonists injected into the area postrema inhibit cisplatin-induced emesis in the ferret. *Br. J. Pharmacol.*, **97**, 247–55.

Hogan, C.M. (1990) Advances in the management of nausea and vomiting. *Nurs. Clin. N. Am.* **25**, 475–97.

Hogan, K., Miyata, K., Kamato, T. *et al.* (1991) Antagonism of the serotonin (5-HT$_3$) receptor by YM060, a novel 4,5,6,7-tetrahydrobenzimidazole derivative and its enantiomer. *FASEB J.*, **5**, A1232.

Hrushesky, W.J.M. and Roemeling, R. (1986) Chemotherapy-induced vomiting: Circadian drug timing as a source of predictable within-patient variability. *Cancer Treat. Rep.*, **70**, 1347–48.

Ison, P.J. and Peroutka, S.J. (1986) Neurotransmitter receptor binding studies predict antiemetic efficacy and side effects. *Cancer Treat. Rep.*, **70**, 637–41.

Ito, T., Yoshida, N., Miura, Y. *et al.* (1990) Antiemetic effects of AS-5370, a novel serotonin 5-HT$_3$ receptor antagonist. *Eur. J. Pharmacol.*, **183**, 1214–15.

Jacobs, L. and Comroe, J.H. (1971) Reflex apnea, bradycardia and hypotension produced by serotonin and phenylbiguanide acting on the nodose ganglia of the cat. *Circ. Res.*, **29**, 145–55.

Janssen, P.A., Niemegeers, C.J., Schellekens, K.H. *et al.* (1963) The pharmacology of dihydrobenzperidol (R-4749), a new potent and short acting neuroleptic agent chemically related to haloperidol. *Arzneimittel-Forsch.*, **13**, 205–11.

Jordan, L.N. (1989) Effects of fluid manipulation on the incidence of vomiting during outpatient cisplatin infusion. *Oncol. Nurs. Forum.*, **16**, 213–18.

Jordan, N.S., Schauer, P.K., Schauer, A. *et al.* (1985) The effect of administration rate on cisplatin-induced emesis. *J. Clin. Oncol.*, **3**, 559–61.

Joss, R.A., Brand, B.C., Buser, G.S. and Cerny, T. (1990) The symptomatic control of cytostatic drug-induced emesis. A recent history and review. *Eur. J. Cancer*, **26** (Suppl 1): S2–S7.

Joss, R.A., Galeazzi, R.L., Bischoff, A.K. and Brunner, K.W. (1985) Alizapride, a new substituted benzamide, as an antiemetic during cancer chemotherapy. *Eur. J. Clin. Pharmacol.*, **27**, 721–25.

Kamato, T., Miyata, K., Nishida, A. *et al.* (1991) Antiemetic effects of YM060, a new serotonin 5-HT$_3$ receptor antagonist and its enantiomer in ferrets receiving cytotoxic drug. *FASEB J.*, **5**, A1232.

Kelley, S.L., Braun, T.J., Meyer, T.J. *et al.* (1986) Trial of droperidol as an antiemetic in cisplatin chemotherapy. *Cancer Treat. Rep.*, **70**, 469–72.

King, F.D. and Sanger, G.J. (1989) 5-HT$_3$ receptor antagonists. *Drugs of the Future*, **14**, 875–89.

King, G.L. and Landauer, M.R. (1990) Effects of zacopride and BMY 25801 (batanopride) on radiation-induced emesis and locomotor behaviour in the ferret. *J. Pharm. Exp. Ther.*, **253**, 1026–33.

King, G.L., Landauer, M., Keiffer, V. *et al.* (1988) Zacopride, a 5-HT$_3$ antagonist, modifies emetic and behavioural responses to radiation in the ferret. *FASEB Monogr.*, **2**, A325.

King, G.L. (1990) Emesis and defecations induced by the 5-hydroxytryptamine ($5\text{-}HT_3$) receptor antagonist zacopride in the ferret. *J. Pharm. Exp. Ther.*, **253**, 1034–41.

Kjellen, E., Wennerberg, J. and Pero, R. (1987) Metoclopramide potentiates the effect of cisplatin on xeno-grafted squamous cell carcinoma of the H&N. Proc. 4th Eur. Conf. Clin. Oncol. Cancer Nursing, Madrid, Abstract, 959, 251.

Kjellen, E., Wennerberg, J. and Pero, R. (1989) Metoclopramide enhances the effect of cisplatin on xenografted squamous cell carcinoma of the head and neck. *Br. J. Cancer.*, **59**, 247–50.

Kobrinsky, N.L., Pruden, P.B., Cheang, M.S. *et al.* (1988) Increased nausea and vomiting induced by naloxone in patients receiving cancer chemotherapy. *Am. J. Pediatric Hemato./Oncol.*, **10**, 206–208.

Kocmierska-Grodzka, D. (1976) The influence of X-rays, vitamin A and protease inhibitor on the hydro-proteolytic activity and serotonin content in pancreas and intestine of rats. *Strahlentherapie*, **151**, 562–70.

Komiya, M., Une, T., Furukawa, K. and Karasawa, T. (1990) Characterization of AS-5370, a new potent serotonin $5\text{-}HT_3$ receptor antagonist by radioligand binding assay. *Eur. J. Pharmacol.*, **183**, 316–17.

Kris, M.G., Gralla, R.J., Clark, R.A. *et al.* (1985) Incidence, course and severity of delayed nausea and vomiting following the administration of high-dose cisplatin. *J. Clin. Oncol.*, **3**, 1379–84.

Krupp, P. and Wesp, M. (1975) Inhibition of prostaglandin synthetase by psychotropic drugs. *Experientia*, **31**, 330–31.

Lattimer, N., Rhodes, K.F. and Saville, V.L. (1989) Possible differences in $5\text{-}HT_3$-like receptors in the rat and the guinea-pig. *Br. J. Pharmacol.*, **96**, 270P.

Laville, C.I. and Margarit, J. (1982) Etude pharmacodynamique de l'alizapride. *Sem. Hôp. Paris.*, **58**, 323–31.

Laszlo, J. (1983) 'Emesis as limiting toxicity in cancer chemotherapy', in *Antiemetics and Cancer Chemotherapy*. (ed J. Laszlo) pp. 1–5. The Williams & Wilkins Co., Baltimore.

Laszlo, J., Clark, R.A., Hanson, D.C. *et al.* (1985) Lorazepam in cancer patients treated with cisplatin: A drug having antiemetic, amnesic and anxiolytic effects. *J. Clin. Oncol.*, **3**, 864–69.

Leslie, R.A., Reynolds, D.J.M., Andrews, P.L.R. *et al.* (1990) Evidence for presynaptic $5\text{-}HT_3$ recognition sites on vagal afferent terminals in the brainstem of the ferret. *Neurosci.*, **38**, 667–73.

Lobbezoo, M.W., Janszen, F.H.A., Tulp, M.T.M. and Zwagemakers, J.M.A. (1985) Differential effects of metoclopramide and zetidoline on gastrointestinal motility. *Eur. J. Pharmacol.*, **108**, 105–12.

London, S.W., McCarthy, L.E. and Borison, H.L. (1979) Suppression of cancer chemotherapy induced vomiting in the cat by nabilone, a synthetic cannabinoid. *Proc. Soc. Exp. Biol. Med.*, **160**, 437–40.

Longo, D.L., Wesley, M., Howser, D. *et al.* (1985) Results of a randomized double-blind crossover trial of scopolamine versus placebo administered by transdermal patch for the control of cisplatin-induced emesis. *Cancer Treat. Rep.*, **66**, 1975–76.

Lucot, J.B. (1989) Blockade of 5-hydroxytryptamine$_3$ receptors prevents cisplatin-induced but not motion- or xylazine-induced emesis in the cat. *Pharmacol. Biochem. Behav.*, **32**, 207–10.

Lybak, S., Kjellen, E., Wennerberg, J. and Pero, R. (1990) Metoclopramide enhances the effect of ionizing radiation on xenografted squamous cell carcinoma of the head and neck. *Int. J. Radiat. Oncol. Biol. Phys.*, **19**, 1419–24.

Magnussen, I. and Nielsen-Kudsk, F. (1979) Pharmacokinetics of intravenously administered L-5-hydroxytryptophan in man. *Acta Pharmacol. Toxicol.*, **44**, 308–314.

Maher, J. (1981) Intravenous lorazepam to prevent nausea and vomiting associated with cancer chemotherapy. *Lancet*, **1**, 91–92.

Malone, J.M., Christensen, C.W., Yashinsky, D. *et al.* (1990) Prochlorperazine and transdermal scopolamine added to metoclopramide antiemetic regimen. *J. Reprod. Med.*, **35**, 932–34.

Marin, J., Ibanez, M.C. and Arribas, S. (1990) Therapeutic management of nausea and vomiting. *Gen. Pharmacol.*, **21**, 1–10.

Mark, A.L. (1983) The Bezold-Jarisch reflex revisited: Clinical implications of inhibitory reflexes originating in the heart. *J. Am. Coll. Cardiol.*, **1**, 90–102.

Martin, M. (1990) LAS 30451. In *Supportive Therapy: Challenges for the '90s*. Perugia International Cancer Conference III: pp. 92–93.

Martin, M., Diaz-Rubio, E., Sanchez, A. *et al.* (1990)

The natural course of emesis after carboplatin treatment. *Acta Oncol.*, **29**, 593–95.

Martin-Jimenez, M. and Diaz-Rubio, E. (1986) Clinical evaluation of the simultaneous blockade of the dopamine D-2, histamine H-1 and muscarinic cholinergic receptors in cancer chemotherapy-induced emesis: Results of a controlled trial. *Cancer Chemother. Pharmacol.*, **18**, 168–71.

Matsuoka, O., Tsuchiya, T. and Furukawa, Y. (1962) The effect of X-irradiation on 5-hydroxytryptamine (serotonin) contents in the small intestines of experimental animals. *J. Radiat. Res.*, **3–2**, 104.

Mechoulam, R. and Feigenbaum, J.J. (1987) 'Towards cannabinoid drugs', in *Prog. Medicinal Chemistry.*, **24**, 159–207.

Meyer, B.R., O'Mara, V. and Reidenberg, M.M. (1987) A controlled clinical trial of the addition of transdermal scopolamine to a standard metoclopramide and dexamethasone antiemetic regimen. *J. Clin. Oncol.*, **5**, 1994–97.

McCarthy, L.E. and Borison, H.L. (1977) Anti-emetic activity of nabilone – a cannabinol derivative, reversed by naloxone in awake cats. *Pharmacologist*, **19**, 230.

McCarthy, L.E. and Borison, H.L. (1981) Antiemetic activity of n-methyl-levonantradol and nabilone in cisplatin-treated cats. *J. Clin. Pharmacol.*, **21**, 30–37.

McRitchie, B., McClelland, C.M., Cooper, S.M. *et al.* (1984) Dopamine antagonists as anti-emetics and as stimulants of gastric motility, in *Mechanisms of Gastrointestinal Motility and Secretion* (eds A. Bennett and G. Velo), pp. 287–301. Plenum Press, New York.

Middlefell, V.C., and Price, T.L. (1991) 5-HT_3 receptor agonists may be responsible for the emetic effects of zacopride in the ferret. *Br. J. Pharmacol.*, **103**, 1011–1–12.

Miner, W.D. and Sanger, G.J. (1986) Inhibition of cisplatin-induced vomiting by selective 5-hydroxytryptamine M-receptor antagonism. *Br. J. Pharmacol.*, **88**, 497–99.

Miner, W.D., Sanger, G.J. and Turner, D.H. (1986) Comparison of the effect of BRL 24924, metoclopramide and domperidone on cisplatin-induced emesis in the ferret. *Br. J. Pharmacol.*, **58**, 374P.

Miner, W.D., Sanger, G.J. and Turner, D.H. (1987) Evidence that 5-hydroxytryptamine$_3$ receptors mediate cytotoxic drug and radiation-evoked emesis. *Br. J. Cancer*, **56**, 159–62.

Miolan, J.P., Lajard, A.M., Rega, P. and Roman, C. (1984) Vagal control of gastrointestinal tract during vomiting, in *Gastrointestinal Motility*, (ed C. Roman) pp. 167–75. MTP Press, Lancaster.

Moertal, C.G., Reitemeier, R.J. and Gage, R.P. (1963) A controlled clinical evaluation of antiemetic drugs. *J. Am. Med. Assoc.*, **186**, 116–18.

Monkovic, I. and Gylys, J.A. (1990) Developments in the antiemetic area: Chemistry, pharmacology and therapy. *Prog. Med. Chem.*, **27**, 297–323.

Morrow, G.R. (1989) Chemotherapy-related nausea and vomiting: Etiology and management. *Cancer J. Clinicians*, **39**, 89–104.

Mott, J.C. and Paintal, A.S. (1953) The action of 5-hydroxytryptamine on pulmonary and cardiovascular vagal afferent fibres and its reflex respiratory effects. *Br. J. Pharmacol.*, **8**, 238–41.

Nelson, D.R. and Thomas, D.R. (1989) [^{3}H]-BRL 43694 (granisetron), a specific ligand for 5-HT_3 binding sites in rat brain cortical membranes. *Biochem. Pharmacol.*, **38**, 1693–95.

Newberry, N.R., Cheshire, S.H. and Gilbert, M.J. (1991) Evidence that the 5-HT_3 receptors of the rat, mouse and guinea-pig superior cervical ganglion may be different. *Br. J. Pharmacol.*, **102**, 615–20.

Olynyk, J.K., Cullen, S.R. and Leahy, M.F. (1989) Midazolam: An effective antiemetic agent for cytotoxic therapy. *Med. J. Aust.*, **150**, 466.

Osborne, R.J., Slevin, M.L., Hunter, R.W. and Hamer, J. (1985) Cardiac arrhythmias during cytotoxic chemotherapy: Role of domperidone. *Human Toxicol.*, **4**, 617–23.

Osieka, R., Glatte, P., Pannenbäcker, R. and Schmidt, C.G. (1986) Enhancement of semustine-induced cytotoxicity by chlorpromazine and caffeine in a human melanoma xenograft. *Cancer Treat. Rep.*, **70**, 1167–71.

Pentilla, A. and Kormano, M. (1971) Effect of X-irradiation of the exteriorized jejunal loop on the morphology and 5-hydroxytryptamine content of the enterochromaffin cells in the mouse. *Strahlentherapie*, **142**, 238–47.

Pentillä, A., Kormano, M. and Ahonen, A. (1975) Effects of 400R whole-body X-irradiation on 5-hydroxytryptamine content of the rat gastrointestinal tract. *Strahlentherapie*, **149**, 426–37.

Peroutka, S.J., U'Prichard, D.C., Greenberg, D.A. and Snyder, S.H. (1977) Neuroleptic drug interactions with norepinephrine alpha receptor binding sites in rat brain. *Neuropharmacol.*, **16**, 549–56.

Peroutka, S.J. and Snyder, S.H. (1982) Antiemetics: Neurotransmitter receptor binding predicts therapeutic actions. *Lancet*, **2**, 658–59.

Perrot, J., Nahas, G., Laville, C. and Debay, A. (1982) 'Substituted benzamides as antiemetics', in *Treatment of Cancer Chemotherapy-induced Nausea and Vomiting* (eds D.S. Poster, J.S. Penta and S. Bruno), pp. 195–207. Mason Publishing, USA.

Peters, C.A.H. (1989) Myths of antiemetic administration. *Cancer Nurs.*, **12**, 102–106.

Peters, J.A. and Lambert, J.J. (1989) Electrophysiology of 5-HT_3 receptors in neuronal cell lines. *Trends in Pharmacol. Sci.*, **10**, 172–75.

Preziosi, P., Ripanti, G., Navarra, P. *et al.* (1989) Comparison among 5-HT_3 antagonists on cisplatin emesis in pigeons. *Arch. Int. Pharmacodyn. Ther.*, **301**, 301.

Racké, K. and Schwörer, H. (1991) Regulation of serotonin release from the intestinal mucosa. *Pharmacological Res.*, **23**, 13–25.

Redd, W.H., Andresen, G.V. and Minagawa, R.Y. (1982) Hypnotic control of anticipatory emesis in patients receiving cancer chemotherapy. *J. Consult. Clin. Psychol.*, **50**, 14–19.

Reiser, G., and Hamprecht, B. (1988) Substance P and serotonin synergistically activate a cation permeability in a neuronal cell line. *Naunyn-Schmiedeberg's Arch. Pharmacol.*, **337** (Suppl): R109.

Reynolds, D.J.M., Leslie, R.A., Grahame-Smith, D.G. and Harvey, J.M. (1989) Localization of 5-HT_3 receptor binding sites in human dorsal vagal complex. *Eur. J. Pharmacol.*, **174**, 127–30.

Reynolds, D.J.M., Barber, N.A., Grahame-Smith, D.G., *et al.* (1991) Cisplatin-evoked induction of **c-fos** protein in brainstem of the ferret: the effect of cervical vagotomy and the anti-emetic 5-HT_3 receptor antagonist granisetron (BRL 43694). *Brain Res.*, **565**, 231–236.

Roberts, D.J. (1982) The pharmacological basis of the therapeutic activity of clebopride and related substituted benzamides. *Curr. Ther. Res.*, **31** (Suppl): S1–S44.

Robertson, D.W., Cohen, M.L., Krushinski, J.H. *et al.* (1990) LY 191617, a 5-HT_3 receptor antagonist which does not cross the blood–brain barrier. *Proc. Second IUPHAR Meeting on Serotonin*, P149, pp. 111.

Robinson, T.W. and Giri, S.N. (1987) Effects of chronic administration of doxorubicin on heart phospholipase A_2 activity and *in vitro* synthesis and degradation of prostaglandins in rats. *Prostaglandins, Leukotrienes Med.*, **26**, 59–74.

Roussak, J.B., Carey, P. and Parry, H. (1984) Cardiac arrest after treatment with domperidone. *Br. Med. J.*, **289**, 1579.

Roylance, R.R., Andrews, P.L.R., Hawthorn, J. *et al.* (1989) The anti emetic effects of atropine sulphate in the ferret. *Br. J. Pharmacol.*, **96**, 330P.

Rudd, J.A. and Naylor, R.J. (1990) Preliminary assessment of feverfew (Tanecetum parthenium) to antagonise cisplatin-induced emesis in the ferret. *Br. J. Pharmacol.*, **39**, 247P.

Sagrada, A., Nicola, M., Micheletti, R. and Templeton, D. (1990) Antiemetic activity of DA 6215 against vomiting induced by different chemotherapeutic agents. *Proc. Second IUPHAR Meeting on Serotonin*, P154, pp. 114.

Sallan, S.E., Zinberg, N.E. and Frei, E. (1975) Antiemetic effect of delta-9-tetrahydrocannabinol in patients receiving cancer chemotherapy. *N. Engl. J. Med.*, **293**, 795–97.

Saller, R. and Hallenbrecht, D. (1985) Comparison of the antiemetic efficacy of two high-dose benzamides, metoclopramide and alizapride against cisplatin-induced emesis. *Cancer Treat. Rep.*, **69**, 1301–303.

Sancilio, L.F., Pinkus, L.M., Jackson, C.B. and Munson, H.R. (1991) Studies on the emetic and antiemetic properties of zacopride and its enantiomers. *Eur. J. Pharmacol.*, **192**, 365–69.

Sanger, G.J. (1990) New antiemetic drugs. *Can. J. Physiol. Pharmacol.*, **68**, 314–24.

Sanger, G.J. and King, F.D. (1988) From metoclopramide to selective gut motility stimulants and 5-HT_3 receptor antagonists. *Drug Des. Delivery*, **3**, 273–95.

Sanger, G.J. and Nelson, D.R. (1989) Selective and functional 5-hydroxytryptamine$_3$ receptor antagonism by BRL 43694 (granisetron). *Eur. J. Pharmacol.*, **159**, 113–24.

Sawika, J. and Sallan, S. (1977) Transdermal therapeutics system, scopolamine (TS): prevention of vomiting associated with cancer chemotherapy. *Soc. Clin. Oncol.*, **18**, 302.

Scogna, D.M. and Smalley, R.V. (1979) Chemotherapy-induced nausea and vomiting. *Am. J. Nurs.*, Sept: 1562–64.

Sepulveda, M.I., Lummis, S.C.R. and Martin, I.L. (1991) 2-Methyl-5-HT is a partial agonist at 5-HT_3 receptors in NIE-115 neuroblastoma cells. *Br. J. Pharmacol.* 102, 138P.

Schimizu, T. and Wolfe, L.S. (1990) Arachidonic acid cascade and signal transduction. *J. Neurochemistry*, **55**, 1–15.

Sicuteri, F. (1968) Sensitization of nociceptors by 5-hydroxytryptamine in man. *Int. Congr. Pharmacol.*, Vol. 9, Pergamon Press, pp. 57–86.

Smaldone, L., Alberts, D., Aapro, M. *et al.* (1990) Randomized double-blind crossover, comparison of batanopride (BMY 25801) and metoclopramide in patients receiving cisplatin-based chemotherapy. *Ann. Oncol.*, **1** (Suppl): W9, 2, p. 109.

Smith, D.B., Newlands, E.S., Spruyt, O.W. *et al.* (1990) Ondansetron (GR 38032F) plus dexamethasone: effective anti-emetic prophylaxis for patients receiving cytotoxic chemotherapy. *Br. J. Cancer.*, **61**, 323–24.

Smith, W.L., Jackson, C.B., Sancilio, L.F. and Alphin, R.S. (1985) Effect of diphenhydramine on the anti-emetic action of metoclopramide against cisplatin-induced emesis in dogs. *Cancer Treat. Res.*, **70**, 934–35.

Smith, W.L., Callahan, E.M. and Alphin, R.S. (1988) The emetic activity of centrally administered cisplatin in cats and its antagonism by zacopride. *J. Pharm. Pharmacol.*, **40**, 142–43.

Smith, W.L., Alphin, R.S., Jackson, C.B. and Sancilia, L.F. (1989) The antiemetic profile of zacopride. *J. Pharm. Pharmacol.*, **41**, 101–105.

Sokoloff, P., Giros, B., Martres, M.P. *et al.* (1990) Molecular cloning and characterization of a novel dopamine receptor (D3) as a target for neuroleptics. *Nature*, **237**, 146–51.

Spiess, J.L., Adelstein, D.J. and Hines, J.D. (1987) Evaluation of ethanol as an antiemetic in patients receiving cisplatin. *Clin. Ther.*, **9**, 400–404.

Stables, R., Andrews, P.L.R., Bailey, H.E. *et al.* (1987) Antiemetic properties of the 5-HT_3 receptor antagonist, GR 38032F. *Cancer Treat. Rev.*, **14**, 333–36.

Stannard, D. (1989) Pressure prevents nausea. *Nursing Times*, **95**, 33–34.

Stefanini, E. and Clement-Cormier, Y. (1981) Detection and characterization of dopamine receptors in dog area postrema. *Eur. J. Pharmacol.*, **74**, 257–60.

Stell, L.K., Sweedler, I.K. and Catravas, G.N. (1983) Effects of ^{60}Co radiation on synthesis of prostaglandins $F_{2\alpha}$, E_2 and thromboxane B_2 in lung airways of guinea-pigs. *Radiat. Res.*, **94**, 156–65.

Stepanovic, S.R. and Nikolic, J.V. (1979) The effect of X-irradiation on the amount of dopamine in corpus striatum of the rat. *Experientia*, **35**, 111–12.

Strohl, R.A. (1983) Nursing management of the patient with cancer experiencing taste changes. *Cancer Nurs.*, **6**, 353–59.

Stryker, J.A., Demers, L.M. and Mortel, R. (1979) Prophylactic ibuprofen administration during pelvic irradiation. *J. Radiat. Oncol. Biol. Phys.*, **5**, 2049–52.

Tattersall, F.D., Dourisch, C.T., Duchnowski, M. *et al.* (1990) The anti-emetic action of the novel 5-HT_3 receptor antagonist L-683–877 in the ferret. *Eur. J. Pharmacol.*, **183**, 1966–67.

Tortorice, P.V. and O'Connell, M.B. (1990) Management of chemotherapy-induced nausea and vomiting. *Pharmacotherapy*, **10**, 129–45.

U'Prichard, D.C., Greenberg, D.A., Sheehan, P.P. and Snyder, S.H. (1978) Tricyclic antidepressants: Therapeutic properties and affinity for alpha-noradrenergic receptor binding sites in the brain. *Science*, **199**, 197–99.

Van Wijngaarden, I., Tulp, M.T.H. and Sondijn, W. (1990) The concept of selectivity in 5-HT receptor research. *Eur. J. Pharmacol.*, **188**, 301–12.

Villalón, C.M., den Boer, M.O., Heiligers, J.P.C. and Saxena, P.R. (1991) Further characterization by use of tryptamine and benzamide derivatives, of the putative 5-HT_4 receptor mediating tachycardia in the pig. *Br. J. Pharmacol.*, **102**, 107–12.

Vincent, B.J., McQuistron, D.J., Einhorn, L.H. *et al.* (1983) Review of cannabinoids and their anti-emetic effectiveness. *Drugs*, **25** (Suppl 1): 52–62.

Vinciguerra, V., Moore, T. and Brennan, E. (1988) Inhalation marijuana as an antiemetic for cancer chemotherapy. *NY State J. Med.*, **88**, 525–27.

Waeber, C., Pinkus, L.M. and Palacios, J.M. (1990)

The (S)-isomer of [^{3}H]-zacopride labels 5-HT_3 receptors with high affinity in rat brain. *Eur. J. Pharmacol.*, **181**, 283–87.

Wallis, D.I. (1989) 'Interaction of 5-hydroxytryptamine with autonomic and sensory neurones', in *The Peripheral Actions of 5-hydroxytryptamine*, (ed J.R. Fozard), pp. 220–46. Oxford Press, Oxford.

Wampler, G. (1983) The pharmacology and clinical effectiveness of phenothiazines and related drugs for managing chemotherapy-induced emesis. *Drugs*, 25 (Suppl 1): 35–51.

Warren, K. (1988) Will I be sick, nurse? *Nursing Times*, **84**, 30–32.

Winningham, M.L. and MacVicar, M.G. (1988) The effect of aerobic exercise on patient reports of nausea. *Oncol. Nurs. Forum.*, **15**, 447–50.

Winter, J. and Hart, L.L. (1987) Transdermal scopolamine in nausea and vomiting. *Drug. Intell. Clin. Pharm.*, **21**, 712–14.

Yamahara, J., Rong, H.Q., Naitoh, Y. *et al.* (1989a) Inhibition of cytotoxic drug-induced vomiting in suncus by a ginger constituent. *J. Ethnopharmacol.*, **27**, 353–55.

Yamahara, J., Rong, H.Q., Iwamoto, M. *et al.* (1989b) Active components of ginger exhibiting anti-serotonergic action. *Phytotherapy Res.*, **3**, 70–71.

Yelnosky, J., Katz, R. and Dietrich, E.V. (1964) A study of some of the pharmacologic actions of droperidol. *Toxicol. Appl. Pharmacol.*, **6**, 37–47.

Yoshida, N., Ito, T., Omoya, H. *et al.* (1990) AS-5370: A potent and long-lasting serotonin 5-HT_3 receptor antagonist. *Proc. Second IUPHAR Meeting on Serotonin*, P151, pp. 112.

Young, R.W. (1986) 'Mechanisms and treatment of radiation-induced nausea and vomiting', in *Nausea and vomiting: Mechanisms and treatment* (eds C.J. Davis, G.V. Lake-Bakaar and D.G. Grahame-Smith), pp. 94–109. Springer-Verlag, Berlin.

10

Psychological effects of anti-cancer therapy

ANN CULL

10.1 INTRODUCTION

Various types of cancer therapy can give rise to nausea and vomiting but the problem is chiefly associated with and best researched in the use of cytotoxic drugs. As well as challenging patients' physical status and promoting further treatment complications, nausea and vomiting disrupt patients' capacity to function in daily living and compromise their emotional well being.

In a much quoted survey Coates *et al.* (1983) found patients ranked 'being sick' and 'feeling sick' as the most troublesome of 45 common chemotherapy side effects. Love *et al.* (1989) also demonstrated a relationship between nausea and vomiting and patient distress but pointed out that the cumulative impact of multiple side effects can outweigh specific effects and that functional disruption and emotional distress are greater when side effects prove resistant to coping efforts. When nausea and vomiting are severe or intractable compliance may be lost. More than 80% of Love's sample experienced nausea and by cycle six 46% had considered stopping treatment. In a study of patients who did stop chemotherapy prematurely Wilcox *et al.* (1982) reported that 71% gave these gastro-intestinal symptoms as their main reason for stopping.

Increasingly it has been recognized that pharmacologically induced side effects may be compounded by psychological factors such that nausea and vomiting similar to that induced by drugs may occur at other times as a result of learning processes.

Conditioned nausea and vomiting occurring during or after drug administration may be difficult to distinguish from drug-induced effects. When sickness occurs prior to treatment it is referred to as anticipatory nausea and/or vomiting (ANV). Although it occurs less frequently than post-treatment nausea and vomiting (PTNV), ANV can be equally troublesome to patients who themselves tend to regard these manifestations with distress as evidence of psychological weakness (Leventhal *et al.*, 1988).

To date, anti-emetic drugs do not appear to control ANV once it has developed (Morrow, 1991) and may on occasion cause a paradoxical worsening of symptoms by process of conditioning (Carey and Burish, 1988).

It has been suggested that improvements in the management of chemotherapy-induced emesis have resulted in a significant reduction in the severity (though not the incidence) of ANV to the point where it no longer constitutes a significant clinical problem (Stefanek *et al.*, 1988). Certainly the need for comparable

Emesis in Anti-cancer Therapy
Mechanisms and treatment
Published in 1993 by Chapman & Hall, London
ISBN 0 412 37250 9

attention to be given to other hitherto neglected side effects of cancer therapy – persistent fatigue, cognitive impairment, sexual dysfunction – is increasingly being recognized.

However, Lindley *et al.* (1989) report that even with anti-emetic medication more than 50% of all chemotherapy patients experience PTNV. Morrow (1991) argues that gains achieved by anti-emetic therapy to date have been offset by the use of more aggressive cytotoxic regimes resulting in no net reduction in patients' experience of PTNV or ANV that are discernible in his large database.

Data are not yet available which reflect the impact of recently introduced 5-HT_3 receptor antagonists on the incidence and severity of ANV. Even with encouraging improvements in emetic control, economic restrictions of prescribing mean complete protection from PTNV is unlikely to be universal and ANV is likely to remain a significant clinical problem for some time to come.

10.2 PREVALENCE

Over the past ten years the prevalence of ANV has been frequently studied but estimates are highly variable: from 14% (Love *et al.*, 1983) to 65% (Coons *et al.*, 1981). Review papers published up to 1986 Burish and Carey (1986) estimated a prevalence rate of 32% in a cumulative sample of 1700 adult patients. When prospective studies only were reviewed (Love *et al.*, 1989; Andrykowski *et al.*, 1985; Jacobsen *et al.*, 1985), the prevalence rate rose to 45%. From his own series of 60 patients, Morrow (1984) reported that approximately one in four patients experiences ANV by the fourth cycle of chemotherapy.

It therefore remains difficult to be precise about the prevalence of ANV among cancer patients receiving chemotherapy. Methodological differences among studies make comparison difficult and potentially crucial intervening variables (e.g. anti-emetic regime) are either not reported or are uncontrolled.

10.3 PROBLEMS OF DEFINITION

Of some importance is the way the phenomena to be studied are defined yet this remains controversial. Andrykowski (1986) identified three classes of definition of anticipatory side effects, as follows:

Nausea and/or vomiting

1. *prior* to a chemotherapy infusion (Nesse *et al.*, 1980; Nicholas, 1982);
2. *pre/during* chemotherapy infusion (Schulz, 1980);
3. either (1) or (2) with some qualifying clause:
   - (a) *before* infusion associated with some *treatment-related stimulus* (Nerenz *et al.*, 1982)
   - (b) *before/during* chemotherapy *without another cause* (Fetting *et al.*, 1983);
   - (c) *prior* to treatment *on day 1* of chemotherapy cycle (Andrykowski, 1986);
   - (d) *before/during* infusion in patients with prior chemotherapy nausea/vomiting (Stefanek *et al.*, 1988);
   - (e) (i) at times other than after an injection; *and*
     - (ii) associated with a chemotherapy-related thought or stimulus; *and*
     - (iii) not attributable to a non treatment-related condition (Leventhal *et al.*, 1988).

Andrykowski *et al.* (1988) has defined anticipatory nausea (AN) as:

- within 24 hours preceding chemotherapy infusion;
- but no continuous nausea since previous infusion;
- no nausea associated with oral medicine in past week.

Three points emerge in defining anticipatory side effects. First, it is important to be clear whether nausea and vomiting are assessed together or separately. Anticipatory vomiting very rarely occurs without prior nausea but nausea will not always be followed by vomiting. Secondly, since nausea and/or vomiting that occur during lengthy infusions may have a pharmacological component, the consensus view now favours restricting the definition of ANV to events preceding the delivery of chemotherapy. This allows a distinction to be made between ANV and any learned component of delayed emesis. Delayed emesis begins 2–3 days after treatment and can persist for 5–7 days. The mechanisms underlying delayed effects are not fully understood and for some patients conditioning may be a contributory factor. Thirdly, it is important for clinicians to be clear that apparent ANV is neither due to organic disease such as brain metastases or gastro-intestinal malignancy nor to the action of other medication.

10.4 METHODOLOGICAL ISSUES

Methodological differences between studies have confounded efforts to arrive at estimates of prevalence and prognostic indices for ANV.

Early estimates of prevalence came largely from retrospective studies. Stunkard *et al.*, (1985) demonstrated the unreliability of such data by comparing concurrent and retrospective assessments of vomiting obtained from patients following gastric surgery. Retrospective accounts significantly exaggerated the frequency of vomiting. Concurrent reporting is therefore preferable.

Sample size has also varied widely and has often been small for the number of variables being assessed. Wide variations in the demographic characteristics of samples are relevant since age and sex have been implicated in susceptibility to treatment side effects. In most studies, data from patients with different diagnoses who are undergoing different chemotherapy with different anti-emetic support are reported together. Since the prevalence of ANV may be expected to vary with patients' experience of PTNV, which is a function of the cytotoxic and anti-emetic agents prescribed, future studies should analyse data from different drug protocols separately and relevant treatment parameter should be specified.

Since the risk of developing ANV increases with successive treatment cycles, the timing of the assessment is critical in cross-sectional studies. More useful data about the development of ANV can be derived from prospective longitudinal studies but in either case the timing of the assessment should be specified.

The method of measurement too has varied from study to study. Several Quality of Life measures with satisfactory psychometric properties have been developed (de Haes *et al.*, 1983; Aaronson *et al.*, 1987) but, typically, these contain a single item each for nausea and vomiting embedded in a lengthier questionnaire. Investigators focussing on nausea and vomiting have generally preferred to develop their own scales, details of which are not always published. Data on the reliability or validity of these measures are rarely offered.

Vomiting has frequently been rated by an observer who scores presence/absence of vomiting or counts number of vomits. Differences arise between studies even in this apparently objective measure, for example, whether or not retching is included.

More commonly, self-report measures of nausea and vomiting have been developed. Visual analogue scales are widely used but Morrow's review cited a range from 3-point to 10-point scales (1984). Different dimensions of the patient's experience have also been assessed, such as frequency, duration and severity, in different studies. Anticipatory and post-treatment effects should be reported separately: it is therefore essential for the time period to which the assessment refers to be clearly defined. The majority of authors report data from their own rating scales but without this information being given in full.

Two scales specifically designed to assess nausea and vomiting have been published, as follows:

1. The Morrow assessment of nausea and emesis, – MANE (Morrow, 1984)
   Frequency of ANV and PTNV are each assessed on a 4-point scale from 'never' to 'every treatment'. Duration is recorded in hours and severity of response is rated on a 6-point scale from 'very mild' to 'intolerable'. Six-point scales are also used to assess when nausea and vomiting were at their worst. Evidence of satisfactory reliability and validity are presented both by the author and independently by Carnike *et al.* (1988). They demonstrated significant correlations between frequency, severity and duration of nausea and vomiting and question whether it is necessary to assess all three dimensions. They also note that the MANE is more reliable in assessing nausea than vomiting. This instrument is in fact increasingly widely used in research in this area.

2. Functional living index: emesis – FLIE (Lindley *et al.*, in press)
   This 18-item scale adopts the format of Schipper's well known Functional Living Index: Cancer (1984). In the FLIE scale, nausea and vomiting are assessed separately by items that focus on the extent of functional disruption and emotional distress caused by these symptoms. Items are scored on a 7-point graded visual analogue scale with end points labelled 'not at all' and 'a great deal'. The scale does not specifically separate ANV from PTNV. Questions refer to 'the past three days'. No data are yet available on the psychometric properties of this instrument. It should be noted that this scale may present some of the problems of administration already ascribed to the FLIC described by Ganz *et al.*, (1988). In this study, significant numbers of patients responded by ringing numbers rather than treating the line as a continuous scale as intended. It may be that the FLIE should also be completed in the presence of a researcher to ensure quality control of the data collected.

10.5 AETIOLOGY AND PROGNOSTIC FACTORS

A variety of models have been proposed to explain ANV. Chang (1981) implicated brain metastases or malignant processes in the gastro-intestinal system in the onset of ANV. While this will explain nausea and vomiting in some cancer patients, the prevalence and time of presentation of symptoms caused by metastatic disease does not fit observations of ANV. Morrow (1991) has reported systematic screening of patients in his ANV studies for brain or GI malignancy. No association was found between metastatic disease and the development of ANV.

Chang's (1981, 1982) psychodynamic interpretation of ANV is harder to test scientifically. There are no data to support his hypothesis that anticipatory side effects represent 'underlying psychological readjustment problems'.

Following observations of the effect of operant conditioning on other aspects of illness behaviour such as complaints of pain maintained by the reinforcing effect of attention and sympathy from others (Fordyce, 1973), Redd and Andrykowski (1982) speculated that ANV in oncology patients might also be maintained by secondary gain. Closer analysis suggests the negative effects of chemotherapy outweigh any such gains (Redd *et al.*, 1985) and that removal of attention does not diminish the symptoms.

Scientific interest has chiefly focussed on the hypothesis that nausea and vomiting become conditioned responses through a learning process which is variously referred to as classical conditioning (Burish and Carey, 1984), respondent learning (Burish and Carey, 1986) or associative learning (Carey and Burish, 1988). Essentially, these conceptualize the same process whereby chemotherapy (the

Table 10.1 Studies of prognostic indices of ANV

I *Before chemotherapy*	
Conditioned stimulus, e.g. nurse, thoughts, smells, tastes	No response/irrelevant response
Unconditioned stimulus i.e. emetogenic chemotherapy	Unconditioned response i.e. nausea/vomiting
II *In context of chemotherapy* (repeated)	
CS + UCS	UCR
III *After association is learned*	
CS e.g. nurse, thoughts, smells, tastes	CR i.e. nausea/vomiting

unconditioned stimulus; UCS) causes nausea and/or vomiting (the unconditioned response; UCR). By repeated administration of chemotherapy, an association is learned between stimuli associated with the chemotherapy setting and drug delivery. Thus, previously neutral stimuli (conditioned stimuli; CS) such as the sight of the chemotherapy nurse, by association with the sequence drug-nausea/vomiting (UCS–UCR), become sufficient in themselves to evoke the conditioned response (CR), that is nausea and/or vomiting, even in the absence of the drug (UCS). (Table 10.1.)

Conditioned stimuli typically are sight, smells or tastes associated with drug infusion but they may also be activated by memory such that the thought of these stimuli is sufficient to evoke the conditioned response.

The Pavlovian model of classical conditioning is often represented mechanistically and some updating of concepts is helpful in understanding the putative mechanism of induction of ANV.

Rescorla (1988) reviewed current thinking about classical conditioning to point out that it is not the simple pairing of events (UCS + CS) which is crucial but that the process involves learning relationships between events. Conventionally, Pavlovian conditioning was conceived of as a slow process emerging from repeated presentations of the stimuli but there are now data which demonstrate that rapid learning can also occur by this means. From the reflex tradition in physiology we have now moved on to appreciate that human learning can combine the individual's preconceptions with his capacity to discriminate logical and perceptual relationships between events to achieve adaptation to a complex world.

Ethically it is not acceptable to induce ANV experimentally to test this hypothesis. Evidence to support the learning model has been drawn from a range of other sources. It has been demonstrated under laboratory conditions that emesis can develop as a CR in dogs to external stimuli that regularly preceded the injection of apomorphine (Pavlov, 1927).

It remains contentious whether the extensive animal work on taste aversion (or 'bait shyness') refers to the same learning process. A variety of experimental animals will develop strong aversions to the taste of food that has been associated with illness. This is an interesting model since the food may have been consumed many hours before the onset of symptoms yet learning can frequently be demonstrated after a single exposure (Robertson and Garcia, 1985). The link between this work and the experience of oncology patients is based on the assumption that the animals would retch if they were forced to ingest the aversive food. This has not been demonstrated and – given that the animals most commonly used in these experiments are rodents which cannot vomit – the assumption remains unproven. Interest in this work has also been fostered by the apparent role of taste sensations associated with chemotherapy in the onset of ANV. Garcia and Koelling (1966) have suggested that taste aversions result from a selective association between taste and gastro-intestinal distress which makes tastes unpalatable. However, Grant's thorough review (1987) presents evidence to suggest that emetic mechanisms are neither necessary nor sufficient to account for all conditioned taste aversions.

Several human studies demonstrate conditioning in chemotherapy patients. Bernstein and Webster (1980) reported taste aversions conditioned to a novel flavour of ice cream eaten just prior to the infusion of emetogenic chemo-therapy. Learning occurred although patients knew the ice cream had not made them sick. Thus, cognitive factors appear insufficient to prevent the development of taste aversion.

The most dramatic examples of conditioning have arisen from patients' reports of the extent of the process of stimulus generalization to the point where previously effective anti-emetic measures become conditioned stimuli capable of evoking the emetic response (Morrow *et al.*, 1982; Redd *et al.*, 1985).

Although it is generally agreed that anticipatory side effects are acquired by an associative learning process it is not clear why some patients develop conditioned responses while others do not nor why some patients suffer ANV after only one or two cycles of chemotherapy while others take much longer. The identification of prognostic factors to discriminate patients most at risk of developing ANV and to chart the course of symptom development is of theoretical as well as clinical significance. If the model is valid, factors predicting the development of ANV should be explicable in terms of learning theory principles. Clinically the aim is to identify patients most in need of prophylactic or at least palliative intervention to minimize anticipatory symptoms.

A range of characteristics has been examined for predictive power and these fall broadly into two categories:

1. variables which directly influence the strength of the conditioning process; and
2. variables reflecting individual differences in susceptibility.

In some cases it remains contentious whether the relationship between the prognostic factor and ANV is direct or indirect.

10.6 POST-TREATMENT NAUSEA AND VOMITING

A general prediction from the learning theory model is that PTNV must be present for ANV to develop. There are no published reports to contradict this.

Learning occurs more rapidly with more intense unconditioned responses. Andrykowski *et al.*, (1985), in a prospective study, found the magnitude of PTN the primary factor contributing to the development of AN, accounting for 24% of the variance between groups. Other studies have demonstrated correlations between frequency, severity and duration of post-treatment side effects and ANV (Morrow, 1982; Cohen *et al.*, 1986).

The emetic potential of cytotoxic drugs used can now be reliably specified (Penta *et al.*, 1983) and ANV is more common with the more emetogenic protocols (Morrow, 1982).

It is generally assumed that PTNV is solely a function of the emetogenicity of chemotherapy moderated by the efficacy of any anti-emetic medication prescribed. These is some evidence that non pharmacological factors – i.e. susceptibility to GI distress, expectation of nausea and anxiety related to infusion – contribute to individual differences in post-treatment emetic response (Jacobsen *et al.*, 1986). These factors might also be relevant to the development of ANV. Although not collected from patients receiving highly emetic chemotherapy, for example, cisplatin, these data make it likely that anti-emetic prescribing based solely on the emetic potential of the cytotoxic drugs administered is likely to be sub-optimal. Since severity of PTNV can vary from cycle to cycle of chemotherapy for the same patient (van Komen and Redd, 1985) optimal supportive intervention will depend on monitoring changing risk factors over the course of treatment.

TREATMENT-RELATED VARIABLES

Other factors related to the delivery of chemotherapy have been investigated. Larger doses of i.v. drugs at first infusion are associated with increased risk of ANV (Andrykowski *et al.*, 1988). Stronger side effects are reported following long infusions compared to short injections (Andrykowski *et al.*, 1985). Longer infusions may facilitate conditioning by offering longer exposure to clinic-related stimuli and, by reducing the time between those stimuli and PTNV but longer infusion may result in greater anxiety, a factor which is also thought to facilitate conditioning.

The learning theory model predicts that the probability of the conditioned response occurring increases with the number of exposures to the learning situation. The incidence of anticipatory symptoms is regularly found to increase with the number of treatment cycles given (Nerenz *et al.*, 1986; Andrykowski and Redd, 1987).

Increasingly, the salience of the conditioned stimulus also strengthens conditioning and awareness of tastes or smells during infusions has been found associated with ANV (Nerenz *et al.*, 1986). van Komen and Redd (1985) asked patients which stimuli elicited their anticipatory symptoms. Anticipatory vomiting was elicited by smells in 40% and by thoughts and sights in 30% of cases. By contrast, 75% of patients experienced anticipatory nausea triggered by thoughts, 22% reported smells and only 3% sights.

Nerenz and his colleagues have reported several studies (1982; 1984; 1986) that show an association between tastes during injections and anticipatory nausea. Since taste sensations are more prevalent among patients receiving nitrogen mustard or platinum-based compounds – that is highly emetogenic drugs – it may be that this effect is mediated by PTNV. Nerenz *et al.* (1986) reported informally that patients who blocked taste sensations – for example, by sucking a flavoured sweet – had a lower incidence of AN than those who did not. More systematic investigation of the value of taste blocking is called for.

TREATMENT CENTRE VARIATION

van Komen and Redd (1985) found a significant difference in prevalence and severity of ANV between two clinic settings. Patients treated in a large room within sight of other patients were more likely to develop ANV than those treated separately. It is not clear how this apparent social facilitation effect operates. Cohen *et al.* (1986), in a multicentre study, found treatment centres to have one of the strongest zero order and unique associations with PTNV and ANV although the centres used comparable treatment protocols. In this study it was not clear whether differences were due to aspects of the physical environment, to treatment practices, or to staff variables.

AGE FACTORS

Younger patients are known to report ANV more frequently than older patients but it is not clear whether particular age ranges are significant. The demarcation of older versus younger age among adult patients varies across studies (Nesse *et al.*, 1980; Morrow *et al.*, 1982; Fetting *et al.*, 1983).

The effect of age may be mediated by disease status and treatment. Nerenz *et al.* (1983) found no relationship between age and development of ANV among women treated for metastatic breast cancer, whereas 60% of younger women, i.e. those under 45, receiving adjuvant chemotherapy, developed ANV. Only 8% of women aged 45–54 and no women under 55 in their sample developed ANV.

An earlier suggestion that younger patients are treated with more aggressive therapy has not been supported (Andrykowski *et al.*, 1985; Cohen *et al.*, 1986; Morrow and Dobkin, 1988) but there is a strong interaction with PTNV such that younger patients with more severe PTNV are particularly likely to develop ANV.

Younger patients may be more susceptible to conditioning. It remains unclear whether or how age might directly influence the acquisition phase of learning but clinical reports of persistent anticipatory symptoms, i.e. resistant to extinction, are more common among younger patients.

Cohen *et al.* (1986) and others have suggested that younger patients may be more anxious and/or more sensitive to unpleasant aspects of treatment. Thus the effect of age on the development of ANV may be indirect.

SUSCEPTIBILITY TO MOTION SICKNESS

Morrow (1985) demonstrated that patients who report susceptibility to motion sickness have more chemotherapy side effects than case-matched controls treated with the same drugs who have no such history. This pattern was found for ANV as well as PTNV.

This association was pursued by Leventhal *et al.* (1988). Using a series of logistic analyses controlling for PTNV, and an event history analysis, they found a history of motion sickness to be independently related to AN with predictive power independent of age, taste during injection or pretreatment anxiety.

Following Seligman's review (1970) of the generality of learning theory, Leventhal suggests motion sickness may represent a marker of 'preparedness' for associative learning such that susceptibility to one type of gastrointestinal distress may facilitate conditioning between PTNV and a variety of other cues. Morrow (1985) suggests chemotherapy patients who are susceptible to motion sickness may be providing additional input to the vomiting centre through the vestibular system and that they may benefit from additional anti-emetic medication, for example Scopalamine, to combat this.

Andrykowski *et al.* (1988) found a more rapid development of AN was related to a history of experiencing nausea across a greater variety of situations. Several studies (Redd *et al.*, 1985; Jacobsen *et al.*, 1986) have discussed the role of constitutional differences in patients' susceptibility to GI distress. More constitutionally vulnerable patients are more likely to experience higher levels of PTNV and hence are at greater risk of developing ANV.

A recent study by Forrest *et al.* (1990) showed nausea and vomiting after general anesthesia were more likely to occur in young healthy females undergoing laparoscopy and the risk was increased fourfold if performed during menstruation. The potential for hormonal effects to interact with other risk factors for ANV in oncology patients has not been examined.

The principal significance of these studies lies in the demonstration that the aetiology of chemotherapy side effects is complex, involving individual differences as well as the pharmacological properties of the drugs administered and calling for greater flexibility in anti-emetic treatment strategy. The physiological mechanisms underlying these individual differences are not completely understood, nor is it clear whether this represents susceptibility to motion sickness *per se*, or, more generally, that it is GI distress in response to a range of stimuli which is important.

ANXIETY

The role of anxiety as a mediating factor in the development of ANV has been a major focus of research effort but the results have been conflicting.

Several authors (Schultz, 1980; Altmaier *et al.*, 1982; Andrykowski *et al.*, 1985) report higher anxiety among patients who develop ANV than among those who do not. This has not been a universal finding (Zook *et al.*, 1983; Andrykowski *et al.*, 1988) and in correlational analysis of retrospective data it is not possible to determine whether anxiety is a cause or a consequence of ANV. More frequently, causal explanations have been sought. Given the physiological arousal associated with anxiety and what is known of the potential psychogenesis of nausea and vomiting, one hypothesis is that ANV can be explained as a symptom of anxiety.

In a prospective study, Nerenz *et al.* (1986) reported a mean incidence of AN of 18% per cycle of chemotherapy among patients who were highly anxious compared with 9.8% among less anxious patients. Andrykowski *et al.* (1985) found anxiety to be the single best predictor of ANV, after PTNV, accounting for 13.6% of the variance between groups.

The evidence does not support the hypothesis that ANV is merely a concomitant of infusion-related anxiety and a better understanding of the role of anxiety has typically been sought through Spence's hypothesis (1958) that anxiety facilitates more rapid conditioning. Anxiety is held to increase the individual's generalized drive which is in turn associated with Pavlovian concepts of increased excitatory potential of the nervous system which are held to facilitate conditioning (Teplov, 1964). In fact, considerable variation can be shown between individuals in performance on experimental conditioning tasks and anxiety may account for only a small proportion of the variance (Spence, 1964).

Dolgin *et al.* (1985) suggest that anxious patients are more vigilant to their environment and hence to stimuli associated with chemotherapy. Anxiety may also increase the salience of these stimuli thereby facilitating conditioning. This has been confirmed in their study of paediatric oncology patients.

Others have argued for a two-stage process (Burish and Carey, 1986) by which anxiety as a conditioned response to chemotherapy becomes a conditioned stimulus to nausea and vomiting. Burish and Carey also discuss Fetting's theory that pharmacologically induced nausea and vomiting lowers the threshold for GI upset in response to other stimuli and that anxiety causes neurotransmitter changes which can induce nausea and vomiting in patients with a lowered threshold. Anxiety, associated with increased noradrenergic activity, may be sufficient to stimulate nausea and vomiting in some patients and clonidine, which reduces noradrenergic activity, has been found to eliminate ANV in 50% of patients after a single cycle.

In the assessment of anxiety there is some controversy over the relative roles of trait and state anxiety. Trait anxiety is generally conceived of as a predisposition to perceive a wide range of circumstances as threatening. van Komen and Redd (1985) reported an association between higher trait anxiety and the development of ANV whereas Andrykowski *et al.* (1985) found no such association.

Transient state anxiety, characterized by perceived feelings of tension, apprehension and heightened autonomic nervous system, has received more attention but the findings are also inconclusive.

Andrykowski and Redd (1987) failed to confirm their hypothesis that ANV would occur more rapidly in highly anxious patients.

In a separate study, Andrykowski *et al.* (1988) found patients with early onset of ANV were not significantly more anxious than those who never developed ANV, suggesting elevated state anxiety is not a necessary precondition. Later onset symptoms were characteristically preceded by an escalation of infusion-related anxiety. It was suggested that increased anxiety could be due to the procedure becoming more aversive – increasing difficulty with venepuncture, for example, or to cognitive concerns such as concern about treatment outcome.

This was only partially supported by Morrow's work (1991). He too found an association between state anxiety and ANV. Over five cycles of chemotherapy he was only able to demonstrate an association between escalating anxiety and ANV when the increment came between cycles one and two stimulating ANV before cycle three.

Andrykowski (1988) emphasizes that assessment of the role of state anxiety is sensitive to differences in the criterion group employed. Patients experiencing pretreatment nausea at other times than 24 hours before chemotherapy were found to be more anxious than patients whose anticipatory symptoms were confined to this time period.

Morrow (1991), in assessing differences among measures of anxiety, points to the inclusion of symptoms of anxiety which may be confounded by drug effects as compared with items assessing cognitive or affective state. He found significant association between ANV and anxiety as measured by the SCL-90 (Derogatis *et al.*, 1979) and Spielberger's State-Trait Inventory (Spielberger *et al.*, 1969) but not as assessed by the anxiety scale of the Profile of Mood States (McNair *et al.*, 1981). This is somewhat surprising given the degree of overlap among items on the latter two measures.

Nerenz *et al.* (1986) attempted by interview to assess predictors of anxiety before injection. Patients who indicated worry about the prospect of intravenous treatment and higher expectations of difficulty with treatment were significantly more likely to be anxious, as were patients receiving adjuvant chemotherapy for breast cancer. The authors suggest these findings may be useful in identifying patients at risk of developing ANV.

The consensus to date suggests that anxiety is not a direct cause of anticipatory symptoms but is more likely to be an important mediating factor. State anxiety does appear to exacerbate post-treatment nausea and vomiting thereby increasing the risk of ANV. The physiological mechanisms by which this occurs are incompletely understood. Anxiety is a useful predictor of patients at risk of ANV with the advantage that a range of effective interventions are available for anxiety management. For a fuller discussion of the role of anxiety see Andrykowski's excellent review (1990).

10.7 PROGNOSTIC INDICES

Prospective studies have increasingly demonstrated that no single factor is as good as several in combination in identifying patients at risk of developing ANV. Different authors have developed different indices and report their predictive power in different ways depending on the statistical model employed (Table 10.2).

Morrow (in press) has recently reported the most comprehensive series to date. In his initial study patients found to experience ANV were significantly more likely to have four of his eight prognostic characteristics than those without ANV. His validation study then attempted to predict the development of ANV prior to the fourth cycle of chemotherapy. The accuracy of prediction was less than in the preceding study and both in this and a second validation study Morrow found his schema more accurate at screening out patients who subsequently did not develop ANV than in predicting those who did. Patients who

Table 10.2 Summary of the major contributions to this field

Author	Sample size	Prognostic factors	Predictive power
1. Andrykowski, Redd and Hatfield, 1985	80	PTN after 1st infusion; Mean length of infusion; State anxiety, after 1st two cycles; Age; Introversion; Trait anxiety	Accounts for 47% of group variance ANV vs no ANV
2. Cohen *et al.*, 1986	149	Age*; Anti-emetic; Drug toxicity; PTNV; Type of cancer; Extent of disease; Treatment centre	49% of group variance
3. Nerenz *et al.*, 1986	192	Preinfusion anxiety; " taste; PTNV; Age	Not reported
4. Andrykowski *et al.*, 1985	80	Trait anxiety; State anxiety*; Mean PTN; Length of infusion; Introversion	25.8% of group variance
5. Andrykowski *et al.*, 1988	64	Severity/duration; PTN after 1st infusion; Expectation of nausea	12% of group variance
6. Morrow, 1984; 1991	176, 355, 297	Age; PTNV; 'warm, hot all over', sweating, generalized weakness } after chemotherapy; Severity of PTNV; Susceptibility to motion sickness	

* denotes single greatest factor

experience fewer than three of Morrow's eight factors are unlikely to develop ANV. He suggests the yield of positive cases may be increased by 15–20% by predicting that patients with four or more of these characteristics will develop ANV.

The refinement of prognostic indices remains an issue of interest not only in predicting patients who will develop ANV and in attempting to understand the course of its development but also clinically in identifying patients who require specific intervention.

10.8 PREVENTIVE INTERVENTION

Results suggest that the development of anticipatory side effects could be avoided or at least significantly reduced by better control of post-treatment nausea and vomiting. The new 5-HT_3 receptor antagonists hold the promise of better emetic control but prescribing policies also require some attention. Waiting until the patient complains of nausea and vomiting before prescribing anti-emetic medication is a poor strategy from the point of view of preventing ANV and greater sensitivity to changing anti-emetic requirements over the course of chemotherapy is required. Provision of optimally effective anti-emetic cover from the outset should be the goal of treatment that aims to prevent the development of ANV.

Greater attention is also beginning to be given to the crucial issue of patient compliance with anti-emetic medication, a factor which has not always been optimal.

Attention to the non pharmacological factors identified as relevant determinants of PTNV suggests that information given to patients may be important in modifying expectations and that anxiety management strategies may facilitate patients' coping. Patients' anxiety mounts during delays experienced waiting for chemotherapy and procedural routines may play a part in differences reported between centres. To the extent that any of these strategies reduces PTNV, they are also relevant to the reduction of anticipatory side effects.

HYPNOSIS

Hypnosis was the first psychological technique to be used in the control of nausea and vomiting. Unfortunately there are more anecdotal reports and case studies than controlled investigations to confirm its efficacy.

Hypnosis appears particularly effective in reducing ANV among children and adolescents (Le Baron and Zeltzer, 1984; Cotanch *et al.*, 1985).

Reeves and colleagues (1983) used hypnosis for pain control in adult cancer patients and observed that these patients also obtained relief of PTNV. To study hypnotic control of ANV they used a multiple baseline design in a series of six single case studies (Redd *et al.*, 1982). Hypnosis eliminated AV for all patients. Anticipatory emesis reappeared when hypnosis was not used and stopped when it was reinstated. Anticipatory nausea was significantly reduced by the introduction of hypnosis. Walker *et al.* (1988) reported significant improvements in both ANV and PTNV when hypnotherapy was offered in 14 patients with particularly severe side effects. Hypnotic control is probably best understood as a self-control technique by which the patient learns to invoke a physiological condition incompatible with nausea and vomiting. Both deep relaxation and distraction techniques are involved and there is evidence that the therapist does not need to be present before or during the chemotherapy, the technique can be self-directed by the patient. Redd and Andrykowski (1982) have pointed out that hypnosis is not universally acceptable and some patients may have misapprehensions about the process. No advantage has been demonstrated for hypnosis relative to other interventions (Carey and Burish, 1988) so reluctant hypnotic subjects may equally be offered an alternative therapy.

RELAXATION TRAINING

In contrast to the more passive relaxation procedures of hypnotic induction, progressive muscle relaxation training (PMRT) is a more active technique involving a series of muscle tensing and relaxing exercises (Jacobsen, 1938; Bernstein and Borkovec, 1973). It is usually supplemented with guided imagery (GI), i.e. thoughts and mental pictures which facilitate relaxation (Turk *et al.*, 1983).

This technique has been widely used in controlled studies which have been well summarized by Carey and Burish (1988). Research shows that quite brief training in PMRT and GI, with practice at home between treatments, can reduce physiological arousal in both patients' and nurses' reports of nausea and anxiety (Lyles *et al.*, 1982; Cotanch, 1983). Data on vomiting are less consistent but start from a low baseline frequency of this symptom in the groups studied.

Burish, who with colleagues has made a major contribution to this field, suggests that relaxation reduces conditioned responses by distracting patients' attention from conditioned stimuli and by reducing autonomic arousal and anxiety thought to mediate the development of ANV (Burish *et al.*, 1985). The emphasis on relaxation as a self-control procedure is seen as beneficial in combating patients' feelings of helplessness in the face of treatment side effects. The effects of PMRT and GI appear strongest during training although modest benefits have been observed during follow-up when patients relaxed themselves. Particularly encouraging is the report from Burish *et al.* (1987) of the value of this technique in preventing or at least delaying development of ANV for patients receiving highly emetogenic therapy. Patients taught to use PMRT and GI before their first cycle of treatment were significantly less likely to have developed ANV by cycle five than no-treatment controls. Levels of PTNV anxiety, depression and hostility were all significantly lower in the treatment group.

Relaxation training is relatively easy to learn (although somewhat expensive of therapist time unless audiotapes are also used), with demonstrable benefits in prophylaxis and treatment of distress and ANV. Thus this is a valuable technique for many patients.

SYSTEMATIC DESENSITIZATION

Systematic desensitization (S.D.) invokes the principles of learning theory to sever a learned association. The patient is taught PMRT and in the relaxed state is gradually exposed to a series of stimuli graded from least to most anxiety provoking. Typically, the stimuli are imaginal although practice *in vivo* can also be used. The object is to have the patient learn a new association between these stimuli and a response incompatible with anxiety, i.e. relaxation. This is classically the treatment approach of choice for combating phobic anxiety and some authors conceptualize ANV as a phobic response to chemotherapy (Raesal *et al.*, 1990).

SD can be a time-consuming procedure but Morrow and Morrell (1982) were able to show a benefit after only two sessions. Desensitized patients showed significantly less ANV than controls who received supportive counselling or no treatment although, interestingly, anxiety was not reduced more in the SD group than for controls.

In a subsequent study comparing these same treatment groups with patients offered PMRT, Morrow (1986) found an advantage to SD over other groups in reduction of AN and anxiety. In a more recent study (Morrow and Dobkin, 1988) he was able to show that medical and nursing staff could use SD to treat patients with ANV as effectively as clinical psychologists.

Having thus overcome the main difficulties with this technique, Morrow and colleagues have demonstrated the utility of systematic desensitization in the treatment of ANV.

OTHER BEHAVIOURAL INTERVENTIONS

Biofeedback has been used by Burish and his colleagues (Burish *et al.*, 1981; Shartner *et al.*, 1985). Both electromyographic and thermal feedback were effective in reducing physiological arousal and patients reported reduction in nausea and negative affect. However, in this study, biofeedback was always used in conjunction with PMRT so no evidence can be obtained on the specific contribution of the biofeedback.

Stress inoculation as a means of helping patients to cope better with unexpected stressors was explored by Moore and Altmaier (1981) but in the absence of objective data its efficacy cannot be evaluated.

There has been considerable interest in the value of external devices such as video games as distractors for paediatric and adolescent patients. Diverting attention from unpleasant sensations and potential conditioned stimuli has proved an effective strategy for reducing anticipatory symptoms and these returned when the distractors were removed (Kolko *et al.*, 1985; Redd *et al.*, 1987). The one published study of distraction in an adult patient (Greene *et al.*, cited in Carey and Burish, 1988) suggested the efficacy of distraction may lessen over time as novelty is lost. Relaxation training introduced at this point was effective and it may be that this self-control technique offers a more enduring response.

INTERVENTION CHOICE

Not all patients will benefit from psychological therapy – as for any intervention – and indeed not all are willing to try. There is a lack of data to identify which patients are more likely to benefit. There is also a lack of comparative studies to determine the relative benefits of different intervention strategies. At present several different therapeutic interventions all appear superior to placebo or no treatment in reducing ANV.

A common theme is the induction of global relaxation, that is a reduction in physiological arousal. The mechanism by which this reduces ANV remains the subject of speculation. However, distraction studies have shown that symptoms can also be reduced without relaxation. All behavioural interventions require the patients' cognitive participation in attending to non-anxiety producing stimuli; this fact has led Carey and Burish (1988) to conclude that cognitive distraction may play an important role in reducing psychological side effects.

10.9 CONCLUSIONS

Anticipatory nausea and vomiting remains a significant clinical problem in patients undergoing cancer therapy. It arises as the result of an associative learning process with a prevalence which reflects those treatment-related factors significant to the learning process and individual differences in susceptibility.

A key factor in the aetiology is the severity of chemotherapy-induced nausea and vomiting. It is hoped that the new 5-HT_3 receptor antagonists will represent a significant advance in anti-emetic control but it is clear that non pharmacological factors are also relevant. Biomedical and psychological research needs to be more closely integrated for optimal clinical management in future.

A number of individual differences are known to be relevant but their physiological basis remains obscure. Anxiety and susceptibility to GI distress seem particularly relevant. Psychological interventions can offer significant relief to the patient suffering from ANV although their mechanisms of action are incompletely understood and the basis for selection of one technique rather than another is likely to be made on pragmatic rather than scientific grounds at present.

REFERENCES

Aaronson, N.K., Bakker, W., Stewart, A.L. *et al.* (1987) 'Multidimensional approach to the measurement of quality of life in lung cancer clinical trials', in *The Quality of Life of Cancer Patients*. (eds N.K. Aaronson and J. Beckmann) Raven Press, New York.

Altmaier, E.M., Ross, W.E. and Moore, K. (1982) A pilot investigation of the psychologic function of patients with anticipatory vomiting. *Cancer*, **49**, 201–4.

Andrykowski, M.A., Redd, W.H. and Hatfield, A.K. (1985) Development of anticipatory nausea: A prospective analysis. *J. Consult. Clin. Psychol.*, **53**, 447–54.

Andrykowski, M.A. (1986) Definitional issues in the study of anticipatory nausea in cancer chemotherapy. *J. Behav. Med.* **9**(1), 33–41.

Andrykowski, M.A. and Redd, W.H. (1987) Longitudinal analysis of the development of anticipatory nausea. *J. Consult. Clin. Psychol.*, **55**(1), 36–41.

Andrykowski, M.A. (1988) Defining anticipatory nausea and vomiting: Differences among cancer chemotherapy patients who report pretreatment nausea. *J. Behav. Med.*, **11**(1), 59–69.

Andrykowski, M.A., Jacobsen, P.B., Marks, E. *et al.*

(1988) Prevalence predictors and course of anticipatory nausea in women receiving adjuvant chemotherapy for breast cancer. *Cancer*, **62**, 2607–13.

Andrykowski, M.A. (1990) The role of anxiety in the development of anticipatory nausea in cancer chemotherapy: a review and synthesis. *Psychosom. Med.*, **52**(4), 458–75.

Bernstein, D.A. and Borkovec, T.D. (1973) Progressive relaxation training: A manual for the helping professions. Research Press, Champaign, IL.

Bernstein, I.L. and Webster, M.M. (1980) Learned taste aversions in humans. *Physiol. Behav.*, **25**, 363–66.

Burish, T.G., Shartner, C.D. and Lyles, J.N. (1981) Effectiveness of multiple site EMG biofeedback and relaxation in reducing the aversiveness of cancer chemotherapy. *Biofeedback Self Regul.*, **6**, 523–35.

Burish, T.G. and Carey, M.P. (1984) 'Conditioned responses to cancer chemotherapy: etiology and treatment', in *Impact of Psychoendocrine Systems in Cancer and Immunity*. (eds B.H. Fox and B.H. Newberry) C.J. Hogrefe, New York.

Burish, T.G., Redd, W.H. and Carey, M.P. (1985) 'Conditioned nausea and vomiting,' in cancer chemotherapy: treatment approaches in *Cancer, Nutrition and Eating Behaviour*. (eds T.G. Burish, S.M. Levy, and B.E. Meyerowitz) Lawrence Earlbaum, New Jersey.

Burish, T.G. and Carey, M.P. (1986) Conditioned aversive responses in cancer chemotherapy patients: Theoretical and developmental analysis. *J. Consult. Clin. Psychol.*, **54**(5), 593–60.

Burish, T.G., Carey, M.P., Krozely, M.G. *et al.* (1987) Conditioned nausea and vomiting induced by cancer chemotherapy. *J. Consult. Clin. Psychol.*, **55**, 42–48.

Carey, M.P. and Burish, T.G. (1988) Etiology and treatment of the psychological side effects associated with cancer chemotherapy: A critical review and discussion. *Psych. Bull.*, **104**(3), 307–25.

Carnrike, C.L.M., Brantley, P.J. and Bruce, B. (1988) Test-retest reliability and concurrent validity of the morrow assessment of nausea and emesis (MANE) for the assessment of cancer chemotherapy related nausea and vomiting. *J. Psychopathol. Behav. Assessment*, **10**(2), 107–16.

Chang, J.C. (1981) Nausea and vomiting in cancer patients: an expression of psychological mechanisms. *Psychosomatics*, **22**, 707–9.

Chang, J.C. (1982) More on psychological mechanisms in patients with nausea and vomiting following chemotherapy. *Psychosomatics*, **23**, 651.

Coates, A., Abraham, S., Kaye, S.B. *et al.* (1983) On the receiving end – patient perception of the side effects of cancer chemotherapy. *Eur. J. Cancer Clin. Oncol.*, **19**(2), 203–8.

Cohen, R.E., Blanchard, E.B., Ruckdeschel, J.C. *et al.* (1986) Prevalence and correlates of post-treatment and anticipatory nausea and vomiting in cancer chemotherapy. *J. Psychosom. Res.*, **30**(6), 643–54.

Coons, H.L. (1981) Conditioned nausea in cancer patients receiving cisplatinum chemotherapy. Unpublished manuscript. University of Wisconsin–Madison. Cited by W.H. Redd and M.A. Andrykowski (1982) in Behavioural intervention in cancer treatment: Controlling aversion reactions to chemotherapy. *J. Consult. Clin. Psych.*, **50**(6), 1018–29.

Cotanch, P. (1983) Relaxation training for control of nausea and vomiting in patients receiving chemotherapy. *Cancer Nurs.*, **6**, 277–83.

Cotanch, P., Hockenberry, M. and Herman, S. (1985) Self hypnosis and antiemetic therapy in children receiving chemotherapy. *Oncol. Nurs. Forum*, **12**, 41–46.

De Haes, J.C.J.M., Pruyn, J.F.A. and Knippenberg, F.C.E. (1983) Klachtenlijst voor kankerpatienten. Eerste ervarigen. *Nederlands Tijdshirift voor de Psychologie*, **38**, 403–22.

Derogatis, L.R., Abeloff, M.D. and Melisaratos, N. (1979) Psychological coping mechanisms and survival time in metastatic breast cancer. *J. Amer. Med. Assoc.*, **242**, 1504–8.

Dolgin, M.J., Siegel, S.E. and Katz, E.R. (1985) Conditioned aversions in paediatric cancer patients receiving chemotherapy. Paper presented to the Society of Behavioural Medicine. Cited in T.G. Burish and M.P. Carey (11), New Orleans.

Fetting, J.H., Wilcox, P.M., Iwata, B.A. *et al.* (1983) Anticipatory nausea and vomiting in an ambulatory oncology population. *Cancer Treat. Reports*, **67**, 1093–98.

Fordyce, W.E. (1973) An operant conditioning method for managing chronic pain. *Post Grad. Medicine*, **53**, 123–24.

Forrest, J.B., Beattie, W.S. and Goldsmith, C.H. (1990) Risk factors for nausea and vomiting after general anaesthesia. *Can. J. Anaesth.*, **37**(4), Part II, 590.

Ganz, P.A., Haskell, C.M., Figlin, R.A. *et al.* (1988) Estimating the quality of life in a clinical trial of patients with metastatic lung cancer using the Karnofsky Performance Status and the Functional Living Index – Cancer. *Cancer*, **61**, 849–56.

Garcia, J., and Koelling, R.A. (1966) Relation of cause to consequence in avoidance learning. *Psychonomic Sci.*, **4**, 123–24.

Grant, V.L. (1987) Do conditioned taste aversions result from activation of emetic mechanisms? *Psychopharmacology*, **93**, 405–15.

Greene, P.G., Seime, R.J. and Smith, M.E. Distraction and relaxation training in the treatment of anticipatory nausea and vomiting: A single subject intervention cited in Carey, M.P. and Burish, T.G. (1988) *Psychol. Bull*, **104**, 307–25.

Jacobsen, E. (1938) Progressive relaxation. Univ. of Chicago, Chicago ILL.

Jacobsen, P.B., Redd, W.H. and Holland, J.C. (1985) Parameters of chemotherapy-induced anticipatory nausea in cancer patients. Paper presented to the Society of Behavioural Medicine, New Orleans. Cited in Burish and Carey (1986).

Jacobsen, P.B., Andrykowski, M.A., Redd, W.H. *et al.* (1986) Non pharmacologic factors in the development of post-treatment nausea with adjuvant chemotherapy for breast cancer. *Cancer*, **61**, 379–85.

Kolko, D.J. and Rickhard-Figueroa, J.L. (1985) Effects of video games on the adverse corollaries of chemotherapy in paediatric oncology patients: A simple case analysis. *J. Consult. Clin. Psychol.*, **53**, 223–28.

Le Baron, S. and Zeltzer, L.K. (1984) Behavioural intervention for reducing chemotherapy related nausea and vomiting in adolescents with cancer. *J. Adolescent Health Care*, **5**, 178–82.

Leventhal, H., Easterling, D.V., Nerenz, D.R. *et al.* (1988) The role of motion sickness in predicting anticipatory nausea. *J. Behav. Med.*, **11**(2), 117–30.

Lindley, C.M., Bernard, S. and Fields, S.M. (1989) Incidence and duration of chemotherapy induced nausea and vomiting in the Outpatient Oncology population. *J. Clin. Oncol.*, **7**, 1142–49.

Lindley, C.M., Hirsch, J.D., O'Neill, C.V. *et al.* (1991) Consequences of chemotherapy induced emesis in an outpatient oncology population. *J. Clin. Oncol.* In press.

Love, R.R., Nerenz, D.R. and Leventhal, H. (1983) Anticipatory nausea with cancer chemotherapy: Development through two mechanisms. *Proc. Am. Soc. Clin. Oncol.*, **242**(67).

Love, R.R., Leventhal, H., Easterling, D.V. *et al.* (1989) Side effects and emotional distress during cancer chemotherapy. *Cancer*, **63**, 604–12.

Lyles, J.N., Burish, T.G., Krozely, M.G. *et al.* (1982) Efficacy of relaxation training and guided imagery in reducing the aversiveness of cancer chemotherapy. *J. Consult. Clin. Psychol.*, **50**, 509–24.

McNair, D.M., Lorr, M. and Doppleman, L.F. (1981) EITS manual for the profile of mood states. Educational and Industrial Testing Service, San Diego.

Moore, K., and Altmaier, E.M. (1981) Stress inoculation training with cancer patients. *Cancer Nurs.*, **4**, 389–93.

Morrow, G.R. (1982) Prevalence and correlates of anticipatory nausea and vomiting in chemotherapy patients. *JNCI*, **68**(4), 585–8.

Morrow, G.R., Arseneau, J.C., Asbury, R.F. *et al.* (1982) Anticipatory nausea and vomiting with chemotherapy. *N. Eng. J. Med.*, **306**, 431–32.

Morrow, G.R. and Morrell, C. (1982) Behavioural treatment for the anticipatory nausea and vomiting induced by cancer chemotherapy. *N. Engl. J. Med.*, **307**, 1476–80.

Morrow, G.R. (1984) The assessment of nausea and vomiting. *Cancer*, **53**(10) (Suppl) 2267–78.

Morrow, G.R. (1984) Clinical characteristics associated with the development of anticipatory nausea and vomiting in cancer patients undergoing chemotherapy treatment. *J. Clin. Oncol.* **2**(10), 1170–76.

Morrow, G.R. (1985) The effect of susceptibility to motion sickness on the side effects of cancer chemotherapy. *Cancer*, **55**, 2766–70.

Morrow, G.R. (1986) Effect of the cognitive hierarchy in the systematic desensitisation treatment of anticipatory nausea, in *Cancer Patients: A Component Comparison with Relaxation Only, Counselling and No Treatment. Cog. Therapy Res.*, **10**, 421–46.

Morrow, G.R. and Dobkin, P.L. (1988) Anticipatory nausea and vomiting in cancer patients undergoing chemotherapy treatment: prevalence aetiology and behavioural interventions. *Clin. Psychol. Rev.*, **8**, 517–56.

Morrow, G. (1991) Anticipatory nausea and emesis: A physiological response or phobia? Paper presented at Emesis Round Table, Chartres. (in preparation).

Morrow, G.R., Lindke, J.L. and Black, P.M. (1991) Predicting development of anticipatory nausea in cancer patients: Prospective examination of eight clinical characteristics. *J. Pain Symptom Management*, **6**, 4, 215–23.

Morrow, G.R., Lindke, J. and Black, P.M. Anticipatory nausea development in cancer patients: Replication and extension of a learning model. *Brit. J. Psych.* (in press).

Nerenz, D.R., Leventhal, H. and Love, R.R. (1982) Factors contributing to emotional distress during cancer chemotherapy. *Cancer*, **50**, 1020–27.

Nerenz, D.R., Leventhal, H. and Love, R.R. (1983) The relationship of age and disease status to emotional distress from chemotherapy for breast cancer. *Proc. Am. Soc. Clin. Oncol.*, **243**, 62.

Nerenz, D.R., Leventhal, H., Love, R.R. *et al.* (1984) Psychological aspects of cancer chemotherapy. *Int. J. App. Psych.*, **30**, 521–29.

Nerenz, D.R., Leventhal, H., Easterling, D.V. *et al.* (1986) Anxiety and drug taste as predictors of anticipatory nausea in cancer chemotherapy. *J. Clin. Oncol.*, **4**, 224–33.

Nesse, R.M., Carli, Curtis, G.C. *et al.* (1980) Pretreatment nausea in cancer chemotherapy: a conditional response. *Psychosom. Med.*, **42**, 33–36.

Nicholas, D.C. (1982) Prevalence of anticipatory nausea and emesis in cancer chemotherapy patients. *J. Behav. Med.*, **5**, 461–63.

Pavlov, I.P. (1927) *Conditioned Reflexes: An Investigation of Physiological Activity of the Cerebral Cortex.* Oxford University Press, Oxford.

Penta, J., Poster, D. and Bruno, S. (1983) The pharmacologic treatment of nausea and vomiting caused by cancer chemotherapy: A review in *Antiemetics and Cancer Chemotherapy.* (ed J. Laszlo) Williams & Wilkins, Baltimore.

Raesal, R.T., Bajramovic, H. and Mai, F. (1990) Anticipatory nausea and vomiting: a form of chemotherapy phobia? *Can. J. Psychiat.* **35**(1), 80–82.

Redd, W.H., Andresen, G.V. and Minagawa, R.Y. (1982) Hypnotic control of anticipatory emesis in patients receiving cancer chemotherapy. *J. Consult. Clin. Psychol.*, **50**, 14–19.

Redd, W.H. and Andrykowski, M.A. (1982) Behavioural intervention in cancer treatment: Controlling aversion reactions to chemotherapy. *J. Consult. Clin. Psychol.*, **50**(6), 1018–29.

Redd, W.H., Burish, T.G. and Andrykowski, M.A. (1985) Aversive conditioning and cancer chemotherapy, in *Cancer Nutrition and Eating Behaviour: A Biobehavioural Perspective.* (eds T.G. Burish, S.M. Levy and B.E. Meyerowitz) Lawrence Earlbaum, New Jersey.

Redd, W.H., Jacobsen, P.B., Die Trill, M. *et al.* (1987) Cognitive attentional distraction in the control of conditioned nausea in paediatric cancer patients receiving chemotherapy. *J. Consult. Clin. Psychol.*, **55**, 391–95.

Reeves, J.L., Redd, W.H., Minagawa, R.Y. *et al.* (1983) Hypnosis in the control of pain during hyperthermia treatment of cancer, in *Advances in Pain Research and Therapy.* (eds J.J. Bonica, U. Lindbland and A. Iggo) Raven Press, New York.

Rescorla, R.A. (1988) Pavlovian conditioning: Its not what you think it is. *Amer. Psychologist*, **43**(3), 151–60.

Robertson, R.G. and Garcia, J. (1985) X-rays and learned taste aversions: Historical and psychological ramifications, in *Cancer Nutrition and Eating Behaviour: A Biobehavioural Perspective.* (eds T.G. Burish, S.M. Levy and B.E. Meyerowitz) Lawrence Earlbaum, New Jersey.

Schipper, H., Clinch, J., McMurray, A. *et al.* (1984) Measuring the quality of life of cancer patients. The functional living index – Cancer: development and validation. *J. Clin. Oncol.*, **2**, 472–83.

Schultz, L.S. (1980) Classical (Pavlovian) conditioning of nausea and vomiting in cancer chemotherapy. *Proc. Am. Soc. Clin. Oncol.*, **21**(C), 244.

Seligman, M.E.P. (1970) On the generality of the laws of learning. *Psych. Rev.*, **77**(5), 406–18.

Shartner, C.D., Burish, T.G. and Carey, M.P. (1985) Effectiveness of biofeedback with progressive muscle relaxation training in reducing the aversiveness of cancer chemotherapy: A preliminary report. *Jpn. J. of Biofeedback Res.*, **12**, 33–40.

Stefanek, M.E., Sheidler, V.R. and Fetting, J.H. (1988) Anticipatory nausea and vomiting: Does it remain a significant clinical problem? *Cancer*, **62**, 2654–57.

Stunkard, A., Foster, G., Glassman, J. *et al.* (1985) Retrospective exaggeration of symptoms: vomiting after gastric surgery for obesity. *Psychosom. Med.*, **47**, 150–55.

Spence, K.W. (1958) A theory of emotionally based drive (D) and its relation to performance in simple learning situations. *Amer. Psychologist*, **13**, 131–41.

Spence, K.W. (1964) Anxiety (drive) level and performance in eyelid conditioning. *Psych. Bull.*, **61**, 129–39.

Spielberger, C.D., Gorlisch, R.L., and Lushene, R.E. (1969) The State–Trait Anxiety Inventory: Manual. Consulting Psychologists, Press Inc., Palo Alto.

Teplov, B.M. (1964) 'Problems in the study of general types of higher nervous activity in man and animals', in *Pavlov's Typology*. (ed J.A. Gray) Pergamon Press, Oxford.

Turk, D.C., Meichenbaum, D. and Genest, M. (1983) Pain and behavioural medicine: a cognitive–behavioural prospective. Guilford, New York.

van Komen, R.W. and Redd, W.H. (1985) Personality factors associated with anticipatory nausea/vomiting in patients receiving cancer chemotherapy. *Health Psychol.*, **4**(3), 198–202.

Walker, L.G., Dawson, A.A., Pollet, S.M. *et al.* (1988) Hypnotherapy for chemotherapy side effects. *Br. J. Exp. Clin. Hypnosis*, **5**(2), 79–82.

Wilcox, P.M., Fetting, J.H., Nettesheim, K.M., *et al.* (1982) Anticipatory vomiting in women receiving cyclophosphamide methotrexate and 5FU adjuvant chemotherapy for breast carcinoma. *Cancer Treat. Rep.*, **66**, 1601–3.

Zook, D.J. and Yasko, J.M. (1983) Psychologic factors: Their effect on nausea and vomiting experienced by clients receiving chemotherapy. *Oncol. Nurs. Forum*, **10**, 76–81.

11

The clinical care of patients receiving chemotherapy

A.L. JONES and D. CUNNINGHAM

11.1 INTRODUCTION

The side-effects of chemotherapy are variable and depend on the drug or combination regimen which is used, however, most cytotoxic drugs cause emesis to some extent. Until recently, despite the widespread use of anti-emetic prophylaxis, up to 30% of patients receiving chemotherapy still experienced nausea or vomiting (Craig and Powell, 1983). Nausea and vomiting are considered by patients as among the most distressing side-effects of chemotherapy (Coates *et al.*, 1983) and have a negative impact on quality of life which is particularly important when chemotherapy is used as palliation in incurable disease. Suboptimal anti-emetic prophylaxis may lead to non-compliance with treatment possibly resulting in the curtailment of potentially curative treatment such as adjuvant chemotherapy. It has been estimated that between 10–15% of patients may delay or stop treatment because of problems with severe emesis.

A large number of anti-emetic drugs with different mechanisms of action are available but, until recently, their use has been somewhat empirical, relying on polypharmacy. The development of more highly emetogenic chemotherapy, including cisplatin-based and high dose drug regimens which are now more widely used, has necessitated new strategies for anti-emetic control. Over the last decade there has been an increased understanding of the physiology that underlies emesis (Borison and McCarthy, 1983). This knowledge, together with the development of methodology to conduct carefully controlled, prospective randomized anti-emetic trials (Willan, 1984; Olver *et al.*, 1976), has allowed a more rational use of the anti-emetic drugs which are already in general use, and has also resulted in the development of newer anti-emetic drugs with specific sites of action, in particular the serotonin receptor (5-HT_3) antagonists.

In this chapter the factors influencing the selection of appropriate anti-emetic prophylaxis based on patient characteristics and the drug regimen concerned are discussed, with particular reference to the problems of delayed and anticipatory emesis. The design of anti-emetic trials is reviewed and the role of oncology nursing staff in the clinical management of cancer patients undergoing treatment is also discussed.

Emesis in Anti-cancer Therapy
Mechanisms and treatment
Published in 1993 by Chapman & Hall, London
ISBN 0 412 37250 9

Table 11.1 Factors affecting emetic responses to chemotherapy

Patient factors	Previous emesis during chemotherapy (poor control → anticipatory vomiting) Age Alcohol intake Emesis during pregnancy Prior history of motion sickness Sex
Chemotherapy	Emetic potential of chemotherapy drug Dose of chemotherapy drug Schedule of chemotherapy drug Combination chemotherapy regimens Route of administration Time of administration
Anti-emetic drug	Dose and schedule Toxicity

11.2 SELECTION OF ANTI-EMETIC SCHEDULES

11.2.1 PATIENT SUSCEPTIBILITY

A number of patient characteristics may be relevant in determining individual susceptibility to emesis following chemotherapy (Table 11.1). In practice these characteristics do not usually influence the choice of anti-emetic drugs as selection is determined by the emetic potential of the chemotherapy regimen under consideration. Age, however, does have an indirect influence on the choice of anti-emetic drugs. This is because of the risk of side-effects of anti-emetic drugs; younger patients (less than 30 years old), for example, are more likely to experience dystonic reactions with dopamine receptor antagonists such as metoclopramide, especially when used at high dose or with the repeated dose schedules (Kris *et al.*, 1983). For metoclopramide, the incidence of *trismus* or *torticollis* has been reported at 27% in patients under the age of 30 compared with only 2% in those over 30 years (op. cit.).

A history of a chronic high alcohol intake (>100 g/day) may predict for successful anti-emetic control: however, it is still essential that adequate anti-emetic schedules are used in these patients (D'Acquisto *et al.*, 1986; Sullivan *et al.*, 1983). Female patients are more susceptible to emesis than men, especially those women who have experienced severe emesis during pregnancy. Patients with a history of motion sickness are also more susceptible to chemotherapy-induced emesis (Morrow, 1984).

A major factor influencing emesis is the degree of emetic control achieved with previous chemotherapy, since those patients who fail to achieve adequate emetic control on one course of chemotherapy are more likely to fail on subsequent courses. This is in part due to the development of anticipatory vomiting and emphasizes the necessity for effective anti-emetic control with the initial cycle of chemotherapy (Morrow, 1982).

Patients receiving chemotherapy may also have concurrent medical problems or cancer-related problems such as subacute intestinal obstruction, metabolic disturbances including hypercalcaemia and renal failure, or brain metastasis – all of these may in themselves cause emesis and require a different approach for symptom control. The use of opiate analgesia and antibiotics may also compound chemotherapy-induced emesis and therefore it is important to consider non-malignant causes of emesis in all cancer patients to ensure optimal control of emesis.

11.2.2 EMETIC CHALLENGE AND ACUTE EMESIS

The emetic potential of cytotoxic drugs varies with different drugs. However, those drugs that most commonly cause emesis are also

Table 11.2 Emetic potential of cytotoxic drugs

Highly emetogenic	Cisplatin Mustine Dacarbazine Cyclophosphamide (i.v. ≥1000 mg/m²) Melphalan (i.v. ≥100 mg/m²)
Moderately emetogenic	Carboplatin Daunorubicin Carmustine Lomustine Dactinomycin Epirubicin Cytarabine Procarbazine Mitoxantrone 5-fluorouracil (i.v. bolus) Etoposide (i.v.)
Low emetic potential	Etoposide (oral) Mitomycin C Methotrexate Bleomycin Chlorambucil 5-fluorouracil (continuous infusion) Melphalan (oral) Vinblastine Vincristine

those that are likely to result in the most severe emesis; these are listed in Table 11.2. Cisplatin and dacarbazine induce emesis which is often severe in over 90% of patients. Most commonly used chemotherapy regimens are considered as moderately emetogenic causing emesis in 30–90% of patients. It has been suggested that the emetogenicity of cytotoxic drugs may depend in part on their ability to damage DNA; hence, drugs which do not affect DNA (e.g. vinca alkaloids) have a very low emetic potential (Carl *et al.*, 1989). The severity of emesis caused by a given cytotoxic drug is also dose-dependent and in combination regimens the individual emetogenic potential of each component drug must be considered when planning anti-emetic prophylaxis.

The acute phase of emesis is described as occurring within the first 24 hours following chemotherapy with the onset of nausea and vomiting usually within 2–4 hours of treatment, with maximum emesis persisting for 6–8 hours. Acute emesis occurs to some degree with all drugs with a moderate or high emetogenic potential. Cyclophosphamide and other pro-drugs which are metabolized to an active form are an exception to this pattern and have a later onset of emesis at 9–18 hours after chemotherapy (Fetting *et al.*, 1982).

11.2.3 DELAYED EMESIS

Acute emesis and its underlying mechanisms are well documented and even with highly emetogenic drugs such as cisplatin, control of acute emesis can now be achieved in 70–80% of patients (Kris *et al.*, 1985). The problem of delayed emesis which starts 24 hours after chemotherapy and may persist for up to seven to ten days has more recently been identified and the underlying mechanisms are less clear (Kris *et al.*, 1985; Lindley *et al.*, 1989). Delayed emesis may occur even when there has been complete control of acute emesis; however, it is more frequently observed in those patients who do not achieve complete control. In the out-patient setting 52% and 33% of patients reported nausea and vomiting only in the delayed period of emesis (Lindley *et al.*, 1989). Delayed emesis is a particular feature of cisplatin therapy with most patients experiencing some degree of emesis 48–72 hours after cisplatin doses in excess of 100 mg/m². Although delayed emesis is generally less severe than acute emesis in terms of vomiting, persistent nausea represents a major cause of morbidity and if severe and prolonged can interfere with the patient's nutritional status.

11.2.4 ANTICIPATORY EMESIS

This represents a conditioned response that occurs in 10–15% with patients who experience nausea and/or vomiting even prior to chemotherapy (Morrow, 1982). Anticipatory emesis is most likely to develop in those patients who have had poor emetic control with previous cycles of treatment and is often difficult to control although centrally acting drugs (the benzodiazepines, for example, which have an amnesic effect) may help especially when given 24 hours before chemotherapy is due. Behavioural therapy and desensitization may also be used.

11.2.5 RADIOTHERAPY

Radiotherapy may also cause nausea and vomiting; the degree of this depends on the site to be irradiated, the volume of the irradiated field, and the fractionation schedule, i.e. the amount of radiation to be given with each treatment. Large fields, for example, total body irradiation, or fields involving the gut, are highly emetogenic and most patients will experience emesis; in contrast, fields involving peripheral limbs or lung have a relatively low emetogenic potential. Lower total doses of radiation or a high dose with a large number of fractions are also less emetogenic.

11.3 ASSESSMENT OF RESPONSE

The assessment of anti-emetic response is complex and, ideally, it should include a separate evaluation of nausea, retching and vomiting both for the acute phase of emesis (first 24 hours) and the delayed phase (day 2 to day 5). Patients in trials should be monitored by a trained observer to record the number, timing and intensity of each emetic response during the acute phase with accurate timing of the onset and termination of symptoms. Anti-emetic trials can also be conducted on outpatients using diary cards filled in by the patients to document emesis. This is particularly useful for assessment of delayed emesis. In both the inpatient and outpatient setting, an oncology nurse is often the most appropriate person to monitor the patients and to ensure accurate administration of the trial drugs and also to monitor compliance if the trial drug is given orally.

Emetic episodes are usually defined as any episode of vomiting or any amount of retching within a five-minute period. Episodes of retching which occur more than five minutes apart are considered as separate emetic episodes. Patients who experience more than five emetic episodes within a 24-hour period are generally considered to have failed treatment and would be considered for 'rescue' medication. The number of episodes defined as 'failure', however, may vary between trials and the criteria should be clearly stated. Nausea may be perceived as one of the worst problems of chemotherapy by patients and should be evaluated separately. Pretreatment and post-treatment nausea can be assessed using a visual analogue scale (VAS), or categorical scale, with the difference between the scores used as a measure of overall nausea.

The toxicity attributed to anti-emetic drugs must be monitored carefully as patient preference, which forms an important component of the assessment of an anti-emetic trial, may be determined as much by toxicity as by anti-emetic efficacy.

11.3.1 ANTI-EMETIC TRIALS

Preclinical data can indicate a likely dose and schedule for anti-emetic drugs, but the lack of a dependable animal model necessitates human studies to determine optimal therapy. With a new anti-emetic agent, uncontrolled trials can determine possible activity, but ultimately controlled trials with comparison against standard therapy are required to define the precise role and usage of an individual drug.

Ideally, anti-emetic trials should employ a prospective randomized double-blind design with careful attention to stratification before randomization to avoid bias due to patient characteristics which affect emesis during chemotherapy – age, alcohol consumption and concurrent drugs, for example (Pater and Willan, 1984; Olver *et al.*, 1976). Patients in anti-emetic trials should be naive to chemotherapy or radiotherapy to avoid any problems of anticipatory vomiting. The emetogenic potential of the chemotherapy regimens must be similar for both arms. A crossover design using patients as their own controls minimizes the variance in results for a given sample size.

This crossover approach can be criticized if the efficacy of treatments varies between the two periods (the so-called 'period' effect) (Olver *et al.*, 1976). This interaction may occur if the emetic stimulus differs between courses or if patients are lost to the study after the first treatment period or if the relative efficacy of the two treatments is different either due to poor control of emesis or to an alteration in the patient's clinical status. Careful statistical analysis of any interaction between treatments and study periods should allow detection of a 'period' effect.

Despite carefully designed trials, the evaluation of efficacy of different drugs is still problematic partly because of variance in criteria of response between different investigators. This may arise when nausea and vomiting are considered together rather than separately and when vomiting and retching are evaluated differently.

11.4 ANTI-EMETIC AGENTS

A number of anti-emetic agents are in common use and their pharmacology has been discussed in previous chapters. The choice of anti-emetic schedule depends on the emetic challenge and patient characteristics. Guidelines about the use of these drugs are given in Table 11.3. No single drug has proven ideal, giving complete control of emesis and no toxicity, and therefore combinations of different anti-emetics are frequently used to improve emetic control.

11.4.1 PHENOTHIAZINES

Phenothiazines are useful anti-emetic agents against motion sickness and other forms of emesis not related to chemotherapy. Although structure-activity studies have suggested that prochlorperazine should be the most active drug in this class, in practice, prochlorperazine is less effective than other non-phenothiazine drugs such as metoclopramide or dexamethasone (Gralla *et al.*, 1981; Markman *et al.*, 1984). Chlorpromazine has been shown to be more effective than prochlorperazine with anti-emetic control in approximately 50% of non-platinum-containing chemotherapy regimens (Cunningham *et al.*, 1987). The dose of all phenothiazines is limited by unpleasant side-effects including sedation, dry mouth and extrapyramidal reactions which are unacceptable to patients.

11.4.2 CORTICOSTEROIDS

Corticosteroids have well defined anti-emetic activity against regimens of moderate emetogenicity (Markman *et al.*, 1984; Cunningham *et al.*, 1987; Aapro *et al.*, 1983; Chiara *et al.*, 1987; D'Olimpio *et al.*, 1985). There are no apparent therapeutic differences between different corticosteroids such as dexamethasone, methylprednisolone; comparative studies, however, have not been conducted. Dexamethasone as an anti-emetic drug is the most commonly used steroid in the United Kingdom. The mechanism of its anti-emetic action is unclear but may involve inhibition of prostaglandin synthesis or alteration of the blood–brain barrier (Livera *et al.*, 1985; Rich *et al.*, 1980). The apparent anti-emetic activity of progestins such as megestrol acetate used to treat cachexia

Table 11.3 Dose and schedule of commonly used anti-emetic drugs

Drug	Route	Dose and schedule	Frequency
Metoclopramide	i.v.	1–2 mg/kg in 100 ml N/saline over 15 minutes	30 minutes before chemotherapy and repeated 2 and 4 hours later
	po	20 mg	q.d.s. 3–4 days
Dexamethasone	i.v.	8 mg in 10 ml N/saline over 2–3 minutes	With chemotherapy
	po	4 mg	t.d.s. 3–4 days
Lorazepam	i.v.	1–2 mg/m^2 in 50 ml N/saline over 15 minutes	30 minutes before chemotherapy and repeat at 2–4 hours
	po	1–2 mg	24 hours and 12 hours prior to chemotherapy (for anticipatory vomiting)
Ondansetron	i.v.	8 mg slow injection*	15 minutes before chemotherapy
	po	8 mg*	b.d. 3–4 days
Chlorpromazine	i.v./i.m.	25 mg	3–6 hours
	po	25–50 mg	3–6 hours
Haloperidol	i.v.	1–3 mg	3-6 hours
	po	1.5–3 mg	b.d. to q.d.s.
Nabilone	po	2 mg	6–12 hours

* local, not manufacturer's recommendations

may suggest a common steroid receptor pathway (Loprinizi *et al.*, 1990). Corticosteroids also have anti-emetic activity against highly emetogenic chemotherapy but in this situation they are usually used in combination with other anti-emetics such as metoclopramide or serotonin receptor antagonists (Kris *et al.*, 1985; Loprinizi *et al.*, 1990; Jones *et al.*, 1991). Although caution is necessary when using steroids in diabetic patients, short courses of steroids are generally well tolerated with minimal problems of fluid retention and dyspepsia.

11.4.3 CANNABINOIDS

There are two cannabinoids in clinical use as anti-emetics, 9 tetrahydrocannabinol (THC) and a semisynthetic agent nabilone which has structural similarities to THC. THC has greater anti-emetic efficacy than prochlorperazine (Sallan *et al.*, 1980) but optimal anti-emetic control with THC is seen at doses which cause dysphoria, hypotension and dizziness in up to 30% of patients. The incidence of these side-effects is higher in elderly patients. Similar side-effects are seen with nabilone although these are less reduced at lower doses in combination with prochlorperazine (Cunningham *et al.*, 1985). Both cannabinoids have unpredictable absorption by the oral route and are lipid-soluble. Consequently they have a long biological half-life and repeated dosing may result in drug accumulation with an increased incidence of side-effects. There is currently relatively little role for cannabinoids in anti-emetic prophylaxis given the wide availability of more active and less toxic drugs.

11.4.4 BUTYROPHENONES

Both droperidol and haloperidol are effective anti-emetic drugs although ideally they should be given by continuous intravenous or subcutaneous infusion because of their extensive first pass metabolism and short half-lives. Their side-effects are similar to those of phenothiazines (dystonia, dry mouth, sedation) and are a consequence of their activity as dopamine receptor antagonists. Anti-emetic activity is dose-dependent and because of increased toxicity at effective doses, their use as prophylaxis in patients receiving chemotherapy is limited (Bakowski, 1984; Grunberg *et al.*, 1984).

11.4.5 BENZODIAZEPINES

The anti-emetic activity of lorazepam was reported in 1981 (Maher, 1985) but the clinical use of lorazepam and other benzodiazepines as anti-emetics is limited by side-effects, including sedation, which may preclude their use in the outpatient setting. The amnesic and anxiolytic properties of lorazepam, however, may be useful to reduce anticipatory vomiting when these drugs are given at least 24 hours prior to chemotherapy (Lazlo *et al.*, 1985). These amnesic properties may have contributed to patient preference for lorazepam rather than metoclopramide in one comparative study (Bowcock *et al.*, 1984). The development of shorter acting oral benzodiapenes could be useful in anti-emetic prophylaxis. Lorazepam can be used in combination with other anti-emetics such as metoclopramide to reduce the severity of extrapyramidal reactions (Kris *et al.*, 1987).

11.4.6 SUBSTITUTED BENZAMIDES

Metoclopramide is the most commonly used drug in this class; however, at conventional oral doses – 10–20 mg three to four times a day – it is has little efficacy as an anti-emetic and activity induced in controlled trials was no more effective than a placebo (Gralla, 1983). When metoclopramide is given as a short intravenous infusion over 15 minutes at higher dose (2 ng/kg) before chemotherapy and a further two times within the first 24 hours, it is effective in the treatment of acute emesis induced by both moderately and highly emetogenic regimens including platinum-based chemotherapy. This schedule has been shown to be superior to phenothiazines, dexamethasone and cannabinoids in controlled trials (Cunningham *et al.*, 1985; Meyer *et al.*, 1984). For patients receiving cisplatin, high-dose metoclopramide affords complete control of emesis in 20–40% of patients, and for those patients receiving moderately emetogenic chemotherapy, control is 60% or greater. This level of control still means that a substantial number of patients experience significant emesis. High dose metoclopramide, however, has been the best single agent available thus far prior to the development of the selective 5-HT_3 receptor antagonists (below).

The efficacy of metoclopramide has been correlated with the attainment of high blood drug levels (> 850 ng/ml) (Meyer *et al.*, 1984) and is also dependent on the maintenance of steady state levels (Kerr *et al.*, 1985). These therapeutic blood levels can also be achieved using high oral doses of metoclopramide (50–100 mg) and in a randomized trial complete or major control of emesis was achieved in two thirds of patients receiving high dose metoclopramide both by the oral and by the intravenous route (Anthony *et al.*, 1986).

Although effective control of emesis can be achieved using high-dose metoclopramide there are a number of side-effects including sedation, akathisia and dystonic reactions which may develop, especially in patients under the age of 30 years (Kris *et al.*, 1983). The overall incidence of extrapyramidal side-effects is 10–15%. Extrapyramidal reactions can be significantly decreased by the concurrent administration of benzotropine or lorazepam although this may be at the expense of increased sedation (Kris *et al.*, 1987). These side-effects are due to dopamine receptor blockade. At high doses the anti-emetic activity of metoclopramide is also due to serotonin receptor blockade (Fozard and Mobarok Ali, 1978) providing a rationale for the development of selective serotonin receptor anta-gonists which would not have unwanted side-effects associated with dopamine receptor antagonism.

11.4.7 SEROTONIN RECEPTOR ANTAGONISTS

The development of selective serotonin receptor antagonists has resulted in a class of drugs which are highly effective anti-emetics but without the classical adverse reactions associated with dopamine receptor blockade. A number of serotonin receptor antagonists have now been studied in clinical trials. These drugs include ondansetron (GR38032F; Glaxo), granisetron (BRL-43694A; SmithKline Beecham), tropisetron (ICS205-930; Sandoz), MDL 72222 (Merrell Dow), batanopride (Bristol-Myers Squibb) and RG12915 (Rhône-Poulenc Rorer). Much of the early work focused on the first available drugs in this class, ondansetron and granisetron, both of which are highly effective anti-emetics. So far there have been no trials published of direct comparative trials between different serotonin receptor antagonists and any differences in potency between these drugs still have to be inferred from preclinical data and individual trials. The available evidence, however, suggests that these drugs appear similar in terms of efficacy and side-effects, although there may be some differences in convenience of use.

In open, uncontrolled studies (Table 11.4'A'), serotonin receptor antagonists were effective in the prophylaxis of platinum-induced emesis with complete or major control in approximately two-thirds of patients. Both ondansetron and granisetron have also been shown to be effective against radiation-induced emesis, including TBI, with over 50% of patients achieving complete control of TBI-induced emesis with a single injection of granisetron (Hunter *et al.*, 1991). Serotonin receptor antagonists have also been shown to be effective in control of emesis induced by moderately emetogenic chemotherapy in up to 20% of patients and also effective in the control of emesis refractory to conventional anti-emetic drugs including dexamethasone and metoclopramide.

Both ondansetron and granisetron have been subject to comparative trials against other anti-emetics (Table 11.4'B', above). When evaluating these trials it is important to ensure that the comparator involved represents optimal conventional anti-emetic prophylaxis as trials using low dose metoclopramide, for example with platinum-based chemotherapy, would not provide a valid basis for comparison. Ondansetron given as a continuous infusion was superior to high dose intravenous metoclopramide (2–3 mg/kg) against acute emesis with cisplatin (50–100 mg/kg), with 70% of patients achieving complete or major control with ondansetron compared with the 40% on metoclopramide (Marty *et al.*, 1990; Hainsworth *et al.*, 1991; De Mulder *et al.*, 1990). There were no differences in the control of delayed emesis measured by vomiting in these studies although control of delayed nausea was superior with metoclopramide. Despite failure to control delayed emesis, patient pre-ference was for ondansetron, probably because of the lower incidence of adverse events such as extrapyramidal reactions. Ondansetron has been shown to be effective against emesis induced by moderately emetogenic chemotherapy with 70–80% complete/major control against cyclophosphamide-containing regimens (Cubeddu *et al.*, 1990) and was more effective than low dose oral metoclopramide (Schmoll, 1989; Bonneterre *et al.*, 1990) although this was not an ideal comparator.

Ondansetron has also been shown to be safe and effective in pediatric patients receiving chemotherapy (Carden *et al.*, 1990).

Comparative studies with granisetron have used a combination of metoclopramide with dexamethasone as the comparator. This has been shown to be an effective combination for both highly and moderately emetogenic chemotherapy and superior to either agent alone, and as such may provide a better basis for comparative studies (Kris *et al.*, 1987; O'Brien *et al.*, 1989). In one study, granisetron was as effective as this combination with 70% complete or major control against high dose cisplatin (>50 mg/m^2) (Chevallier, 1990). For moderately emetogenic chemotherapy, granisetron was superior to a combination of chlorpromazine and dexamethasone (70% versus 49% complete/major control) with fewer side-effects (Marty, 1990). Another serotonin receptor antagonist, tropisetron, has also been shown to be more effective than haloperidol against emesis induced by high-dose alkylating therapy (Bregini *et al.*, 1991). Both ondansetron and granisetron remain effective during repeated courses of chemotherapy.

There are fewer reported trials using serotonin receptor antagonists for emesis induced by radiotherapy; again, however, both ondansetron and granisetron appear to be equally effective (Priestman, 1989; Hunter *et al.*, 1991). Comparative studies have only used a low dose of metoclopramide as a comparator and therefore the relative potency of these drugs with respect to radiation-induced emesis needs further evaluation.

Initial studies with ondansetron used infusional i.v. therapy at doses of 0.04–0.35 mg/kg over a 24-hour period because of the short half-life (approx. 3 hours) of the drug. Subsequent studies have used short i.v. infusions of ondansetron or bolus doses followed by repeat i.v. or oral doses. Oral ondansetron has been shown to be effective against non-platinum-based chemotherapy. Efficacy may be dose-related with optimal control in one study at 8 mg t.d.s. (Fraschini *et al.*, 1991). There have been reports, however, that efficacy of ondansetron may in fact decline at higher intravenous doses which would limit its use in patients refractory to conventional doses (Gronberg *et al.*, 1989).

Granisetron is more potent than ondansetron with maximal efficacy at a single dose of 3 mg i.v. (compared with 24–32 mg for ondansetron); this difference, however, may have little clinical importance unless there are differences in side effect or ease of administration. An oral form of granisetron has been developed but is not in widespread use yet. Both drugs are widely distributed and eliminated by non-renal mechanisms. Granisetron has a longer half-life (10 hours) than ondansetron and biological activity is still evident 24 hours after a single dose (Upward *et al.*, 1990). This difference may affect ease of administration as granisetron can be given as a single injection whereas ondansetron is recommended in multiple-dosing schedules which vary for different chemotherapy regimens. Clinical practice, however, suggests that prescription of ondansetron above twice or thrice daily may not be necessary.

Both ondansetron and granisetron are effective against drugs such as cisplatin or ifosfamide given in fractionated schedules over several days; this suggests that patients do not develop tolerance to these drugs (Sledge *et al.*, 1990; Hainsworth *et al.*, 1991). Despite their role in control of acute emesis, the evidence for the value of serotonin receptor antagonists in delayed emesis is less clear. Up to 70% of patients achieve complete or major control of acute emesis with ondansetron, but this number decreases for delayed emesis for both platinum- and non-platinum-containing regimens and any superiority over conventional anti-emetics is less apparent with respect to delayed emesis. In one study there was no difference between ondansetron and metoclopramide in delayed emesis following

Table 11.4 Results of uncontrolled (A) and controlled (B) trials using 5-HT_3 receptor antagonists in the prophylaxis of platinum-induced emesis

Drugs	Dose/schedule	Emetic challenge	Emetic control(%)*	Reference
A: Uncontrolled trials				
Ondansetron*	0.18 mg/kg q6–8h	Cisplatin	63/83 (75)	Hesketh *et al.*, 1989
	0.04–0.35 mg/kg i.v. infusion	Cisplatin	18/19 (95)	Kris *et al.*, 1988
	0.15 mg/kg i.v. q8h	Cisplatin (over 5 days)	27/35 (77)	Einhorn *et al.*, 1990
	0.18 mg/kg q2h q4h 0.4 mg/kg q24h 0.15 mg/kg q2h	Cisplatin ≥100 mg/m^2	5/10 (50) 6/10 (60) 1/8 (13) 11/12 (92)	Kris *et al.*, 1989
	8–12 mg i.v. stat + 1–3 mg/h for 24h i.v.	Melphalan ≥120 mg/m^2	14/33 (42)	Viner *et al.*, 1990
	4 mg i.v. q6h × 7 doses	Ifosfamide (1st course and refractory)	10/12 (83)	Green *et al.*, 1989
	5 mg/m^2 then 2–4 mg po q8h 5 days	Moderately emetogenic/ refractory (children)	26/30 (87)	Pinkerton *et al.*, 1990
	4 mg i.v. stat 4 mg po b.d. (24h)	Refractory emesis	14/15 (93)	Cunningham *et al.*, 1987
	8 mg i.v. stat then 1 mg/kg 24h	Cisplatin ≥70 mg/m^2	18/26 (69)	Marty *et al.*, 1989
	4–8 mg po q6–8h	Radiation (8–10 Gy upper abd)	(71–91)	Priestman, 1989
Granisetron	40–80 μg/kg i.v.	Cisplatin or Cy/Dox	12/22 (55)	Addelman *et al.*, 1990
	40 μg/kg i.v.	Cisplatin or Dox/Cy	11/20 (55)	Cassidy *et al.*, 1988
ICS-205–930	5–20 mg/m^2 before chemotherapy	Cisplatin plus 5-fluorouracil plus Cy (refractory)	20/22 (91)	Seinen *et al.*, 1989
	20–40 mg i.v. × 2	Cisplatin (refractory)	9/11 (81)	Leibundgut and Lancranjan, 1987
Ondansetron plus	4 mg i.v. stat, 4 mg po q8h for 5 days	Moderately emetogenic	Improved emesis score in 8/8	Cunningham *et al.*, 1989
Dexamethasone	8 mg i.v. stat, 4 mg–1 mg po q8h (5 days)			

Ondansetron plus Dexamethasone	8 mg q8h 5 days 8 mg q8h 3 days	Refractory emesis	9/14 (64)	Smith *et al.*, 1990
B: Comparative trials				
Ondansetron versus Dexamethasone	4 mg i.v. stat 4 mg po q6h 5 days 8 mg i.v. stat 4 mg reducing to 6 mg q6h over 5 days	Moderately emetogenic	83/100 (83) Acute 63/87 (73) Delayed 79/100 (79) Acute 76/87 (85) Delayed	Jones *et al.*, 1991
Ondansetron versus	8 mg po q8h 3–5 days	Moderately emetogenic (3 studies)	(86) (80) (72)	Schmoll, 1989
Metoclopromide	20 mg po q8h 3–5 days		(42) (62) (61)	
Ondansetron versus	0.15 mg/kg i.v. q4h 3 days	Cisplatin ≥20 mg/m² for 5 days	18/23 (78)	Sledge *et al.*, 1990
Metoclopramide	1 mg/kg i.v. q4h 3 days		3/22 (14)	
Ondansetron versus	8 mg stat, 1 mg/h infusion 24h	Cisplatin	57/76 (77)	Marty *et al.*, 1990
Metoclopramide	3 mg/kg stat, 0.5 mg/kg infusion 8h		32/76 (42)	
Ondansetron versus Placebo	0.15 mg/kg. i.v. q6h	Cisplatin ≥50 mg/m²	11/14 (79) 0/14 (0)	Cubeddu *et al.*, 1990
Ondansetron versus	8 mg po q8h	Radiation (8–10 Gy upper abdomen)	37/38 (99)	Priestman, 1989
Metoclopramide	10 mg po q8h		31/44 (70)	
Ondansetron versus Placebo	0.15 mg/kg	Cy + Dox or 5-fluorouracil	7/10 (70)	Cubeddu *et al.*, 1990
Ondansetron and Dexamethason versus	O–8 mg i.v. stat 1 mg/h 24h then 8 mg t.d.s. days 2–6	Cisplatin	49/71 (69)	Smyth *et al.*, 1991
Ondansetron and Placebo	D–20 mg i.v. stat		40/71 (56)	
Ondansetron and Dexamethasone versus	O–0.15 mg/kg stat T + 2h T + 4h	Cisplatin	81/89 (91)	Roila *et al.*, 1991
Ondansetron and Placebo	D–20 mg i.v stat		57/59 (64)	

* complete or major control of emesis Cy = cyclophosphamide Dox = doxorubicin

high dose cisplatin (>50 mg/m^2) (Deriulder *et al.*, 1990) and indeed metoclopramide was significantly better in control of nausea. In another study, dexamethasone was equally effective as ondansetron in control of delayed emesis after moderately emetogenic chemotherapy (Jones *et al.*, 1991). Although it has been shown that a single i.v. dose of granisetron could control emesis in 40–44% of patients for up to seven days after platinum, this figure still represents a significant number of patients failing to achieve control of delayed emesis. Further doses of granisetron may re-establish control in most patients; the efficacy of granisetron, however, against delayed emesis warrants further evaluation when the oral preparation becomes more widely available.

5-HT_3 receptor antagonists are generally well tolerated and do not cause the central nervous system side-effects such as the severe sedation or extrapyramidal side-effects associated with dopamine receptor blockade. The main side-effects include mild or moderate headache (which is reported in up to 15% of patients and is readily controlled with paracetamol), a feeling of flushing and fatigue, and also asymptomatic reversible increases in hepatic transaminase concentrations. Ondansetron is known to increase large bowel transit time and has been reported to cause diarrhoea in approximately 1% of patients. Constipation has also been reported in approximately 3% of patients. There have been isolated reports of hypersensitivity reactions and extrapyramidal reactions with ondansetron (Coupe, 1987).

11.5 COMBINATION THERAPY AND RECOMMENDATIONS

Despite the advent of 5-HT_3 receptor antagonists, approximately 20% of patients receiving moderately emetogenic chemotherapy and up to 40% of patients receiving platinum-based therapy will still experience a degree of acute and/or delayed emesis. Delayed emesis is now recognized as a major problem in cancer care and may occur even when anti-emetic drugs are administered for several days.

When anti-emetic drugs with different mechanisms of action are used in combination there is usually improved control of acute emesis, although not necessarily any reduction in delayed emesis. For example, the combination of dexamethasone and metoclopramide or the addition of metoclopramide to lorazepam and dexamethasone significantly improves anti-emetic control (Kris *et al.*, 1987; O'Brien *et al.*, 1989). In addition, lorazepam may reduce the likelihood of extrapyramidal reactions with dopamine receptor antagonists. However, improvement in anti-emetic control may be at the expense of increased toxicity, in particular sedation and drug interactions. It is important to develop single schedules suitable for outpatient use.

In uncontrolled studies dexamethasone enhanced the efficacy of ondansetron in patients with refractory emesis (Cunningham *et al.*, 1989; Smith *et al.*, 1990). This interaction was predicted from the ferret model of chemotherapy-induced emesis (Hawthorne and Cunningham, 1990). In comparative trials against platinum-based chemotherapy regimens in chemotherapy, naive dexamethasone contributed significantly to the anti-emetic control offered by ondansetron in both the acute and delayed phases of emesis. There was no excess of side-effects with the combination and patient preference was significantly greater for the combination treatment (Smyth *et al.*, 1991; Rolla *et al.*, 1991; Smith *et al.*, 1991). A combination of a 5-HT_3 receptor antagonist together with a corticosteroid offers the optimal anti-emetic control currently available for highly emetogenic regimens.

Table 11.5 Suggested anti-emetic schedules

Moderately emetogenic chemotherapy:	
1	Dexamethasone 8 mg with chemotherapy then 4 mg oral t.d.s. for 3 days
or	
2	Ondansetron 8 mg i.v. 15 minutes before chemotherapy then 8 mg once or b.d. or Granisetron 3 mg i.v. before chemotherapy.
Highly emetogenic chemotherapy:	
1	Metoclopramide 2 mg/kg i.v. 15 minutes before chemotherapy and 2 and 4 hours after then 20 mg orally q.d.s. for 3–4 days
plus	dexamethasone 8 mg i.v. with chemotherapy then 4 mg orally t.d.s. for 3 days
or	
2	As schedule 1 but add lorazepam 1–2 mg 30 minutes before chemotherapy and repeat at 2–4 hours (NB: causes sedation but useful in patients at high emetic risk)
or	
3	As schedule 1 but add procylidine 50 mg orally t.d.s. or diphenyldramine 50 mg i.v. to prevent extrapyramidal reactions (patients ≤30 years)
or	
4	Ondansetron 8 mg i.v. and dexamethasone 8 mg before chemotherapy then ondansetron 8 mg oral once or b.d. for 1 day and dexamethasone 4 mg q.d.s. 4–5 days or Granisetron 3 mg i.v. before chemotherapy.
Anticipatory emesis	
1	Lorazepam 1–2 mg orally 24 hours before chemotherapy plus appropriate schedule as above

11.5.1 RECOMMENDATIONS FOR ANTI-EMETIC THERAPY

Although 5-HT_3 receptor antagonists are very effective anti-emetic drugs, the high current costs may dictate other priorities for resource allocation to ensure the most cost-effective management of cancer (Rees, 1991). There is no proven advantage for serotonin receptor antagonists against conventional anti-emetic drugs for prophylaxis of emesis induced by moderately emetogenic chemotherapy in terms of efficacy although the side-effect profile of serotonin receptor antagonists may be favourable. Even for those patients receiving platinum-based chemotherapy, high dose metoclopramide in combination with dexamethasone achieves emetic control in 60–70% of cases. Guidelines for anti-emetic therapy are given in Table 11.5.

In view of the high incidence of extrapyramidal reactions in children and younger patients (≤30 years) with dopamine receptor antagonists, the use of serotonin receptor antagonists can be advocated in this patient population and these drugs have been shown to be safe and effective in children (Pinkerton *et al.*, 1990). Serotonin receptor antagonists are also recommended for patients who fail to achieve anti-emetic control or who experience unacceptable toxicity with other drugs.

It is important to administer anti-emetic drugs for an adequate period (i.e. for several days after moderately and high emetogenic regimens) to minimize problems of delayed emesis; ondansetron, however, may be less effective for delayed emesis than for acute emesis even when administered over several days (Jones *et al.*, 1991; Einhorn *et al.*, 1990). The role of granisetron, which has a longer duration of action, requires further investigation but at best it only achieves partial control of delayed emesis. It appears that the anti-emetic properties of dexamethasone may have advantages for control of delayed emesis and this drug may be used in combination with a serotonin receptor antagonist for optimal control.

Anticipatory emesis develops as a conditioned response in 10–20% of patients who have experienced previous emesis (Morrow, 1982; Devlen *et al.*, 1987) and once it is established poses a difficult management problem. Behavioural therapy, including relaxation techniques and hypnosis, has been used with some success but is not widely available (Burishand Lyles, 1981). Benzodiazepines and other anti-emetics given 24 hours prior to chemotherapy may also reduce the problem (Lazlo *et al.*, 1985) but prevention of anticipatory emesis by effective anti-emetic control with the first course of chemotherapy is of paramount importance.

11.6 THE ROLE OF THE ONCOLOGY NURSE

The control of chemotherapy-induced nausea and vomiting require close collaboration between the oncologist and nurse. The oncology nurse needs an understanding of the available anti-emetic drugs in order to allay patient anxiety and to be able to administer the drugs safely and effectively and to evaluate the anti-emetic response. It is clearly essential that these are administered regularly rather than on an 'as required' basis and the oncology nurse has an important role in patient education to ensure effective use of anti-emetics by outpatients. With highly emetogenic regimens it may be better to administer chemotherapy late in the day as patients' perception of emesis is less severe at night than in the morning (Headley, 1987). Certainly the initiation of anti-emetic prophylaxis 24 hours prior to chemotherapy has been shown to reduce emesis (Willans *et al.*, 1989). In the trial setting the oncology nurse is often the most appropriate person to act as a trained observer, monitoring the patient and documenting emetic response and drug compliance.

11.7 CONCLUSIONS

Both the clinical care and symptomatic control of cancer patients undergoing chemotherapy has improved over the last decade. This is a consequence of a better understanding of the physiology of emesis and the identification and pharmacological evaluation of new active drugs. Careful prospective clinical research has resulted in the use of safe and effective anti-emetic drugs, either alone, or in combination, for all patients undergoing chemotherapy, including those who pose special problems such as children and young adults. 5-HT_3 receptor antagonists represent an important and useful new class of drug having low toxicity and are a major advance against acute platinum-induced emesis. Despite these advances, complete or major control of emesis is still not achieved universally and the problems of delayed emesis warrant special recognition in the future. While further improvements in emetic control may be possible with the drugs currently available, further research is necessary to identify other mechanisms involved in the physiology of emesis and thereby afford the opportunity to optimize anti-emetic control and improve the quality of life for cancer patients undergoing treatment.

REFERENCES

Aapro, M.S., Plozia P.M., Alberts, D.S. *et al.* (1983) Double-blind crossover study of the antiemetic efficacy of high-dose dexamethasone vs high-dose metoclopramide. *J. Clin. Oncol.*, **2**, 466–71.

Addelman, M., Erhickman, C., Fine, S. *et al.* (1990) Phase I/II trial of granisetron: a novel 5-hydroxytryptamine antagonist for the prevention of chemotherapy-induced nausea and vomiting. *J. Clin. Oncol.*, **8**, 337–41.

Anthony, L.B., Krozeley, M.G., Woodward, N.J. *et al.* (1986) Anti-emetic effect of oral versus intravenous metoclopramide in patients receiving cisplatin. A randomised double-blind trial. *J. Clin. Oncol.*, **4**, 94–103.

Bakowski, M.T. (1984) Advances in anti-emetic therapy. *Cancer Treat. Rev.*, II, 237–56.

Bonneterre, J., Chevalier, B., Metz, R. *et al.* (1990) A randomised double-blind comparison of ondanstron and metoclopramide in the prophylaxis of emesis induced by cyclophosphamide, fluorouracil and doxorubicin or epirubicin chemotherapy. *J. Clin. Oncol.* **8**, 1063–69.

Borison, H.L. and McCarthy, C.E. (1983) Neuropharmacology of chemotherapy induced emesis. *Drugs*, **25**, 8–17.

Bowcock, S.J., Stockdale, A.D., Bolton, J.A.R. *et al.* (1984) Anti-emetic prophylaxis with high dose metoclopramide or lorazepam and vomiting induced by chemotherapy. *Br. Med. J.*, **288**, 1879.

Bregini, M., Siena, S., Di-Nicola, M. *et al.* (1991) Tropisetron plus haloperidol to ameliorate nausea and vomiting associated with high dose alkylating agent cancer chemotherapy. *Eur. J. Cancer*, **27**, 561–65.

Burish, T.G. and Lyles, J.N. (1981) Effectiveness of relaxation training in reducing adverse reactions to cancer chemotherapy. *J. Behav. Med.*, **4**, 65–78.

Carden, P.A., Mitchell, S.L., Waters, K.D. *et al.* (1990) Prevention of cyclophosphamide/cytarabine-induced emesis with ondansetron in children with leukaemia. *J. Clin. Oncol.*, **8**, 1531–35.

Carl, P.L., Cubeddu, L.X., Lindley, C. *et al.* (1989) Do humoral factors mediate cancer chemotherapy-induced emesis? *Drug Metab. Rev.*, **21**, 319–33.

Cassidy, J., Raina V., Lewis, C. *et al.* (1988) Pharmacokinetics and anti-emetic efficacy of BRL-43694A, a new selective 5HT-3 antagonist. *Br. J. Cancer*, **58**, 651–53.

Chevallier, B. (1990) Efficacy and safety of granisetron compared with high-dose metoclopramide plus dexamethasone in patients receiving high-dose cisplatin in a single-blind study. The Granisetron Study Group. *Eur. J. Cancer*, **26**, 533–36.

Chiara, S., Campora, E., Lionetto, R. *et al.* (1987) Methylprednisolone for the control of CMF-induced emesis. *Am. J. Clin. Oncol.*, **10**, 264–67.

Coates, A., Abraham, S., Kaye, S.B. *et al.* (1983) On the receiving end – patients perception of the side-effects of cancer chemotherapy. *Eur. J. Cancer Clin. Oncol.*, **19**, 203–8.

Coupe, M. (1987) Adverse reaction to 5-HT3 antagonist ICS 205930. *Lancet*, **i**, 1494.

Craig, J.B. and Powell, B.L. (1983) Review: The management of nausea and vomiting in clinical oncology. *Am. J. Med. Sci.*, **293**, 34–44.

Cubeddu, L.X., Hoffman, I.S., Fuenmayor, N.T. and Finn, A.L. (1990, a) Antagonism of serotonin S3 receptors with ondansetron prevents nausea and emesis induced by cyclophosphamide-containing regimens. *J. Clin. Oncol.*, **8**, 1721–27.

Cubeddu, L.X., Hoffman, I.S., Fuenmayor, N.T. and Finn, A.L. (1990, b) Efficacy of ondansetron (GR38032F) and the role of serotonin in cisplatin induced nausea and vomiting. *N. Eng. J. Med.*, **322**, 810–16.

Cunningham, D., Evans, C., Gazet, J.-C. *et al.* (1987) Comparison of antiemetic efficacy of domperidone, metoclopramide and dexamethasone in patients receiving outpatient chemotherapy regimens. *Br. Med. J.*, **295**, 250.

Cunningham, D., Forrest, G.J., Soukop, M. *et al.* (1985) Nabilone and prochlorperazine: a useful combination for emesis induced by cytotoxic drugs. *Br. Med. J.*, **24**, 864–65.

Cunningham, D., Hawthorn, J., Pople, A. *et al.* (1987) Prevention of emesis in patients receiving cytotoxic drugs by GR38032F, a selective 5HT3 receptor antagonist. *Lancet*, **i**, 1461–63.

Cunningham, D., Soukop, M., Gilchrist, N.L. *et al.* (1985) Randomised trial of intravenous high dose metoclopramide and intramuscular chlorpromazine in controlling nausea and vomiting induced by cytotoxic drugs. *Br. Med. J.*, **290**, 604–5.

Cunningham, D., Turner, A., Hawthorn, J. and Rosin, R.D. (1989) Ondansetron with and without dexamethasone to treat chemotherapy-induced emesis *Lancet*, **i**, 1323.

D'Acquisto, R.W., Tyson, L.B., Gralla, L.J. *et al.* (1986) The influence of a chronic high alcohol intake on chemotherapy-induced nausea and vomiting. *Proc. Am. Soc. Clin. Oncol.*, **5**, 257.

De Mulder P.H., Seynaeve, C., Vermorken, J.B. *et al.* (1990) Ondansetron compared with high dose metoclopramide in prophylaxis of acute and delayed cisplatin induced nausea and vomiting. A multicentre randomised double-blind crossover study. *Ann. Intern. Med.*, **113**, 834–40.

Devlen, J., Maguire, P., Phillips, P. *et al.* (1987) II prospective study. *Br. Med. J.*, **295**, 955–7.

D'Olimpio, J.T., Carnacho, F., Chandra, P. *et al.* (1985) Antiemetic efficacy of high-dose dexamethasone versus placebo in patients receiving cisplatin-based chemotherapy: a randomised double-blind controlled trial. *J. Clin. Oncol.*, **3**, 1133–35.

Einhorn, L.E., Nagy, C., Berner, K. and Finn, A.L. (1990) Ondansetron: a new anti-emetic for patients receiving cisplatin chemotherapy. *J. Clin. Oncol.*, **8**, 731–35.

Fetting, J.H., Grochow, L.B., Felstein, M.F. *et al.* (1982) The course of nausea and vomiting after high dose cyclophosphamide. *Cancer Treat. Rep.*, **66**, 1487–93.

Fozard, J.R. and Mobarok Ali, A.T.M., (1978) Blockade of neuronal tryptamine receptors by metoclopramide. *Eur. J. Pharmacol.*, **49**, 109–12.

Fraschini, G., Ciociola, A., Esparza, L. *et al.* (1991) Evaluation of three oral doses of ondansetron in the prevention of nausea and emesis associated with cyclophosphamide-doxorubicin chemotherapy. *J. Clin. Oncol.*, **9**, 1268–74.

Gralla, R.J. (1983) Metoclopramide – a review of anti-emetic trials. *Drugs*, **25**, 63–73.

Gralla, R.J., Itri, L.M., Pisto, S.E. *et al.* (1981) Antiemetic efficacy of high-dose metoclopramide: Randomised trials with placebo and prochlorperazine in patients with chemotherapy-induced nausea and vomiting. *N. Engl. J. Med*, **305**, 905–9.

Green, J.A., Watkin, S.W., Hammond, P. *et al.* (1989) The efficacy and safety of GR38032F in the prophylaxis of ifosfamide-induced nausea and vomiting. *Cancer Chemother. Pharmacol.*, **24**, 137–9.

Grunberg, S.M., Stevenson, L.L., Russel, C.A. *et al.* (1989) Dose ranging Phase I study of the serotonin receptor antagonist GR38032F for prevention of cisplatin-induced nausea and vomiting. *J. Clin. Oncol.*, **7**, 1137–41.

Grunberg, S.N., Gala, K.V., Lampenfeld, M. *et al.* (1984) Comparison of the anti-emetic effect of high-dose intravenous metoclopramide and high-dose intravenous haloperidol in a randomised double blind crossover study. *J. Clin. Oncol.*, **2**, 782–87.

Hainsworth, J., Harvey, W., Prendergrass, K. *et al.* (1991) A single-blind comparison of intravenous ondansetron, a selective serotonin antagonist with intravenous metoclopramide in the prevention of nausea and vomiting associated with high dose cisplatin chemotherapy. *J. Clin. Oncol.*, **9**, 721– 8.

Hainsworth, J.D., Omura, G.A., Khojasteh, A. *et al.* (1991) Ondansetron (GR38032F) a novel anti-emetic effective in patients receiving a multiple day regimen of cisplatin chemotherapy. *Am. J. Clin. Oncol.*, **14**, 336–40.

Hawthorne, J. and Cunningham, D. (1990) Dexamethasone can potentiate the anti-emetic action of a 5HT3 receptor antagonist on cyclophosphamide induced vomiting in the ferret. *Br. J. Cancer*, **61**, 56–60.

Headley, J.A. (1987) The influence of administration time on chemotherapy-induced nausea and vomiting. *Oncol. Nurs. Forum*, **14**, 43–47.

Hesketh, P.J., Murphy, W.K., Lester, E.P. *et al.* (1989) GR38032F (GR-C705/75): a novel compound effective in the prevention of acute cisplatin-induced emesis. *J. Clin. Oncol.*, **7**, 700–5.

Hunter, A.E., Prentice, H.G., Pothecary, K. *et al.* (1991) Granisetron, a selective 5HT3 receptor antagonist for the prevention of radiation induced emesis during total body irradiation. *Bone Marrow Transplant*, **7**, 439–41.

Jones, A.L., Cunningham, D., Soukop, M. *et al.* (1991) Comparison of dexamethasone and ondansetron in the prophylaxis of emesis induced by moderately emetogenic chemotherapy. *Lancet*, **338**, 483–87.

Kerr, P.J., Graham, J., McGovern, E. *et al.* (1985) The relationship between steady state metoclopramide levels and control of emesis during treatment with cis-platinum. *Br. J. Clin. Pharm.*, **20**, 426–27.

Kris, M.G., Tyson, L.B., Gralla, R.J. *et al.* (1983) Extrapyramidal reactions with high dose metoclopramide. *N. Engl. J. Med.*, **309**, 443.

Kris, M.G., Gralla, K.J., Clark, R.A. *et al.* (1985) Incidence, course and severity of delayed nausea and vomiting following the administration of high-dose cisplatin. *J. Clin. Oncol.*, **3**, 1379–84.

Kris, M.G., Gralla, R.J., Tyson, L.B. *et al.* (1985) Improved control of cisplatin-induced emesis with high dose metoclopramide and with combinations of metoclopramide, dexamethasone and diphenhydramine; results of consecutive trials in 255 patients. *Cancer*, **55**, 527–34.

Kris, M.G., Gralla, R.J., Clark, R.A. *et al.* (1987) Antiemetic control and prevention of side-effects of anticancer therapy with lorazepam or diphenhydramine when used in combination with metoclopramide plus dexamethasone. A double-blind randomised trial. *Cancer*, **60**, 2816–22.

Kris, M.G., Gralla, R.J., Clarke, R.A., Tyson, L.B.

(1988) Dose-ranging evaluation of the serotonin antagonist GR-C507/75 (GR38032F) when used as an anti-emetic in patients receiving anticancer chemotherapy. *J. Clin. Oncol.*, **6**, 659–62.

Kris, M.G., Gralla, R.J., Clark, R.A. *et al.* (1989) Phase II trials of the serotonin antagonist GR38032F for the control of vomiting caused by cisplatin. *J. Natl. Cancer Inst.*, **81**, 42–46.

Lazlo, J., Clark, R.A., Hanson, D.C. *et al.* (1985) Lorazepam in cancer patients treated with cisplatin: a drug with anti-emetic, amnesic and anxiolytic effects. *J. Clin. Oncol.*, **3**, 864–69.

Leibundgut, U. and Lancranjan, I. (1987) First results with ICS205-930 (5HT3 receptor antagonist) in prevention of chemotherapy-induced emesis. *Lancet*, **i**, 1198.

Lindley, C.M., Bernard, S. and Fields, S.M. (1989) Incidence and duration of chemotherapy-induced nausea and vomiting in the outpatient oncology population. *J. Clin. Oncol.*, **7**, 1142–49.

Livera, P., Trojano, M., Simone, I.L. *et al.* (1985) Acute changes in blood CSF barrier permselectivity to serum proteins after intrathecal methotrexate and CNS irradiation. *J. Neurol.*, **231**, 336–39.

Loprinizi, C.L., Ellison, N.M., Schaid, D.J. *et al.* (1990) Controlled trial of megestrol acetate for the treatment of cancer anorexia and cachesxia, *J. Natl. Cancer Inst.*, **82**, 1127–32.

Maher, J. (1981) Intravenous lorazepam to prevent nausea and vomiting associated with cancer chemotherapy. *Lancet*, **i**, 91–92.

Markman, M., Scheidler, V., Ettinger, D.S. *et al.* (1984) Antiemetic efficacy of dexamethasone: randomised double-blind crossover study with prochlorperazine in patients receiving cancer chemotherapy. *N. Engl. J. Med.*, **311**, 549–52.

Marty, H. (1990) A comparative study of the use of granisetron, a selective 5HT3 antagonist, versus a standard anti-emetic regimen of chlorpromazine plus dexamethasone in the treatment of cytotoxic-induced regimens. The Granisetron Study Group. *Eur. J. Cancer* **26**, 528–32.

Marty, M., Droz, J.P., Pouillant, P. *et al.* (1989) GR38032F, a 5HT3 receptor antagonist, in the prophylaxis of acute cisplatin-induced nausea and vomiting. *Cancer Chemother. Pharmacol.*, **23**, 389–91.

Marty, M., Pouillart, P. and School, S. (1990) Comparison of the 5-hydroxytryptamine (serotonin) antagonist ondansetron (GR38032F) with high-dose metoclopramide in the control of cisplatin-induced emesis. *N. Engl. J. Med.*, **322**, 816–21.

Meyer B.R., Levin, M., Draper, D.E. *et al.* (1984) Optimising metoclopramide control of cisplatin-induced emesis. *Ann. Intern. Med.*, **100**, 393–95.

Morrow, G.R. (1982) Prevelance and correlates of anticipatory nausea and vomiting in chemotherapy patients. *J. Natl Cancer Inst.*, **68**, 585–88.

Morrow, G.R. (1984) Susceptibility to motion sickness and the development of anticipatory nausea and vomiting in cancer patients undergoing chemotherapy. *Cancer Treat. Rep.*, **68**, 1177–78.

O'Brien, M.E.R., Cullen, M.H., Woodroffe, C. *et al.* (1989) The role of metoclopramide in acute and delayed chemotherapy induced emesis: a randomised double-blind trial. *Br. J. Cancer*, **60**, 759–63.

Olver I.N., Simon, R.H. and Aisner, J. (1976) Anti-emetic studies: a methodological discussion. *Cancer Treat. Rep.*, **70**(5), 555–63.

Pater, J. and Willan, A. (1984) Methodologic issues in trials of anti-emetics. *J. Clin. Oncol.*, **2**, 484–87.

Pinkerton, C.R., Williams, D., Wooton, C. *et al.* (1990) 5-HT3 antagonist ondansetron – an effective out-patient anti-emetic in children with cancer. *Archives Dis. Child.*, **65**, 822–25.

Priestman, T.J. (1989) Clinical studies with ondansetron in the control of radiation-induced emesis. *Eur. J. Cancer Clin. Oncol.*, **25**(suppl 1), 529–33.

Rees, G.J.G. (1991) Cancer treatment: deciding what we can afford. *Br. Med. J.*, **302**, 799–800.

Rich, W.M., Abdulhayoqlu, G. and Disaia, P.J. (1980) Methylprednisolone as an antiemetic drug during cancer chemotherapy: a pilot study. *Gynaecol. Oncol.*, **9**, 193–98.

Roila, F., Tonato, M., Cognetti, F. *et al.* (1991) Prevention of cisplatin-induced emesis: a double-blind multicentre randomised crossover study comparing ondansetron and ondansetron plus dexamethasone. *J. Clin. Oncol.*, **9**, 675–78.

Sallan, S.E., Zimberg, N.E. and Frei, E. (1980) Anti-emetic effect of delta-9-tetrahydrocannabinol and prochlorperazine. *N. Engl. J. Med.*, **302**, 135–38.

Schmoll, H.J. (1989) The role of ondansetron in the treatment of emesis induced by non-cisplatin-containing chemotherapy regimens. *Eur. J. Cancer Clin. Oncol.*, **25**, 535–39.

Seinen, H., Zonnenberg, B.A., Tjia, P. and Neijt, J. (1989) The effect of three dose levels of ICS 205–930 (a selective 5HT-3 antagonist) on cisplatin-induced nausea and vomiting. *Eur. J. Cancer Clin. Oncol.*, **9**, 1333–35.

Sledge, G.N., Einhorn, L.H., Nagy, C. and Finn, A.L. (1990) Randomised trial of ondansetron (OND) and metoclopramide (MCP) as antiemetic therapy for cisplatin-based chemotherapy. *Proc. Am. Soc. Clin. Oncol.*, **9**, 323.

Smaldone, L., Plozia, P., Alberts, D. *et al.* (1990) Batanopride (BMY-25801): a new 5HT3 receptor antagonist for the prevention of cancer chemotherapy induced emesis. *Cancer Treat. Rev.*, **17**, 319–27.

Smith, D.B., Newlands, E.S., Sprugt, O.W. *et al.* (1990) Ondansetron (GR38032F) plus dexamethasone: effective anti-emetic prophylaxis for patients receiving cytotoxic chemotherapy. *Br. J. Cancer*, **61**, 323–24.

Smith, D.B., Newlands, E.S. and Rustin, G.J.S. (1991) Comparison of ondansetron and ondansetron plus dexamethasone as antiemetic prophylaxis during cisplatin-containing chemotherapy. *Lancet*, **338**, 487–90.

Smyth, J.F., Coleman, R.F., Nicolson, M. *et al.* (1991) Does dexamethasone enhance control of acute cisplatin induced emesis by ondansetron? *Lancet*, **303**, 1423–26.

Sullivan J.R., Leydon M.J. and Bell, R. (1983) Decreased cisplatin induced nausea and vomiting with alcohol ingestion. *N. Engl. J. Med.*, **309**, 796.

Upward, J.N., Arnold, B.D, Link, C. *et al.* (1990) The clinical pharmacology of granisetron (BRL43694) a novel specific 5HT3 antagonist. *Eur. J. Cancer*, **26**, 512–15.

Viner, C.V., Selby, P.J., Zulian, G.B. *et al.* (1990) Ondansetron – a new safe and effective anti-emetic in patients receiving high dose melphalan. *Cancer Chemother. Pharmacol.*, **25**, 449–53.

Williams, C.J., Davies, C., Raval, M. *et al.* (1989) Comparison of starting antiemetic treatment 24 hours before or concurrently with cytotoxic chemotherapy. *Br. Med. J.*, **298**, 430–31.

Afterword: Unresolved issues and future prospects

G.J. SANGER and P.L.R. ANDREWS

The discovery and clinical application of 5-HT_3 receptor antagonists has transformed the treatment of emesis induced by anti-cancer therapies and as a result dramatically improved the quality of life of a growing number of patients. However, there are a number of fundamental and clinical problems outstanding in this field that require investigation to further improve therapy. Some of these are highlighted below:

1. While the principal pathways (e.g. vagal afferent nerves, area postrema) by which cytotoxic drugs and ionizing radiation induce emesis have been identified, the precise cellular mechanisms by which these pathways are activated are still largely unknown. If, for example, the release of 5-HT from the enterochromaffin cell is a critical step in the induction of emesis, then what feature of this cell makes it so sensitive and what is the sub-cellular target that induces the release of 5-HT? Is the rank order of emetic potential of the cytotoxic drugs related to their ability to release 5-HT and if so could this system be used as a predictive assay of the emetic activity of novel cytotoxic drugs?

2. Although 5-HT_3 receptor antagonists can block emesis, the precise role of 5-HT remains to be defined. Does it actually drive the response or act as a sensitizing agent for other agents released by the same stimuli? If the latter, then identification of the other agents may offer an alternative approach to anti-emesis, provided a major candidate can be found. A related question is what is the site of action of the 5-HT_3 receptor antagonists? 5-HT_3 receptors are located on both the peripheral (gut) and central (medulla) ends of the vagal afferents. Attention has focused on the peripherally located receptors as the most likely site but the role (if any) of the central receptors on the vagal afferents or the area postrema has yet to be defined. Are they functionally relevant? Alternatively, could the 5-HT_3 receptors on the area postrema offer a therapeutic target for any of the other side effects of anti-cancer therapy such as loss of appetite?

3. Animal studies have accurately predicted the general efficacy of 5-HT_3 receptor antagonists in humans. However, whereas these agents are consistently and totally

Emesis in Anti-cancer Therapy
Mechanisms and treatment
Published in 1993 by Chapman & Hall, London
ISBN 0 412 37250 9

effective in animals, in man their use as single agents provides complete protection in only 70% of patients. This does not appear to be a problem of the potency of the drugs and suggests that in some (but not all) patients, additional mechanisms operate. Is this a reflection of the psychological effects of the clinical experience of anti-cancer therapy, a reflection of previous emetic experience resulting in plastic changes in the pathways, a reflection of disease factors or is it simply due to a species difference?

4. The incidence of anticipatory emesis can be expected to decrease because fewer patients will have emesis during their therapy and there will be a diffusion of information about improved treatment of emesis through patient self-help groups. However, because it is not yet possible to guarantee complete protection throughout the course of therapy there is still a need to understand the fundamental mechanisms of anticipatory emesis so that appropriate treatment can be given; in the case of patients in which psychotherapy fails, this will probably involve the use of drugs. The psychological effects of the non-emetic effects of anti-cancer therapy (e.g. hair loss) should also not be minimized.

5. The problem of delayed emesis has been brought into greater prominence because of the efficacy of the 5-HT_3 receptor antagonists in the acute phase. Several questions relating to delayed emesis need to be studied:
   (a) Why don't the current animal models of emesis, which are sensitive to 5-HT_3 receptor antagonists, have a delayed phase of emesis?
   (b) What is the impact of blocking the acute phase of emesis on the delayed phase; are the two related in any way?
   (c) Delayed emesis does not occur in all patients; is there any reliable predictive marker?
   (d) What is the mechanism of delayed emesis and does the effectiveness of steroids give an important insight into a therapeutic approach?

6. Studies of the pharmacokinetics and pharmacodynamics of cytotoxic drugs have rightly tended to focus on optimizing the dose for tumour toxicity and have paid less attention to the relationship between these parameters and emesis. Even when careful pharmacokinetic studies have been undertaken it is difficult to look at the relationship with emesis due to the lack of adequately quantified data on the pattern of emesis. Such combined studies may not only have a direct clinical relevance but also would be useful in aiding the identification of basic mechanisms, particularly in elucidating the factors contributing to the latency of emesis. These studies may also identify the optimal time for anti-emetic drug administration.

7. Pharmacokinetic studies have shown differences in distribution and clearance of 5-HT_3 receptor antagonists between cancer patients and healthy subjects. How can this be explained and does it influence drug efficacy and duration of action in patients? In addition, there also appear to be gender differences, with 5-HT_3 receptor antagonists being less effective in women than men. While this may to some extent reflect diseases and chemotherapy differences, the factors contributing should be investigated, particularly in view of the unfortunately large number of patients with breast cancer.

8. The mechanism by which the sensation of nausea is induced are not known and it is fortunate that 5-HT_3 receptor antagonists are almost as effective in combating nausea

as vomiting. One particularly puzzling aspect is the role of the very high levels of vasopressin and whether this is influenced by 5-HT_3 receptor antagonism.

9. Although 5-HT_3 receptor antagonists are highly effective and there is likely to be a plethora of 'me too' compounds available over the next few years we should not be blind to other equally innovative approaches. As new cytotoxic drugs and radiotherapy regimes are continually under development it would be unwise not to explore other approaches as these may induce emesis by different mechanisms and hence not be amenable to treatment with 5-HT_3 receptor antagonists.

10. While this book has focused on the problem of emesis induced by anti-cancer therapies the other side-effects of such therapies should not be neglected as they also have a considerable impact upon quality of life. These include anorexia and conditioned taste aversions. Animal studies have demonstrated an involvement of the area postrema in the mechanism of these symptoms and as 5-HT_3 receptors are present in the area postrema it could be that 5-HT_3 receptor antagonists might alleviate these problems. Long-term effects of anti-cancer therapy also include fatigue, weakness and memory impairment. Because emesis has been such a major problem these tend to have been overlooked but are now likely to move up the list of problems of most concern to patients, unless suitable therapy can be identified.

Index